THE
MERCK
MANUAL

THIRTEENTH EDITION

★

1st Edition – 1899
2nd Edition – 1901
3rd Edition – 1905
4th Edition – 1911
5th Edition – 1923
6th Edition – 1934
7th Edition – 1940
8th Edition – 1950
9th Edition – 1956
10th Edition – 1961
11th Edition – 1966
12th Edition – 1972
13th Edition – 1977

THIRTEENTH EDITION

THE

MERCK
MANUAL

OF

DIAGNOSIS AND THERAPY

Robert Berkow, M.D., *Editor*

John H. Talbott, M.D., *Consulting Editor*

Published by
MERCK SHARP & DOHME RESEARCH LABORATORIES

Division of
MERCK & CO., INC.
Rahway, N.J.

1977

MERCK & CO., INC.
Rahway, N.J.
U.S.A.

MERCK SHARP & DOHME
West Point, Pa.

MERCK SHARP & DOHME RESEARCH LABORATORIES
Rahway, N.J.   *West Point, Pa.*

MERCK SHARP & DOHME INTERNATIONAL
Rahway, N.J.

MERCK CHEMICAL DIVISION
Rahway, N.J.

MERCK CHEMICAL MANUFACTURING DIVISION
Rahway, N.J.

MERCK ANIMAL HEALTH DIVISION
Rahway, N.J.

BALTIMORE AIRCOIL COMPANY, INC.
Baltimore, Md.

CALGON CORPORATION
Pittsburgh, Pa.

HUBBARD FARMS, INC.
Walpole, N.H.

KELCO DIVISION
San Diego, Calif.

Library of Congress Catalog Card Number 1-31760
ISBN Number 911910-02-6
ISSN Number 0076-6526

First Printing—September 1977
Second Printing—December 1977
Third Printing—February 1978
Fourth Printing—August 1978
Fifth Printing—November 1979

Copyright © 1977 by MERCK & CO., INC.
All rights reserved. Copyright under the Universal Copyright
Convention and the International Copyright Convention.
Copyright reserved under the Pan-American Copyright
Convention.

Printed in the U. S. A.

FOREWORD

Under the wise direction of Charles E. Lyght, M.D., who was Editor from 1947 to 1966, THE MERCK MANUAL became established as one of the world's most widely used medical textbooks. The tradition, quality, and success of the book were upheld in the Twelfth Edition under the direction of David N. Holvey, M.D., who guided the initial processes of this edition until his untimely accidental death in 1973. The Thirteenth Edition is respectfully dedicated to Dr. Holvey.

MERCK'S MANUAL OF THE MATERIA MEDICA first appeared in 1899 as a slender 262-page text. It was expressly designed to meet the needs of general practitioners in selecting medications, noting that "memory is treacherous" and even the most thoroughly informed physician needs a reminder "to make him at once master of the situation and enable him to prescribe exactly what his judgment tells him is needed for the occasion." By the Sixth Edition (1934) the book was a 1379-page text widely used and known as THE MERCK MANUAL OF THERAPEUTICS AND MATERIA MEDICA. Since the Eighth Edition (1950), the title has been THE MERCK MANUAL OF DIAGNOSIS AND THERAPY. In order to keep pace with new knowledge and changing needs, much more than the name of the book has changed. However, its purpose remains the same—to provide useful information to practicing physicians.

Today, fewer physicians attempt to manage the whole range of medical disorders that can occur in infants, children, and adults, but those who do must have available a broad spectrum of current and accurate information. Further, the more specialized physician requires precise information about subjects outside his area of greatest expertise. All physicians need ever more information, and review of large areas of subject matter covered succinctly and completely is increasingly required. THE MERCK MANUAL continues to try to meet these needs, excluding mainly details of surgical procedures.

This edition of THE MERCK MANUAL follows the basic format of its immediate predecessor, but it has been almost completely rewritten and the content has been increased by more than 50%. While emphasis remains on diagnosis and treatment, the discussions of basic physiologic, pathologic, and other factors essential to rational diagnostic reasoning and effective therapy have been enriched. More discussions of symptoms and signs have been added, as have suggestions for approaching the problems that patients present to their doctors. Almost every section is larger (e.g., the Cardiovascular Disorders section has twice the content of the Twelfth Edition and the Pediatrics and Genetics section has been more than doubled). A new section has been added to reflect advances in Clinical Pharmacology, and some sections, such as Immunology and Allergic Disorders, have been totally redone and greatly expanded.

Owing to the extensive subject matter covered and a successful tradition, the style and organization of THE MERCK MANUAL differ somewhat from most other texts. Many readers are not fully aware of either the scope of the symptoms, disorders, tests, reference tables, etc. that are covered or their interrelationships. Therefore, to expedite and enhance consultation of the book, readers are urged to spend a few minutes reviewing the Guide for Readers (p. viii), the table of contents at the beginning of each section, and the index (p. 2081).

By definition, a "manual" is a small book—one that can be carried in the hand. By implication, it should be a book that one wishes to carry about and use frequently. Although managing the size of the Thirteenth Edition has been a challenge, the book is only a fraction of an inch taller, broader, and thicker than its predecessor. There are approximately 200 additional pages, but the type is slightly larger than in the last edition.

More important than the quantitative aspects of the book are those relating to quality. We have had contributions from more than 250 authors from the United States, Canada, England, and other countries, as well as guidance and review by an outstanding editorial board. Our debt of gratitude cannot be fully paid, but, for the first time, contributors have been identified and are listed in the front of the book. I wish also to express appreciation and pay special tribute to my Consulting Editor, John H. Talbott, M.D., to my Senior Manuscript Editor, Gloria R. Hamilton, and to my other manuscript editors—Mariam A. Cohen, Doris C. Ferguson, Ruth M. Heckler, Miriam P. Kepner, Frank E. Manson, and Barbara D. Markey—all of whom have worked hard and long with devotion and skill to create this book. Finally, our entire effort could not have succeeded without the experience, patience, and remarkable skills of my secretary, Catherine J. Humber, and the cooperation and proficiency of my format coordinator, Sandra K. Vitale.

We hope that this edition of THE MERCK MANUAL will be a welcome visitor to you, our readers—cordial to your needs and worthy of frequent return invitations. Discussions relating to the next edition have begun and suggestions for improvement or additions will be warmly welcomed and carefully considered.

Robert Berkow, M.D., *Editor*
MERCK SHARP & DOHME RESEARCH LABORATORIES
WEST POINT, PA. 19486

CONTENTS

GUIDE FOR READERS

- The **Contents** (p. vii) shows the pages where readers will find names of contributors, abbreviations and symbols, titles of sections (groupings of related chapters), and the index. **Thumb-tabs** with appropriate abbreviations and section numbers mark each section and the index.

- Each **Section,** designated by the symbol §, begins with its own table of contents, listing the chapters and subchapters in that section.

- **Chapters** are not numbered serially from the beginning to the end of the book; rather, each chapter is numbered according to its order in each section.

- The **Index** contains many cross-entries; page numbers in bold type signify major discussions of the topics. In addition, the text in THE MANUAL gives numerous cross-references to other sections and chapters.

- Each **Page Head** carries (1) the page number (page numbers run serially from the beginning to the end of the book); (2) if space permits, the titles of the relevant chapter and the last subchapter on that page; and (3) the section identification number (on left-hand pages) or chapter number (on right-hand pages).

- **Abbreviations and Symbols,** used liberally as essential space savers, are listed on pp. ix and x.

- The **Tables** and **Figures** found throughout the text are referenced appropriately in the index but are not listed in a table of contents.

- Commonly used **Clinical Procedures** and an extensive discussion of **Laboratory Medicine,** as well as **Ready Reference Guides,** are found in the section under the thumb-tab **REF.**

- **Drugs** are designated in the text by generic (nonproprietary) names. In the last chapter of the Clinical Pharmacology section, most of the drugs mentioned in the book are listed alphabetically with each generic term followed by one or more trademarks.

- The authors, reviewers, editors, and publisher of this book have made extensive efforts to ensure that treatments, drugs, and dosage regimens are accurate and conform to the standards accepted at the time of publication. However, constant changes in information resulting from continuing research and clinical experience, reasonable differences in opinions among authorities, unique aspects of individual clinical situations, and the possibility of human error in preparing such an extensive text require that the reader exercise individual judgment when making a clinical decision and, if necessary, consult and compare information from other sources. In particular, the reader is advised to check the product information included in each package of drug before prescribing or administering it, especially if the drug is unfamiliar or is used infrequently.

ABBREVIATIONS AND SYMBOLS

ACTH	adrenocorticotropic hormone	ft	foot; feet (measure)
ADH	antidiuretic hormone	FUO	fever of unknown origin
ADP	adenosine diphosphate	GFR	glomerular filtration rate
ASO	antistreptolysin O (titer)	GI	gastrointestinal
ATP	adenosine triphosphate	Gm	gram(s)
BCG	Bacillus Calmette-Guerin (vaccine)	G6PD	glucose-6-phosphate dehydrogenase
b.i.d.	2 times a day	GU	genitourinary
BMR	basal metabolic rate	h	hour(s)
BP	blood pressure	HA	hemagglutination, hemagglutinating
BSA	body surface area		
BSP	sulfobromophthalein	Hb	hemoglobin
BUN	blood urea nitrogen	HCl	hydrochloric acid; hydrochloride
C	centigrade		
CBC	complete blood count	HCO_3	bicarbonate
CF	complement fixation, fixating	Hct	hematocrit
		Hg	mercury
Ch.	chapter	HI	hemagglutination-inhibition, inhibiting
Ci	curie		
Cl	chloride, chlorine	Hz	hertz (cycles/second)
cm	centimeter(s)	IgA, etc.	immunoglobulin A, etc.
CNS	central nervous system	IM	intramuscular(ly)
CO	carbon monoxide	in.	inch(es)
CO_2	carbon dioxide	IPPB	inspiratory positive pressure breathing
CPK	creatine phosphokinase		
CSF	cerebrospinal fluid	IU	international unit(s)
cu	cubic	IUD	intrauterine device
cu mm	cubic millimeter(s)	IV	intravenous(ly)
CVA	cerebrovascular accident	IVP	intravenous pyelogram
CVS	cardiovascular system	kcal	kilocalorie (food calorie)
D & C	dilation and curettage	kg	kilogram(s)
DDT	chlorophenothane (dichlorodiphenyl-trichloroethane)	17-KGS	17-ketogenic steroids
		17-KS	17-ketosteroids
		L	liter
dl	deciliter(s)	lb	pound(s)
DNA	deoxyribonucleic acid	LDH	lactic dehydrogenase
DTP	diphtheria-tetanus-pertussis (toxoids/vaccine)	LE	lupus erythematosus
		m	meter(s)
		M	molar
D/W	dextrose in water	mCi, mc	millicurie(s)
ECG	electrocardiogram	MCH	mean corpuscular hemoglobin
EEG	electroencephalogram		
ENT	ear, nose, and throat	MCHC	mean corpuscular hemoglobin concentration
ESR	erythrocyte sedimentation rate		
		MCV	mean corpuscular volume
F	Fahrenheit	mEq	milliequivalent(s)
FDA	U.S. Food and Drug Administration	mg	milligram(s)
		Mg	magnesium
FEV	forced expiratory volume	min	minute(s)
Fr	French (catheter size)	mIU	milli-international unit(s)

ml	milliliter(s)	Sa$_{O_2}$	arterial oxygen saturation
MLD	minimum lethal dose	SBE	subacute bacterial
mm	millimeter(s)		endocarditis
mM	millimole(s)	s.c.	subcutaneously
mo	month(s)	SGOT	serum glutamic
mol wt	molecular weight		oxaloacetic
mOsm	milliosmole(s)		transaminase
N	nitrogen; normal (strength of solution)	SGPT	serum glutamic pyruvic transaminase
ng	nanogram (=millimicrogram)	SLE	systemic lupus erythematosus
nm	nanometer (=millimicron)	sp gr	specific gravity
NPH	neutral protein Hagedorn (insulin)	sq	square
		sq m	square meter
17-OHCS	17-hydroxycorticosteroids	STS	serologic test(s) for
oz	ounce(s)		syphilis
P	phosphorus, pressure	TB	tuberculosis
P$_{CO_2}$	carbon dioxide pressure (or tension)	tbsp	tablespoon(s)
		t.i.d.	3 times a day
P$_{O_2}$	oxygen pressure (or tension)	tsp	teaspoon(s)
		u.	unit(s)
Pa$_{CO_2}$	arterial carbon dioxide pressure	URI	upper respiratory infection
		USPHS	United States Public
Pa$_{O_2}$	arterial oxygen pressure		Health Service
PA$_{O_2}$	alveolar oxygen pressure	WBC	white blood cell
PBI	protein-bound iodine	wk	week(s)
pg	picogram (=micromicrogram)	wt	weight
		yr	year(s)
pH	hydrogen-ion concentration	μ	micro-, micron(s)
		mμ	millimicron(s) (=nanometer)
p o	orally		
PPD	Purified Protein Derivative (tuberculin)	μCi, μc	microcurie(s)
		μg, mcg	microgram(s)
ppm	parts per million	mμg	millimicrogram(s) (=nanogram)
p.r.n.	as needed		
psi	pounds per square inch	$\mu\mu$g	micromicrogram(s) (=picogram)
PSP	phenolsulfonphthalein		
pt	pint(s)	μmol	micromole(s)
q	every	μOsm	micro-osmole(s)
q 4 h, etc.	every 4 hours, etc.	/	per
q.i.d.	4 times a day	<	less than
qt	quart(s)	>	more than
R, r	roentgen(s)	$\leq$	equal to or less than
RA	rheumatoid arthritis	$\geq$	equal to or more than
RBC	red blood cell	$\approx$	approximately equal
RF	rheumatoid factor	$\pm$	plus or minus
RNA	ribonucleic acid	§	section

CONTRIBUTOⱤ

George N. Abraham, M.D.
Associate Professor of Medicine and Microbiology, University of Rochester

William Curtis Adams, M.D.
Medical Director, Emergency Department, SE Alabama General Hospital

James K. Alexander, M.D.
Professor of Medicine, Baylor College of Medicine

Chloe G. Alexson, M.D.
Assistant Professor of Pediatrics, University of Rochester

David G. Ashbaugh, M.D.
Boise, Idaho

Paul C. Atkins, M.D.
Assistant Professor of Medicine; Chief, Allergy Clinic, University of Pennsylvania

Hugh Auchincloss, M.D.
Associate Clinical Professor of Surgery, Columbia University; Associate Attending, Surgery, Presbyterian Hospital in New York

Robert Austrian, M.D.
Chairman of the Department of Research Medicine, University of Pennsylvania

Hervy E. Averette, M.D.
Professor and Director, Division of Gynecologic Oncology, University of Miami

Richard F. Bakemeier, M.D.
Associate Professor of Oncology in Medicine; Associate Director, Cancer Center for Educational Programs, University of Rochester

Gerald L. Baum, M.D.
Professor of Medicine, Tel Aviv University, Israel

Laurence H. Beck, M.D.
Assistant Professor of Medicine; Education Officer, Department of Medicine, University of Pennsylvania

Peter Beighton, M.D., Pʰ. D.C.H.
Professor, Department of h. University of Cape Town, Repu. Africa

Nathaniel I. Berlin, M.D.
Director, Cancer Center; Teuton Professor of Medicine, Northwestern University

Don Carl Bienfang, M.D.
Assistant Professor of Ophthalmology, Harvard University

Harvey Blank, M.D.
Professor and Chairman, Department of Dermatology, University of Miami

Sidney Blumenthal, M.D.
Director, Division of Heart and Vascular Diseases, National Heart, Lung, and Blood Institute

Donald C. Bondy, M.D.
Professor of Medicine, University of Western Ontario, London, Canada

Philip K. Bondy, M.D., F.R.C.P.
Cancer Research Campaign Professor of Medicine, Institute of Cancer Research in association with the Royal Marsden Hospital, London, United Kingdom

Susan Jones Boulay, B.S., R.N.
Nursing Advisor, Greater Rochester Spina Bifida Association; Committee on the Handicapped, Pittsford, New York Central School District

William A. Briscoe, M.D.
Professor of Medicine, Cornell University

Bernard B. Brody, M.D.
Director of Clinical Laboratories, Genesee Hospital

F. E. Bruckner, M.B., M.R.C.P.
Consultant in Rheumatology, St. George's Hospital, London, United Kingdom

Ralph E. Cutler, M.D.
Professor of Medicine, University of Washington

Ronald G. Davidson, M.D., F.R.C.P. (C)
Professor of Pediatrics; Director, Program in Human Genetics, Department of Pediatrics, McMaster University, Hamilton, Ontario, Canada

David O. Davis, M.D.
Professor of Radiology, George Washington University

W. Howard Davis, D.D.S.
Clinical Professor of Oral Surgery, University of Southern California; Consultant, Oral Surgery, Long Beach VA Hospital and Naval Regional Medical Center

Kenneth A. Day, M.B., Ch.B., M.R.C. Psych., D.P.M.
Consultant Psychiatrist, Northgate Hospital, Morpeth, Northumberland, United Kingdom

Roger M. Des Prez, M.D.
Professor of Medicine, Vanderbilt University; Chief of Medical Service, VA Hospital, Nashville

Victor G. deWolfe, M.D.
Head, Department of Peripheral Vascular Disease, Cleveland Clinic Foundation

Preston V. Dilts, Jr., M.D.
Professor and Chairman, Department of Obstetrics and Gynecology, University of Tennessee

Gerald S. Dowdy, Jr., M.D.
Baylor College of Medicine; University of Texas

Eugenie F. Doyle, M.D.
Director of Pediatric Cardiology, New York University

Joseph T. Doyle, M.D.
Professor of Medicine; Head, Division of Cardiology, Albany Medical College

Edmund L. Dubois, M.D.
Clinical Professor of Medicine, Director of the Lupus Clinic, University of Southern California

Howard A. Eder, M.D.
Professor of Medicine, Albert Einstein College of Medicine

Edward R. Eichner, M.D.
Professor of Medicine; Chief of Hematology/ Oncology, Department of Medicine, Louisiana State University

Elliot F. Ellis, M.D.
Professor and Chairman, Department of Pediatrics, State University of New York at Buffalo

Kent Ellis, M.D.
Professor of Radiology, Columbia University

Karl Engelman, M.D.
Associate Professor of Medicine and Pharmacology; Chief, Hypertension and Clinical Pharmacology Section; Director, Clinical Research Center, University of Pennsylvania

Carl D. Enna, M.D.
Chief, Clinical Branch and Surgical Department, USPHS Hospital (National Leprosarium)

Harvey Feigenbaum, M.D.
Professor of Medicine; Senior Research Associate, Krannert Institute of Cardiology, Indiana University

Alvan R. Feinstein, M.D.
Professor of Medicine and Epidemiology, Yale University

F. Robert Fekety, Jr., M.D.
Professor of Internal Medicine, Physician-in-Charge, Section of Infectious Diseases, University of Michigan

W. Jeffrey Fessel, M.D., F.R.C.P.
Kaiser-Permanente Medical Centers; Associate Clinical Professor of Medicine, University of California, San Francisco

Stuart C. Finch, M.D.
Professor of Medicine, Yale University

Norman L. Fine, M.D.
Chief of Respiratory Services, Griffin Hospital; Assistant Clinical Professor of Medicine, Yale University

Gerald A. M. Finerman, M.D.
Associate Professor of Surgery, Orthopaedic Surgery, University of California, Los Angeles

Murray M. Fisher, M.D., Ph.D.
Sunnybrook Medical Centre, University of Toronto, Ontario, Canada

Lawrence Fleckenstein, Pharm.D.
Director, Drug Information Service, Alta Bates Hospital

Emil Frei, III, M.D.
Director and Physician-in-Chief, Sidney Farber Cancer Center; Professor of Medicine, Harvard University

Eugene P. Frenkel, M.D.
Professor of Internal Medicine; Chief, Section of Hematology-Oncology, University of Texas, Dallas

Gerald Friedman, M.D., Ph.D.
Associate Attending Physician; Assistant Clinical Professor of Medicine, Mt. Sinai School of Medicine

Peter L. Frommer, M.D.
Associate Director for Cardiology, Division of Heart and Vascular Diseases, National Heart, Lung, and Blood Institute

Timothy S. Gee, M.D.
Director, Bone Marrow Laboratory, Memorial Hospital for Cancer and Allied Diseases; Associate, Memorial Sloan-Kettering Cancer Center; Assistant Professor, Cornell University

William Patrick Gideon, M.D.
Assistant Professor of Gynecology and Obstetrics, University of Oklahoma; Director, Medical and Child Health for Oklahoma City Area of Indian Health Service

Ray W. Gifford, Jr., M.D.
Head, Department of Hypertension and Nephrology, Cleveland Clinic Foundation

James F. Glenn, M.D.
Professor and Chief of Urology, Duke University

Martin Goldberg, M.D.
Professor of Medicine; Chief, Renal Electrolyte Section, University of Pennsylvania

Bruce N. Goldreyer, M.D.
San Pedro and Peninsula Hospital

M. Jay Goodkind, M.D.
Clinical Associate Professor of Medicine, University of Pennsylvania

Robert A. Goodwin, Jr., M.D.
Chief, Pulmonary Disease Section, VA Hospital, Nashville; Professor of Medicine, Vanderbilt University

Edgar S. Gordon, M.D. *(Deceased)*
Professor of Medicine, University of Wisconsin

Dov Gorshein, M.D.
Associate Professor of Medicine, Hahnemann Medical College and Hospital of Philadelphia

Edward A. Graykowski, M.D., D.D.S.
Medical Director, Public Health Service, National Institute of Dental Research

Alan B. Gruskin, M.D.
Director, Pediatric Nephrology, St. Christopher's Hospital for Children; Associate Professor of Pediatrics, Temple University

Rolf M. Gunnar, M.D.
Professor of Medicine; Chief, Section of Cardiology, Loyola University

G. Peter Halberg, M.D.
Director, Contact Lens Service, St. Vincent's Hospital and Medical Center of New York; Director, Glaucoma Service, New York Eye and Ear Infirmary; Professorial Lecturer (Clinical Professor) Ophthalmology, State University of New York Downstate Medical Center

Caroline Breese Hall, M.D.
Assistant Professor of Pediatrics and Medicine, University of Rochester

William J. Hall, M.D.
Associate Professor of Medicine and Pediatrics, University of Rochester

Robert W. Hamilton, M.D.
Assistant Professor of Medicine/Nephrology; Medical Director, Hemodialysis Section, Bowman Gray School of Medicine

James P. Harnisch, M.D.
Instructor of Medicine, University of Washington

Jack Hartstein, M.D.
Assistant Professor of Clinical Ophthalmology, Washington University

Herbert B. Hechtman, M.D.
Associate Professor of Surgery, Boston University

Stephen E. Hedberg, M.D.
Senior Endoscopist and Associate Visiting Surgeon, Massachusetts General Hospital; Assistant Clinical Professor of Surgery, Harvard University

Werner Henle, M.D.
Professor of Virology in Pediatrics, University of Pennsylvania; Director, Division of Virology, Children's Hospital of Philadelphia

Albert V. Hennessy, M.D.
Professor of Pediatrics and Epidemiology, University of Michigan

D. Wilson Hess, Ph.D.
Associate Professor of Pediatrics, Psychiatry (Psychology) and Education, University of Rochester

Roland G. Hiss, M.D.
Associate Professor of Medicine, University of Michigan

Christopher H. Hodgman, M.D.
Associate Professor of Psychiatry and Pediatrics, University of Rochester

Robert A. Hoekelman, M.D.
Professor of Pediatrics, University of Rochester

Paul D. Hoeprich, M.D.
Professor of Medicine and Pathology; Chief, Section of Infectious and Immunologic Diseases; Department of Internal Medicine, University of California, Davis

Joseph H. Holmes, M.D.
Professor of Medicine and Radiology, University of Colorado

Sam V. Holroyd, D.D.S.
Captain, Dental Corps, U.S. Navy, Naval Graduate Dental School, National Naval Medical Center

Edward H. Hon, M.D.
Doré Professor of Obstetrics and Gynecology, University of Southern California

Richard B. Hornick, M.D.
Professor of Medicine, University of Maryland

Dorothy M. Horstmann, M.D.
Professor of Epidemiology and Pediatrics, Yale University

Charles S. Houston, M.D.
Professor of Environmental Health and Professor of Medicine, University of Vermont

Kenneth A. Hubel, M.D.
Professor of Medicine, University of Iowa

Douglas W. Huestis, M.D.
Professor of Pathology, University of Arizona; Medical Director, Southern Arizona Red Cross Blood Center

Michael Hume, M.D.
Professor of Surgery, Tufts University

Daniel A. Hussar, Ph.D.
Dean of Faculty, Philadelphia College of Pharmacy and Science

Frank L. Iber, M.D.
Professor of Medicine; Chief, Gastroenterology Division, University of Maryland and VA Hospital, Baltimore

Harold L. Israel, M.D.
Honorary Professor of Medicine, Thomas Jefferson University

John C. Ivins, M.D.
Professor of Orthopedic Surgery, Mayo Medical School

George Gee Jackson, M.D.
Professor of Medicine; Chief, Section of Infectious Diseases, University of Illinois

Harry S. Jacob, M.D.
Chief, Section of Hematology; Professor of Medicine, University of Minnesota

Ralph F. Jacox, M.D.
Professor of Medicine, University of Rochester

Mary Jane Jesse, M.D.
Professor of Pediatric Cardiology, University of Miami

John S. Johnson, M.D.
Associate Professor of Clinical Medicine, Vanderbilt University

Pieter H. Joubert, M.B., B.Ch., F.C.P. (S.A.)
University of Rochester; Pharmacology Department, University of the Orange Free State, Republic of South Africa

Karl D. Kappus, Ph.D.
Chief, Neurotropic Virus Surveillance, Bureau of Epidemiology, Center for Disease Control, U.S. Public Health Service

Fred E. Karch, M.D.
Assistant Professor of Pharmacology and Toxicology and of Medicine, University of Rochester

Simon Karpatkin, M.D.
Professor of Medicine, New York University

Stephen I. Katz, M.D., Ph.D.
Senior Investigator, Dermatology Branch, National Cancer Institute

T. A. Kerr, M.D., M.R.C.Psych.
Consultant Psychiatrist, University of Newcastle upon Tyne, United Kingdom

Boris Kerzner, M.D.
Assistant Chief of Ambulatory Medicine, Sinai Hospital of Baltimore, Inc.; formerly, Fellow in Clinical Pharmacology, University of Rochester

Thomas Killip, M.D.
Professor of Medicine and Associate Dean, Northwestern University; Chairman, Department of Medicine, Evanston Hospital

L. G. Kiloh, M.D., F.R.C.P., F.R.C.Psych., F.A.N.Z.C.P.
Professor of Psychiatry, University of New South Wales, Sydney, Australia

Robert R. Kirby, M.D.
Associate Professor of Anesthesiology and Surgery, University of Miami

Arthur E. Kopelman, M.D.
Director of Neonatology, Department of Pediatrics, University of Rochester

Morris N. Kotler, M.B., Ch.B., M.R.C.P. (Ed.)
Associate Professor of Medicine, Hahnemann Medical College and Hospital of Philadelphia

The Rev. Edward H. Lanphier, M.D.
Senior Scientist in Mechanical Engineering, University of Wisconsin

Carl L. Larson, M.D.
Director and Professor of Microbiology, Stella Duncan Memorial Research Institute, University of Montana

Daniel M. Laskin, D.D.S.
Professor and Head, Department of Oral and Maxillofacial Surgery, University of Illinois

Ruth A. Lawrence, M.D.
Associate Professor of Pediatrics and of Obstetrics and Gynecology, University of Rochester

James B. Lee, M.D.
Professor of Medicine, State University of New York at Buffalo

Michael D. Levitt, M.D.
Professor of Medicine, University of Minnesota

Robert I. Levy, M.D.
Director, National Heart, Lung, and Blood Institute

Steven Levy, M.D.
Co-Director, Pulmonary Department, Dr. David M. Brotman Memorial Hospital; Clinical Professor of Medicine, University of California, Los Angeles

Edward B. Lewin, M.D.
Assistant Professor of Pediatrics and Medicine; Director, Pediatric Infectious Disease Unit, University of Rochester

Harold I. Lief, M.D.
Professor of Psychiatry; Director, Division of Family Study, University of Pennsylvania

Larry I. Lipshultz, M.D.
Assistant Professor, Division of Urology, Department of Surgery, University of Texas, Houston

Henry S. Loeb, M.D.
Program Director in Cardiology, VA Hospital, Hines, Illinois; Professor of Medicine, Loyola University

Asger Lunn, M.D.
Air Training Command Surgeon/ret., R.D.A.F.; Medical Advisor, Scandinavian Airlines System, Region Denmark

Joel H. Manchester, M.D.
Newport Beach, California

Leon Marder, M.D.
Associate Professor of Psychiatry and Medicine, University of Southern California; Director, Drug Treatment Center, Rancho Los Amigos Hospital

Richard G. Masson, M.D.
Chief, Pulmonary Medicine, Framingham Union Hospital, Assistant Professor of Medicine, Boston University

John M. Mazzullo, M.D.
Assistant Professor of Pharmacology and Toxicology and Medicine, University of Rochester

Elizabeth R. McAnarney, M.D.
Assistant Professor of Pediatrics, Psychiatry and Medicine; Director, Adolescent Program, University of Rochester

Hamish A. McClelland, M.B., F.R.C.Psych., F.R.C.P., D.C.H.
Consultant Psychiatrist, University of Newcastle upon Tyne, United Kingdom

John H. McClement, M.D.
Director, Chest Service, Bellevue Hospital Center; Professor of Medicine, New York University

Victor A. McKusick, M.D.
Chairman, Department of Medicine, Johns Hopkins University; Physician-in-Chief, Johns Hopkins Hospital

Donald S. McLaren, M.D., Ph.D.
Department of Physiology, University Medical School, Edinburgh, United Kingdom; formerly Professor of Clinical Nutrition, School of Medicine, American University of Beirut, Lebanon

Edwin M. Meares, Jr., M.D.
Professor and Chairman, Department of Urology, Tufts University; Urologist-in-Chief, New England Medical Center Hospital

James Metcalfe, M.D.
Oregon Heart Association Professor of Medicine, University of Oregon

August Miale, Jr., M.D.
Director, Division of Nuclear Medicine; Professor of Radiology and Oncology, University of Miami

Daniel R. Mishell, Jr., M.D.
Professor and Associate Chairman, Department of Obstetrics and Gynecology, University of Southern California

John A. Moncrief, M.D.
Professor of Surgery and Vice Chairman, Medical University of South Carolina

John P. Morgan, M.D.
Assistant Professor of Pharmacology and Internal Medicine, Department of Pharmacology and Toxicology, University of Rochester

Roland W. Moskowitz, M.D.
Professor of Medicine, Case Western Reserve University

Catherine L. Myers, R.N., F.P.N.P.
Family Planning Coordinator, St. Paul-Ramsey Hospital and Medical Center; Chairman, Dist. 6 Nurses Association, American College of Obstetrics and Gynecology

Gary J. Myers, M.D.
Assistant Professor of Pediatrics and Neurology, University of Rochester

Don H. Nelson, M.D.
Professor of Medicine, University of Utah

John B. Nettles, M.D.
Professor and Chairman, Department of Obstetrics and Gynecology, University of Oklahoma

William S. Nevin, M.D.
Director of Pulmonary Medicine, Pima County General Hospital; Associate Staff, University of Arizona

Robert L. Ney, M.D.
Professor and Chairman, Department of Medicine, University of North Carolina

C. Alvin Paulsen, M.D.
Professor of Medicine, University of Washington

Carl M. Pearson, M.D.
Professor of Medicine; Director, Division of Rheumatology, University of California, Los Angeles

John A. Penner, M.D.
Professor of Internal Medicine, University of Michigan

Joseph K. Perloff, M.D.
Professor of Medicine and Pediatrics; Chief, Cardiovascular Section, University of Pennsylvania

Hart deC. Peterson, M.D.
Director, Pediatric Neurology, New York Hospital-Cornell Medical Center

Marjorie Pfaudler, R.N.; B.S., M.A., Nursing Education
Associate Professor of Nursing and Preventive Medicine and Community Health, University of Rochester

Sidney F. Phillips, M.D.
Consultant in Gastroenterology, Mayo Clinic; Professor of Medicine, Mayo Medical School

Nathaniel F. Pierce, M.D.
Associate Professor of Medicine, Johns Hopkins University

Ivan B. Pless, M.D., F.R.C.P.(C)
Associate Professor of Pediatrics and Epidemiology and Health, McGill University, Montreal, Quebec, Canada

James J. Plorde, M.D.
Chief, Microbiology; Chief, Infectious Disease Service, VA Hospital, Seattle; Associate Professor of Medicine, University of Washington

Fred Plum, M.D.
Professor and Chairman, Department of Neurology, New York Hospital-Cornell Medical Center

Ronald C. Pruett, M.D.
Clinical Instructor in Ophthalmology, Harvard University; Assistant Surgeon in Ophthalmology, Massachusetts Eye and Ear Infirmary; Clinical Senior Scientist, Eye Research Institute, Retina Foundation

Eric L. Radin, M.D.
Associate Professor of Orthopedic Surgery, Harvard University

C. George Ray, M.D.
Professor of Pathology and Pediatrics, University of Arizona

Nathaniel Reichek, M.D.
Director, Noninvasive Laboratory, University of Pennsylvania

Eric Reiss, M.D.
Professor of Medicine, University of Miami

Hal B. Richerson, M.D.
Professor of Internal Medicine, University of Iowa

Harold Rifkin, M.D.
Clinical Professor of Medicine, Albert Einstein College of Medicine; Chief, Division of Diabetes, Montefiore Hospital and Medical Center

B. Lawrence Riggs, M.D.
Chairman, Division of Endocrinology and Metabolism, Mayo Clinic and Foundation

Leonor T. Rivera-Calimlim, M.D.
Associate Professor, Department of Pharmacology and Toxicology; Assistant Professor in Medicine, University of Rochester

Gerald P. Rodnan, M.D.
Professor of Medicine, University of Pittsburgh

Robert M. Rogers, M.D.
Professor of Medicine; Associate Professor of Physiology; Chief, Pulmonary Disease Section, University of Oklahoma

Norman Rosenberg, M.D.
Director, Department of Surgery, Middlesex General Hospital; Clinical Professor of Surgery, Rutgers Medical School

Harold P. Roth, M.D.
Chief of Gastroenterology, VA Hospital, Cleveland; Associate Professor of Medicine, Case Western Reserve University

Professor Sir **Martin Roth,** M.D., F.R.C.P.
Professor of Psychiatry, Department of Psychological Medicine, The Royal Victoria Infirmary, Newcastle upon Tyne, United Kingdom

Findlay E. Russell, M.D., Ph.D.
Director, Laboratory of Neurological Research; Professor of Neurology, Physiology, and Biology, University of Southern California

Paul S. Russell, M.D.
John Homans Professor of Surgery, Harvard University; Massachusetts General Hospital

Edwin A. Rutsky, M.D.
Associate Professor of Medicine, University of Alabama, Birmingham

David B. Sachar, M.D.
Associate Professor of Medicine, Mount Sinai School of Medicine

Jay P. Sanford, M.D.
Professor of Medicine and Dean, School of Medicine, Uniformed Services University of the Health Sciences

James W. Sayre, M.D.
Associate Professor of Pediatrics, University of Rochester

Kurt Schapira, M.D.
University of Newcastle upon Tyne, United Kingdom

Albert P. Scheiner, M.D.
Associate Professor of Pediatrics, University of Massachusetts

H. Ralph Schumacher, Jr., M.D.
Associate Professor of Medicine, University of Pennsylvania

Robert H. Schwartz, M.D.
Associate Professor of Pediatrics, University of Rochester

William R. Shapiro, M.D.
Associate Professor of Neurology, Department of Neurology, Cornell University; Chief, Laboratory of Neurological Oncology, Memorial Sloan-Kettering Cancer Center

James Christie Shelburne, M.D.
Director, Cardiology Division, Cardiopulmonary Department, Hoag Memorial Hospital Presbyterian

Paul Sherlock, M.D.
Chief, Gastroenterology Service, Memorial Sloan-Kettering Cancer Center; Professor of Medicine, Cornell University

Harry Shwachman, M.D.
Professor of Pediatrics, Emeritus, Harvard University; Children's Hospital Medical Center

F. A. Simeone, M.D.
Professor of Medical Science, Brown University; Surgeon-in-Chief, Miriam Hospital

Jerome B. Simon, M.D., F.R.C.P.(C)
Associate Professor of Medicine, Queen's University; Head, Division of Gastroenterology, Kingston General Hospital, Ontario, Canada

David P. Simpson, M.D.
Professor of Medicine, University of Wisconsin

John G. Simpson, M.B., Ch.B., Ph.D., M.R.C.Path.
Lecturer in Pathology, Department of Pathology, University of Aberdeen, United Kingdom

Arthur T. Skarin, M.D.
Assistant Professor of Medicine, Harvard University; Division of Oncology, Sidney Farber Cancer Institute

J. Donald Smiley, M.D.
Professor of Internal Medicine, University of Texas, Dallas

Charles B. Smith, M.D.
Associate Professor of Medicine and Microbiology, University of Utah

Jackson A. Smith, M.D.
Professor and Chairman, Department of Psychiatry, Loyola University

Lloyd H. Smith, Jr., M.D.
Professor and Chairman, Department of Medicine, University of California, San Francisco

Helen L. Smits, M.D.
Assistant Professor of Medicine and Associate Administrator, University of Pennsylvania

Gordon L. Snider, M.D.
Professor of Medicine and Chief, Pulmonary Medicine Section, Boston University; Chief, Pulmonary Medicine Section, VA Hospital, Boston

James B. Snow, Jr., M.D.
Professor and Chairman, Department of Otorhinolaryngology and Human Communication, University of Pennsylvania

Selma E. Snyderman, M.D.
Professor of Pediatrics, New York University

P. Frederick Sparling, M.D.
Professor and Chief, Division of Infectious Diseases, University of North Carolina

Gabriel Spergel, M.D.
Physician-in-Charge, Metabolic Research Unit, Jewish Hospital and Medical Center of Brooklyn; Associate Professor of Medicine, State University of New York, Downstate Medical Center; Chief of Endocrinology, Greenpoint Hospital

Wesley W. Spink, M.D.
Emeritus Regents' Professor of Medicine and Comparative Medicine, University of Minnesota

John A. Spittell, Jr., M.D.
Consultant, Internal Medicine and Cardiovascular Diseases, Mayo Clinic; Professor of Medicine, Mayo Medical School

Nigel N. Stanley, M.D.
Assistant Professor of Medicine, University of Pennsylvania

Myron Stein, M.D.
Clinical Professor of Medicine, University of California, Los Angeles; Co-Director, Pulmonary Department, Dr. David M. Brotman Memorial Hospital

Morton A. Stenchever, M.D.
Professor and Chairman, Department of Obstetrics and Gynecology, University of Utah

Marvin J. Stone, M.D.
Charles A. Sammons Cancer Center, Baylor University Medical Center at Dallas; Clinical Professor of Internal Medicine, University of Texas

D. E. Strandness, Jr., M.D.
Professor of Surgery, University of Washington

P. R. Sundaresan, M.D., Ph.D.
Fellow, Clinical Pharmacology Unit, University of Rochester

Borys Surawicz, M.D.
Professor of Medicine; Director, Cardiovascular Division, University of Kentucky

Richard D. Sweet, M.D.
Associate Professor, New York Medical College; Chief, Neurology Service, Metropolitan Hospital Center

Jan P. Szidon, M.D.
Director, Pulmonary Medicine Division, Department of Medicine, Michael Reese Hospital and Medical Center

Alvin S. Teirstein, M.D.
Director, Pulmonary Division; Professor of Medicine, Mount Sinai School of Medicine

Raymond C. Terhune, D.M.D., M.S.D.
Neptune Beach, Florida

Richard A. Thoft, M.D.
Assistant Professor of Ophthalmology, Harvard University; Massachusetts Eye and Ear Infirmary

Marvin Turck, M.D.
Professor of Medicine, University of Washington

Gerard M. Turino, M.D.
Professor of Medicine, Columbia University

John P. Utz, M.D.
Professor of Medicine, Georgetown University

Paul P. VanArsdel, Jr., M.D.
Professor of Medicine, University of Washington

Ralph O. Wallerstein, M.D.
Clinical Professor of Medicine, University of California, San Francisco

W. M. Wardell, D.M., D.Phil.
Associate Professor of Pharmacology and Toxicology and of Medicine; Director, Center for the Study of Drug Development, University of Rochester

Hans Weill, M.D.
Professor of Medicine, Tulane University

M. Weintraub, M.D.
Assistant Professor of Pharmacology and Toxicology and of Medicine, University of Rochester

Harvey J. Weiss, M.D.
Professor of Medicine, Columbia University

William Weiss, M.D.
Professor of Medicine, Hahnemann Medical College and Hospital of Philadelphia

Thomas H. Weller, M.D.
Professor and Head, Department of Tropical Public Health, Harvard School of Public Health

Nanette Kass Wenger, M.D.
Professor of Medicine (Cardiology), Emory University

Stanford Wessler, M.D.
Professor of Medicine, New York University

Sidney J. Winawer, M.D.
Director, Diagnostic Gastrointestinal Laboratory, Memorial Sloan-Kettering Cancer Center; Associate Professor of Medicine, Cornell University

Howard J. Winer, D.D.S.
Los Alamitos, California

Francis C. Wood, Jr., M.D.
Associate Professor of Medicine, University of Washington

Walter S. Wood, M.D.
Professor and Chairman, Department of Community and Family Medicine, Loyola University

Robert Zeppa, M.D.
Professor and Chairman, Department of Surgery, University of Miami

Morton M. Ziskind, M.D.
Professor of Medicine; Director, Pulmonary Diseases Section, Department of Medicine, Tulane University

C. Gordon Zubrod, M.D.
Professor and Chairman, Department of Oncology, University of Miami; Director, Comprehensive Cancer Center for the State of Florida

Burton Zweiman, M.D.
Professor of Medicine, University of Pennsylvania

§1. INFECTIOUS AND PARASITIC DISEASES

---

1. INTRODUCTION

A healthy individual lives in harmony with his normal body flora, but this balance may be disturbed by disease. **Host defenses** are an important factor in determining whether or not infection will occur. These include anatomic barriers, such as intact skin and the ciliated respiratory mucosa; physiologic barriers, such as gastric acid; immune factors, such as specific antibodies; and phagocytic cells, such as polymorphonuclear neutrophils and macrophages of the reticuloendothelial system. Unknown factors are also presumably involved.

The **microbes that cause disease** are sometimes members of the normal flora. For example, *Streptococcus pneumoniae* and the β-hemolytic *S. pyogenes,* which cause pneumococcal pneumonia and streptococcal pharyngitis, respectively, can exist as part of the normal throat flora. Disease can also be caused by microorganisms which are usually harmless or even beneficial members of the normal flora. An example of this is *Streptococcus viridans* endocarditis in a patient with a heart valve damaged by acute rheumatic fever.

Disease may be caused by a microorganism with a particular virulence for man. Most highly virulent pathogens (e.g., *Yersinia [Pasteurella] pestis,* the causative organism of plague, and *Rickettsia rickettsii,* the causative organism of Rocky Mountain spotted fever) are not part of the normal body flora and predictably will cause disease in man.

Some of the more likely causative pathogens of some common bacterial infections are shown in TABLE 1-1.

Many **manifestations** of infections are not due to a direct action of the infecting organism and its products but reflect the response of the infected host, and may not appear in patients with impaired host defense mechanisms. They include inflammation at the site of the infection (absent in patients who lack polymorphonuclear leukocytes) and systemic manifestations such as malaise, fever, and chills. Breakdown of local defense barriers around a local inflammatory process may permit dissemination of infection or absorption of toxic material sufficient to cause constitutional symptoms. This occurs when infection spreads from a local focus, either (1) along the lymphatics to the lymph nodes and through the thoracic duct into the bloodstream, or (2) from entry into the bloodstream directly from an extravascular focus. Bacteria, viruses, rickettsias, parasites, and fungi all can cause disseminated infection. Individuals with disseminated or generalized infections nearly always present with systemic symptoms if host responses are intact.

Laboratory findings in infections usually include an elevated leukocyte count and an increased ESR. Recovery of a microorganism from a site where it is not a normal resident is strong evidence for ascribing the etiology of an infection to that

TABLE 1-1. CAUSATIVE PA[T]

	Bronchitis	Cellulitis	Cystitis	Endocarditis	Furuncles & Carbuncles	Impetigo	Meningitis	Osteomyelitis	Otitis Media	Pneumonia	Prostatitis	Pyelonephritis	Septicemia	Sinusitis	Tonsillitis & Pharyngitis
Enterobacter spp.....			X									√	X	X	
Enterococcus		√	√									√	√		
Escherichia coli......			X				√				√	X	X	X	
Haemophilus influenzae........	X						X		X	√				√	√
Klebsiella spp.			X							√	√	X	X		
Meningococcus......							X						X		
Pneumococcus	X						X		X	X			X	X	
Proteus spp.........			X								√	X	X	X	
Pseudomonas aeruginosa........			√									√	√		
Staphylococcus aureus..........		X		X	X	X	√	X	√	√	√		X	X	
Staph. epidermidis (albus)..........		√		√	√	√						√	√	√	
α-Hemolytic streptococcus				X											
β-Hemolytic streptococcus		X				√	X	√	√	√	√		√	√	X

X = Commonly encountered pathogens; √ = Less commonly encountered pathogens.

organism. For example, isolation of enterococci from the urine is presumptive evidence of enterococcal urinary infection, while isolation of the same organism from the stool is of little significance. A heavy growth of a certain organism in association with a specific clinical syndrome (e.g., large numbers of pneumococci in the sputum of a patient with pneumonia) is also presumptive evidence of etiology. Serologic studies on acute and convalescent serums may show a rise in the titer of antibodies to a specific organism; the procedure is well described under Laboratory Diagnostic Tests in STREPTOCOCCAL INFECTIONS, in §1, Ch. 5.

FEVER AND CHILLS

Fever: *An elevation of body temperature above the normal range.* Oral temperatures above 37.0 C (98.6 F) in persons confined to bed, and above 37.2 C (99.0 F) in persons who are moderately active, usually constitute fever. Rectal temperatures are usually 0.3 to 0.6 C (0.5 to 1 F) higher.

Fever may be (1) **hyperthermic:** temperature of 40.5 C (105 F) or above; (2) **sustained:** temperature constantly above normal; (3) **intermittent:** temperature falling to normal or below each day, then rising again; (4) **remittent:** daily rise and fall of temperature, but without return to normal; (5) **hectic (septic):** marked temperature swings, frequently with chills and sweats; (6) **relapsing:** febrile episodes alternating with one or more days of normal temperature.

Chill: *An attack of shivering with a sense of coldness and pallor of the skin.* Chills are usually followed by fever.

Etiology

A thermoregulatory center in the hypothalamus controls the temperature of the body by altering skin circulation, sweating, and muscle activity. Fever associated with bacterial infection may be due to the action of endogenous **pyrogen** (a protein substance released by leukocytes following contact with bacterial endotoxin or other inflammatory stimuli), which acts directly on the thermoregulatory center. Injury to the hypothalamic heat-dissipating center (e.g., from a CVA or head trauma) can cause the heat-conserving mechanisms to overact. Neurogenic pyrexia is rare except with acute brain injuries and practically never is the cause of FUO.

Low-grade fever may accompany thyrotoxicosis, probably due to increased heat production from an increased metabolic rate. Hyperpyrexia through restriction of heat loss may occur when environmental temperatures and humidity are high and the air stagnant, in ichthyosis and other generalized skin diseases, and with congenital absence of sweat glands. Dehydration in infants may result in hyperpyrexia. Severe trauma, myocardial infarction, cerebral hemorrhage or thrombosis, peripheral arterial occlusion, and malignant neoplasms may cause fever. The fever and chills sometimes seen with hypernephroma may simulate an infectious disease. Massive intravascular hemolysis (e.g., from hemolytic transfusion reactions, drug-sensitivity reactions, or crises in sickle cell anemia), serum sickness, polyarteritis, rheumatic fever, rheumatoid arthritis, and erythema nodosum also cause fever.

Chills are a mechanism for raising body temperature to a new level set by the "thermostat" in the hypothalamus. Shaking chills are seen in many acute bacterial infections, but are by no means specific for them. Pneumococcal pneumonia and gram-negative bacteremia are two conditions characteristically associated with chills. A chill may also be seen with other bacterial infections, fever due to allergic reactions, transfusion reactions, viral infections, and malignancy. In a febrile patient, ingestion of aspirin may cause chills.

Diagnosis

The type of temperature curve may give a clue to the underlying disease. Untreated typhoid fever is characteristically associated with sustained fever (and a pulse rate that is slow for the degree of fever). A hectic type of fever is often seen in localized infections (e.g., acute osteomyelitis, empyema, or intra-abdominal abscess). A relapsing type of fever is seen in malaria, ratbite fever, relapsing fever (due to *Borrelia recurrentis*), and chronic meningococcemia.

Extremely high temperatures (above 41.4 C, or 106.5 F) are rare and are usually neurogenic (following head injury, massive cerebral hemorrhage, or brain surgery) or follow in the wake of heatstroke.

The **differential diagnosis of fever** depends in part on the age of the patient. Causes of fever and their diagnosis in **infants and children** are discussed in §10, Ch. 4.

In adults, an infection, especially TB or occult infections of kidney, brain, liver, or abdominal cavity (with or without abscess formation), are the most likely cause of FUO (see also Etiology, above). A number of febrile diseases (e.g., RA, SLE, regional enteritis, SBE) may be difficult to identify because characteristic or localizing symptoms or signs are minimal or lacking. The collagen vascular diseases and certain neoplastic diseases (particularly leukemia, lymphomas, and hypernephroma) may present solely with high fever.

The history often gives important clues (e.g., a history of drinking contaminated water suggests typhoid; of employment in meat-packing plants, brucellosis; of proximity to rats, typhus or leptospirosis; of being bitten by a rat, ratbite fever).

Frequent physical examinations, x-ray studies, blood cultures, blood counts, and urinalyses may yield a new finding which leads to the diagnosis. Blood cultures should be taken in groups of 1 to 3/day for several days. Serologic tests should be repeated if typhoid, brucellosis, certain virus diseases, or a rickettsial disease is suspected, since a rise in titer as the disease progresses is more significant than a single titer. Malarial parasites must be sought. Antimicrobial therapy may cause drug fever, and sometimes stopping therapy may be followed by a rapid defervescence. X-ray studies may disclose a neoplastic process; scans of the liver, spleen, or bone may show infiltrative processes. Biopsy of enlarged lymph nodes, subcutaneous nodules, chronic skin lesions, or tender muscles frequently permits specific diagnosis.

Treatment

General principles: Basic treatment of fever must be directed to its cause. In serious infections, antibiotics should be started before the results of culture and sensitivity studies are known, but this is rarely necessary in FUO.

Sometimes it is necessary to treat fever symptomatically, but suppression of fever by antipyretic measures impairs a valuable indicator of the disease course. This must be weighed against the desirability of temperature reduction. It must first be decided whether the pyrexia is harmful. Prolonged fever may be debilitating, since the associated increase in metabolism may not be matched by the necessary intake of food (particularly protein), fluid, and electrolytes.

Antipyresis should be considered when fever is debilitating or discomforting or when it affects CNS function.

Antipyretics such as aspirin and acetaminophen act on the thermoregulatory centers to increase heat loss by resetting the hypothalamic "thermostat" at a lower level, thus inducing cutaneous vasodilation and increasing perspiration. These drugs do not alter the course of febrile illnesses, but simply reduce fever. Both are also analgesic, and aspirin is anti-inflammatory. When used as antipyretics, the average oral adult doses are: aspirin 300 to 600 mg q 3 h, acetaminophen 300 to 600 mg q 4 to 6 h. In an occasional patient with high fever, antipyretics may cause a sudden fall of temperature and general circulatory collapse. For this reason, they should be given around the clock. Since pyrazolone compounds (e.g., aminopyrine, dipyrone) occasionally cause fatal agranulocytosis, **they should not be used as antipyretics.**

The oral temperature should be reduced slowly to 38 C (100.5 F) or less. When heroic measures are indicated, as in heat hyperpyrexia (heatstroke), immersion of the patient's trunk and extremities in ice water is necessary. The ice water should be stirred and the patient massaged steadily. The tubbing should be discontinued when rectal temperature falls to 38.5 C (101 F); otherwise, hypothermia and shock may result. A good response can be expected in 10 to 40 min (see also Heat Hyperpyrexia in §20, Ch. 3).

Antipyretic drugs are generally ineffective in the rare neurogenic hyperpyrexia due to damage to the hypothalamus (e.g., following a CVA or head trauma). To control acute neurogenic hyperpyrexia, sodium pentobarbital 100 to 200 mg orally or slowly IV, or sodium phenobarbital 75 to 100 mg orally or IM, can be given, as these drugs are thought to paralyze the overacting heat-conserving center. Doses may be repeated at intervals as indicated by the response.

Special care: Maintaining fluid and electrolyte balance is usually more important than reducing the temperature. Since fluid loss is increased in fever, the patient should be induced to drink adequate amounts of liquids, or fluids should be given parenterally. If fluid loss is excessive and salt intake low, supplementary sodium chloride 1 to 2 Gm t.i.d. should be given. Nutrition should be maintained by a high-vitamin, high-protein diet given in frequent small feedings. Multivitamin preparations may be given daily in prolonged febrile diseases. If fever is prolonged, parenteral hyperalimentation should be considered.

Nursing care in prolonged fever: Patients require scrupulous attention to oral hygiene in order to prevent stomatitis and parotitis. Daily soap-and-water bed baths, followed by a back rub with cool saline, contribute to comfort and morale as well as providing ordinary cleanliness. Meticulous skin care and relief of pressure by frequent turning in bed (together with adequate protein intake) provide the best prophylaxis against decubitus ulcers.

CELLULITIS

Any spreading infection with inflammation of the soft or supporting tissues. Cellulitis usually affects the skin and subcutaneous structures, but deeper tissues may also be involved (as in pelvic or periurethral cellulitis). Erysipelas, a form of cellulitis, is discussed in §16, Ch. 4.

Etiology

Spread of infection may be due to the inherent virulence of the infecting organism, to manipulation of or other trauma to an infected lesion, or to impairment of host defense mechanisms. Streptococci and staphylococci are the most common pathogens, but any organism capable of invading tissue may produce cellulitis. Anaerobic bacteria (particularly *Clostridium perfringens* [*C. welchii*]) may produce a characteristic cellulitis in which gas is present under the skin.

Symptoms and Signs

Fever, chills, malaise, and headache may be present. Leukocytosis usually develops. The area is red, swollen, painful, and warm, with poorly defined borders. Deep cellulitis is characterized by generalized symptoms, local discomfort, and acute pain on palpation of the affected area. With cellulitis caused by gas-forming or other anaerobic organisms, the outstanding features are pain and tenderness of the involved area and crepitation due to the gas in the subcutaneous tissue; usually, more purulent lesions are foul-smelling.

Diagnosis

Ordinarily, superficial cellulitis can be readily identified. However, deep (e.g., pelvic) cellulitis is identifiable only by careful history and thorough physical examination, and appropriate x-ray, radioisotope scan, and ultrasound diagnostic procedures.

Course and Prognosis

Lymphangitis, with lymphadenitis of the regional nodes, usually develops. Bacteremia occurs in some cases. Abscess formation and destruction of tissue may occur. Cellulitis of the scalp may produce intracranial complications by spread through the emissary and diploic veins. Cellulitis of the floor of the mouth and neck is often due to oral anaerobic organisms. It is a serious condition that may require surgery if it causes airway obstruction, but usually responds to antibiotics, most often penicillin. Cellulitis is always serious in very young children and the elderly; the prognosis is relatively good in individuals with normal host defenses.

Treatment

General: The involved part should be rested, and elevated when possible. If severe systemic symptoms are present, bed rest is indicated. Local application of heat or wet dressings may be helpful, but care must be taken not to macerate the skin.

Specific: Since β-hemolytic streptococci and staphylococci are the most frequent causative organisms, a penicillinase-resistant penicillin (e.g., methicillin, oxacillin, nafcillin) or cephalothin, with or without penicillin G, should be given until the results of culture and sensitivity studies are known. If the patient is allergic to penicillin, erythromycin or lincomycin should be given. A cephalosporin may be used **with caution.** For cellulitis due to mixed anaerobes, clindamycin or chloramphenicol should be used. Treatment should be continued until signs of inflammation are subsiding. Treatment of anaerobic cellulitis due to clostridia is discussed under HISTOTOXIC CLOSTRIDIAL DISEASE in §1, Ch. 5.

LYMPHADENITIS

Inflammation of one or more lymph nodes.

Etiology

Any pathogen can produce lymphadenitis—bacteria, viruses, rickettsias, protozoa, fungi. Streptococci and staphylococci are most frequently responsible. The condition is usually secondary to a primary focus elsewhere, usually the skin or subcutaneous tissue.

Symptoms and Signs

Single nodes or groups of nodes may be affected, or involvement may be widespread. Superficial nodes may enlarge greatly. They are often tender and painful, and the overlying skin is inflamed; motion of adjacent structures is inhibited voluntarily because of pain. Systemic symptoms may be minimal or severe. Cellulitis and pronounced swelling of the surrounding tissue often occur, and suppuration with abscess formation may develop. Low-grade or chronic infections may produce firm, nontender nodes that may persist indefinitely, or (as with tuberculosis and certain fungus infections) may caseate and form cold abscesses, or may erode through the surface to create draining sinuses. However, even massive, acutely inflamed nodes may subside completely without sequelae, or may leave only small, firm, palpable (shotty) nodes.

Diagnosis

Diagnosis of lymphadenitis is usually easy. A primary infection is often first indicated by regional lymphadenitis. For example, pediculosis capitis in children may be disclosed by the finding of enlarged posterior cervical nodes, or an abscessed molar by submaxillary lymphadenopathy. Lymph node aspiration, biopsy, or excision may be needed to make the precise etiologic diagnosis.

Treatment

Successful treatment of the underlying cause usually results in prompt regression of secondary lymphadenitis. Appropriate antimicrobials should be given.

Either hot, wet applications or ice packs help to relieve pain; heat may aid in localizing the infection. Abscesses should be incised and drained.

LYMPHANGITIS

An acute or chronic inflammation of the superficial or deep lymphatic channels, usually caused by streptococci or staphylococci.

Symptoms and Signs

Acute lymphangitis: Fever (39 to 40.5 C; 102 to 105 F), chills, malaise, generalized aching, and headache are usually present. Leukocytosis (WBC count 15,000 to 30,000) with a preponderance of neutrophils is common. Patchy areas of inflammation along the path of a lymphatic vessel resemble cellulitis (e.g., erysipelas). Lymphangitis occurring as a complication of a hand or foot infection presents as irregular, pink, tender, linear streaks extending up the limb toward the regional lymph nodes.

Chronic lymphangitis: The lesion appears as a firm cord in or under the skin leading from the site of initial infection (tuberculous, syphilitic, or fungous). The cord may be tender and may have abscesses, ulcers, areas of infection, or healed scars along its course where secondary foci have been established.

Course and Prognosis

Lymphangitis is almost invariably followed by lymphadenitis. Bacteremia is a constant threat. Cellulitis with suppuration, necrosis, and necrotizing ulcers may develop along the course of the involved lymph channel. The outlook is often serious for the very young, aged, or debilitated patient.

Treatment

Care of the original infection is of prime importance. Aerobic and anaerobic blood cultures should be made routinely. For antibiotic therapy of acute lymphangitis, see CELLULITIS, Treatment, above. Antibiotics should be continued until the temperature has been normal for 72 h and acute inflammation is subsiding. For severe cases, bed rest is indicated, with elevation of the affected part. Manipulation of the lesion is contraindicated, and surgery should usually be withheld until localization and suppuration are evident.

With chronic lymphangitis, control of the underlying infection often halts further extension, but residual infection may result in chronic swelling **(lymphedema)** which may require surgical intervention.

BACTEREMIA

The presence of bacteria in the circulating blood. There are several very different circumstances in which bacteremia is found. It is a common transient accompaniment of various surgical manipulations (e.g., incision of an abscess); treatment is usually not necessary since the bacteremia abates spontaneously. Bacteremia is also seen with indwelling IV devices or indwelling urethral catheters, and usually disappears following their removal.

Bacteremia is a common finding in systemic infections. Transient bacteremia probably occurs frequently even with mild infections. Bacteremia is also seen at the onset of pneumococcal pneumonia, usually disappearing when the pneumonia is treated. In patients with SBE, by contrast, bacteremia is constant and is eradicated only by prolonged therapy with bactericidal antibiotics.

Symptoms and Signs
Few symptoms or signs are unique to bacteremia. Fever, though variable in type, is almost always present. It is sometimes intermittent, with wide diurnal variations (septic, "spiking"). Chills are common at the onset. Skin eruptions are common and are usually petechial or purpuric, though papular, pustular, or vesicular lesions may also appear. Secondary infection of the meninges or of serous cavities, such as the pericardium or larger joint cavities, may occur. Endocarditis occurs occasionally if the pathogen is a streptococcus or a staphylococcus; it is rare with gram-negative organisms. Metastatic abscesses may occur almost anywhere and, when sufficiently extensive, produce symptoms and signs characteristic of inflammation in the organ affected. Especially with staphylococcal infections, metastatic abscesses may appear in great numbers throughout the body. Bacteremia (especially gram-negative) may cause shock with hypotension, vascular collapse, renal failure, and death. Severe meningococcal infections may induce the **Waterhouse-Friderichsen syndrome,** a rapidly overwhelming bacteremia with hemorrhagic manifestations and collapse from hemorrhage into adrenal glands.

Urinalysis usually shows albumin and, at times, erythrocytes and leukocytes. Blood counts may show anemia and leukocytosis or leukopenia, depending on the type and duration of infection.

Diagnosis
This is established by blood cultures, which should always be for both aerobic and anaerobic organisms. Repeated cultures (usually not > 6) may be necessary. A single negative culture does not exclude bacteremia; moreover, in some patients with symptoms of bacteremia, cultures never do become positive. Blood is preferably obtained as soon as possible after the onset of a chill, since the chill usually follows endotoxemia or bacteremia by 30 to 60 min. When multiple organisms are cultured, contamination must be suspected. If this finding is repeated on subsequent culture, or if contamination does not seem to be present, then a polymicrobial infection such as an intra-abdominal abscess should be suspected as the source of the bacteremia.

Prognosis
In any infection, sustained bacteremia is a dangerous development. The formation of multiple embolic abscesses is extremely serious and affords a poor prognosis. Bacteremia that is unresponsive to treatment (due to inadequate antibiotic therapy or poor host resistance) is usually fatal.

Treatment
Unless transient, bacteremia indicates lowered resistance in the patient or heightened virulence of the organism, and requires vigorous therapy. Supportive measures are of the utmost importance. Hospitalization is imperative and the patient with shock should be in an intensive care unit. Adequate nutrition must be maintained. Fluid intake should ensure a urinary output of 1500 to 2000 ml/day, and electrolyte balance must be maintained.

Specific treatment of bacteremia is the same as that of the primary infection, but in an intensified form. Antibiotics should be given parenterally. An effective regimen for bacteremia of unknown etiology before sensitivities are known is gentamicin 3 to 5 mg/kg body wt/day IM plus either methicillin 6 to 12 Gm/day IV or cephalothin 6 to 8 Gm/day IV. Carbenicillin 30 Gm/day IV may be added. Prompt, adequate drainage of pus is necessary. Response to therapy is primarily determined clinically and abatement of symptoms and signs is the best guide to the outcome. Therapy should be continued for at least several days after symptoms have subsided.

2. VIRAL DISEASES

GENERAL

Viruses: *The smallest of parasites; intracellular molecular particles, in some instances crystallizable, with a central core of nucleic acid and an outer cover of protein; wholly dependent on cells (bacterial, plant, or animal) for reproduction.* The nucleic acid core (RNA or DNA) represents the basic infectious material, being able in many cases to penetrate susceptible cells and initiate infection alone.

Though most viruses are invisible in the light microscope (size variation, about 0.02 to 0.3μ), they can be seen by electron microscopy and measured by various biophysical and biochemical methods. Like most other parasites, animal viruses stimulate host antibody production.

Several hundred different viruses may infect man. Many have been recognized only recently, so their clinical effects or even relationships are not fully delineated. Many viruses usually produce inapparent infections and only occasionally overt disease; nevertheless, because of their wide (sometimes universal) prevalence and their numerous distinct serotypes, they create important medical and public health problems.

The viruses occurring primarily in man are spread chiefly by man himself, mainly via respiratory and enteric excretions. Such viruses (see TABLE 1-2) are found in all parts of the world, their spread being limited by inborn resistance, prior immunizing infections or vaccines, sanitary and other public health control measures, and, in a few instances, by chemoprophylactic agents.

Many viruses pursue their chief biologic cycle in animals, man being only a secondary or accidental host. The zoonotic viruses (see TABLE 1-3), in contrast to the specifically human agents, are limited to those geographic areas and environments able to support their extrahuman natural cycles of infection (vertebrates or arthropods, or both).

Two properties of certain viruses are noteworthy because of their implications: (1) oncogenicity and (2) a prolonged incubation period. (1) Oncogenic properties of some animal viruses are well known (e.g., Rous sarcoma of chickens, Shope rabbit papilloma, murine leukemia viruses), but as yet no virus has been identified as the primary cause of human malignancy. However, some human viruses (e.g., adenovirus Type 12) can induce tumors in hamsters, particles resembling viruses have been observed by electron microscopy in certain human malignant cells, and Epstein-Barr virus has been found in association with some lymphoid tissue malignancies, such as Burkitt's lymphoma. (2) Kuru, a rare disease confined to natives of New Guinea and characterized by chronic degeneration of the CNS, has been transmitted and passed in primates. Symptoms appear after a prolonged incubation period of about 18 mo; hence the agent has been termed a **"slow"** **virus.** Slow viruses have also been found in sheep and other animals. The implications for man are clear: some of the chronic degenerative diseases, previously with no known etiology, now appear to be due to slow virus infections. Besides Kuru, these include subacute sclerosing panencephalitis (probably measles), progressive multifocal leukoencephalopathy (possibly a papovavirus), and Creutzfeldt-Jakob disease ("transmissible agent"). It is probable that other human diseases will also be linked to slow viruses in the future.

Diagnosis of Viral Infections

In theory, most viral infections can, by some means, be recognized; in practice, diagnosis often remains difficult. A few viral diseases can be diagnosed accurately on clinical and epidemiologic grounds (e.g., several well-known exanthems), but many diagnoses depend on retrospective tests (e.g., serologic examination of acute and convalescent serums), unless an adequately equipped diagnostic virology

TABLE 1-2. HUMAN VIRAL DISEASES: NATURAL CYCLE CHIEFLY IN MAN; PERSON-TO-PERSON SPREAD*

Virus Groups & Categories	No. Known Serotypes	Most Important Syndromes	Serotypes	Prevalence, Distribution	Diagnostic Leads	Specific Therapy	Specific Prophylaxis
Respiratory Influenza A, B, & C	3	Influenza; AFRD; acute bronchitis & pneumonia; croup	A (with many possible subtypes), B, C	Epidemic, occasionally pandemic (A, B); endemic (C)	Clinical & epidemiologic features; serologic; virus isolation	None	Vaccine (moderately effective) Amantadine (A)
Parainfluenza 1–4	4	AFRI (children); acute bronchitis & pneumonia; croup	1 (Sendai, HA-2) 2 (CA, SV-5) 3 (HA-1, SF-4)	1: Local epidemic; 1 & 3: widely in children	Clinical not defined; serologic; virus isolation	None	Vaccines under study
Mumps	1	Parotitis, orchitis, meningoencephalitis	1	Global; most children; some adults	Clinical features; serologic; virus isolation	None	Vaccine
Adenoviruses	33	AFRD (children); ARD (adults); APCF; EKC; viral pneumonia; acute follicular conjunctivitis	1–10, 14, 21	1–3, 5–7: Children 4, 7, 14, 21: Adults 8: Local EKC	APCF, EKC: Clinical features Most: Serologic & virus isolation	None	Vaccine (4,7) for military epidemic situations
Reoviruses	3	Mild RI	(?)	Widely in children; may be same as in animals	Serologic; virus isolation	None	None
Respiratory syncytial	1 (3 subtypes)	U & L RI (infants); mild URI (adults)	1 (?)	Pediatric clinics & hospital wards	Serologic & isolation & identification of viruses	None	None
Infectious mononucleosis	1	Infectious mononucleosis	Epstein-Barr virus	Widespread; apparent chiefly in young adults	Heterophil agglut.; diff. WBC count; fluorescent antibody	None	None

Rhinoviruses	(?)	Common cold; acute coryza with or without fever	>95; probably 100's	Universal; especially in cold months	None	None	None
Enteric Polioviruses	3	Poliomyelitis (paralytic); aseptic meningitis; AFRD (children)	1, 2, & 3	Almost universal; + in warm months; + at younger ages	Paralysis typical; serologic; virus isolation	None	Vaccines: Live (oral) Killed (injected)
Coxsackieviruses	30 (A's: 24; B's: 6)	Herpangina; epidemic pleurodynia; aseptic meningitis; myocarditis; pericarditis; AFRD (children); paralytic disease; fever & exanthem	A's: 2, 4-10, 16, 21, 23 B's: 1-6	Varies with types; most persons infected; + in warm months; + in children	Virus isolation; serologic difficult, due to so many serotypes	None	None
Echoviruses	31**	Aseptic meningitis; fever & exanthem; meningoencephalitis with rash; diarrhea neonatorum; paralytic disease; myocarditis; pericarditis; ARD	4, 6, 8, 11, 14, 16, 18, 20, 30	As for coxsackieviruses	As for coxsackieviruses	None	None
Epidemic gastroenteritis	3 (?)	Epidemic nausea & vomiting	Orbiviruses; "adenolike;" "parvo/ picorna-like"	Local epidemics (children); + in colder months; + in neonates	Clinical & epidemiologic features, electron microscopy of diarrheal stools	None	None

(Continued)

* Developments are so rapid that no summary can be fully up to date. Main abbreviations: **AFRD**, acute febrile respiratory disease; **APCF**, acute pharyngo-conjunctival fever; **ARD**, acute respiratory disease; **EKC**, epidemic keratoconjunctivitis; **LRI**, lower respiratory illness; **URI**, upper respiratory illness.
** Types 9, 10, and 28 have been reclassified; these numbers are not now used.

TABLE 1-2. HUMAN VIRAL DISEASES: NATURAL CYCLE CHIEFLY IN MAN; PERSON-TO-PERSON SPREAD *(Cont'd)*

Virus Groups & Categories	No. Known Sero-types	Most Important		Prevalence, Distribution	Diagnostic Leads	Specific	
		Syndromes	Serotypes			Therapy	Prophylaxis
Exanthems							
Rubeola	1	Measles; encephalomyelitis	1 known	Almost universal; monkeys also infected; CNS involvement rare	Clinical features; serologic; virus isolation	None	Vaccines
Rubella	1	German measles	1 (?)	Universal; birth defects from infection during 1st trimester of pregnancy	Clinical & epidemiologic features; serologic	None	Vaccines
Varicella-zoster	1	Chickenpox	1 known	Almost universal (children); occasionally in adults	Clinical features; serologic; virus isolation	None	γ-Globulin
	Same	Herpes zoster	Same	Common in adults; reactivation or reinfection	Same	None	None
Herpes simplex	2	Herpes labialis; herpetic gingivo-stomatitis; eczema; keratoconjunctivitis; encephalitis; vulvovaginitis	2 established	Recurrent labial, almost universal; gingivo-stomatitis frequent in infants & children; others rare	Clinical features; serologic; virus isolation	Idoxuridine (IDU) under study	None
Roseola infantum	1 (?)	Rose rash, infants (Exanthem subitum)	Not isolated	Widespread; early childhood	Clinical features	None	None
Variola	1	Smallpox	1 known	Formerly epidemic & endemic (unless vaccinated)	Clinical features	None	Vaccine

Erythema infectiosum	2 (?)	"Fifth" disease; rash, malaise	Not isolated	Sporadic outbreaks	Atypical exanthems	None	None
Persistent (Latent) Cytomegaloviruses (salivary gland)	1	Congenital defects (cytomegalic inclusion disease); hepatitis (CMV mononucleosis)	1 established	Virus widespread; recognized disease uncommon	Clinical features; serologic; virus isolation	None	None
Hepatitis 1. Type A	1	Hepatitis A	1 established	Widespread; often epidemic	Clinical & epidemiologic features	None	γ-Globulin; vaccine under study
2. Type B	1	Hepatitis B	1 established	Widespread; may follow use of whole blood & derivatives or contaminated equipment	Clinical features; serologic	None	Strict aseptic precautions; screening for hepatitis B surface antigen; vaccine and γ-globulin under study
Papovavirus	1	Warts (Verrucae)	Not definitely established	Universal; common; often recurrent	Clinical examination & biopsy	None	None
Molluscum contagiosum	1	Molluscum contagiosum tumors	1 established	Infrequent	Clinical examination & biopsy	None	None

TABLE 1-3. VIRUSES TRANSMITTED FROM NATURE TO MAN (ZOONOSES)

Virus Groups & Categories	No. Known Serotypes	Most Important Syndromes	Serotypes	Prevalence, Distribution	Diagnostic Leads	Therapy	Prophylaxis
Arboviruses* Group A	>250	1. Western equine encephalitis (WEE)	Same designations as clinical syndromes	1. N. & S. America	Serologic; pathologic; virus isolation	None	Effective vaccines can be made; except for yellow fever, none in general use
		2. Eastern equine encephalitis (EEE)		2. N. & S. America			
		3. Venezuelan equine encephalitis (VEE)		3. Gulf states to S. America			
		4. Chikungunya encephalitis		4. Africa, S.E. Asia, India			
		5. Mayaro disease		5. S. America, Trinidad			
Group B		1. Yellow fever		1. Africa, Cen. & S. America			
		2. Dengue 1–4		2. Tropics & subtropics worldwide			
		3. Japanese encephalitis		3. Asia, Australia, New Zealand			
		4. Murray Valley encephalitis		4. Australia, New Guinea			
		5. St. Louis encephalitis		5. N. & S. America			
		6. Russian spring-summer encephalitis		6. USSR, E. Central Europe, Malaya			
		7. Omsk hemorrhagic fever		7. USSR			
		8. Kyasanur Forest disease		8. India			
		9. Powassan		9. N. America			
Group C (Bunyamwera supergroup)		1. Bunyamwera and 13 others		1. Africa, S. America, Finland, USA			
		2. Marituba and 12 others		2. S. America, Central America			
		3. California encephalitis and 8 related types		3. Probably worldwide; common in midwest USA			

Group	No.	Diseases	Antigenic types	Distribution	Diagnosis	Treatment	Immunization
Phlebotomus fever group		1. Naples, Sicilian fevers 2. Punta Toro, Chagres fevers 3. Candiru fever		1. Italy, India, Egypt 2. Panama 3. Brazil		None	None
Ungrouped		1. Rift Valley fever 2. Crimean-Congo hemorrhagic fever		1. E. Africa 2. USSR, Central Africa, W. Pakistan		None	Effective vaccines available
Diplornavirus (Reovirus-like)	1	Colorado tick fever	1 known	Western USA	Serologic; virus isolation	None	None
Rabies	1	Rabies (Hydrophobia)	1 known	Worldwide; domestic & wild animals; infrequent in man	Hist'y, clin. & path. findings; virus isolation	None	None
Herpesvirus simiae (B virus)	1	Encephalomyelitis	1 known	Chiefly lab. workers exposed to monkeys, simian tissue cultures	Virus isolation	None	None
Arenaviruses*	≥11	1. Lassa fever 2. Machupo (Bolivian hemorrhagic fever) 3. Junin (Argentinian hemorrhagic fever) 4. Lymphocytic choriomeningitis	Same designations as clinical syndromes	1. Africa 2. S. America 3. S. America 4. Worldwide; chief reservoir: rodents	Virus isolation, serology	None	None

*See also TABLE 1-8 in ARBOVIRUS AND ARENAVIRUS DISEASES, below. Arthropod vectors of most arboviruses are one or more genera and species of mosquito, ticks (Russian spring-summer encephalitis, Crimean hemorrhagic fever) and sandflies (Phlebotomus fever). Arbovirus Groups A and B are now reclassified as Togaviruses.

laboratory is available in the community for more rapid diagnosis by such procedures as culture or immunofluorescence microscopy. During large epidemics (e.g., of influenza), laboratory diagnosis of early cases may aid in recognizing and managing those occurring subsequently. Many state health laboratories and the National Center for Disease Control can also offer diagnostic assistance.

Viruses of man and animals are isolated from secretions, excretions, and tissues by inoculating susceptible animals, chick embryos, and cultures of living cells. Presence of the virus is usually indicated by disease and antibody responses in the animals or by cytopathogenic effects and antigen production in tissue cultures.

Prophylaxis and Treatment

Viral diseases are not susceptible to antibiotics. In certain viral illnesses, particularly those liable to superinfection with bacterial pathogens, antibiotics have been used in an attempt to prevent complications. The efficacy of such treatment is debatable; moreover, indiscriminate use of antibiotics in viral infections (e.g., measles) may be harmful.

Results from the laboratory and from clinical trials hold out hope that the barriers—chiefly intracellular multiplication—to the effective use of chemotherapeutic or chemoprophylactic drugs against viruses and viral diseases may soon be breached, if not broken. Examples are idoxuridine (IDU) and its derivatives for herpes simplex keratitis, methisazone for smallpox, amantadine for influenza A, and exogenous or endogenous interferon, a protein of low molecular weight which is produced by certain cells when stimulated by a variety of substances (e.g., bacteria, some viruses, nucleic acids) and which nonspecifically inhibits replication of a wide range of viruses in the cells of the host producing it. (See also ANTIVIRAL DRUGS in §22.)

In many common, undifferentiated illnesses—the most frequent manifestations of prevalent viruses—decisions concerning the use of chemotherapeutic agents or antibiotics are often complicated by the difficulties of making a definitive diagnosis. In such instances, the best guides are the severity and course of the illness, blood and x-ray findings, and clinical judgment. Because antibiotics cannot be expected to influence most viral illnesses favorably, lack of response should suggest the need for suspending their use and seeking a more specific therapy, if such exists.

Effective prophylactic virus vaccines available for general use include those for influenza, measles, mumps, poliomyelitis, rabies, rubella (German measles), smallpox, and yellow fever. An adenovirus vaccine is available and effective, but should be used only in population groups subject to high risk, such as military recruits. Other vaccines are being developed.

EXANTHEMATOUS VIRAL DISEASES

MEASLES
(Rubeola; Morbilli; Nine-Day Measles)

A highly contagious acute disease characterized by fever, cough, coryza, conjunctivitis, eruption **(Koplik's spots)** *on the buccal or labial mucosa, and a spreading maculopapular cutaneous rash.*

Etiology and Epidemiology

Measles is caused by a paramyxovirus and is spread largely by droplets from the nose, throat, and mouth of persons in the prodromal or early eruptive stages of the disease, or by airborne droplet nuclei. Indirect spread by uninfected persons or by objects is unusual. The period of communicability begins 2 to 4 days before the rash appears and continues during the acute stages of the disease. The virus disappears from nose and throat secretions by the time the rash clears. The mild desquamation that follows the rash is not infective.

Measles and chickenpox appear to be the most readily transmitted of all infectious diseases. Before widespread immunization programs began, measles epidemics occurred every 2 or 3 yr with small localized outbreaks during intervening years. In urban areas, measles occurs mainly in young children. An infant whose mother had measles receives transplacental passive immunity lasting most of the first year of life. Thereafter, susceptibility is high; about 98% of adults have had frank measles, usually during early childhood. One attack of measles confers lifelong immunity.

Symptoms and Signs

After a 7- to 14-day incubation period, prodromal fever, coryza, hacking cough, and conjunctivitis develop. The pathognomonic **Koplik's spots** appear 2 to 4 days later, usually on the buccal mucosa opposite the 1st and 2nd upper molars. These resemble tiny grains of white sand surrounded by an inflammatory areola. If the spots are numerous, the entire background may be a mottled erythema. Pharyngitis and inflammation of the laryngeal and tracheobronchial mucosa develop. Characteristic multinucleated giant cells appear in the nasal secretions, the pharyngeal and buccal mucosa, and often the urinary sediment.

The characteristic rash appears 3 to 5 days after onset of symptoms, usually 1 to 2 days after the appearance of Koplik's spots. It begins in front of and below the ears and on the side of the neck as irregular macules which soon become maculopapular and spread rapidly (within 24 to 48 h) to the trunk and extremities, at which time they begin to fade on the face. Petechiae or ecchymoses may be present with particularly severe rashes.

At the peak of the illness, the temperature may exceed 40 C (104 F), and periorbital edema, conjunctivitis, photophobia, a hacking cough, extensive rash, and mild itching are present. Leukopenia with a relative lymphocytosis is usual. The constitutional symptoms and signs parallel the severity of the eruption and vary with the epidemic. In 3 to 5 days, the fever falls by lysis, the patient feels more comfortable, and the rash begins to fade rapidly, leaving a coppery-brown discoloration followed by a branny desquamation.

Prognosis and Complications

Measles is usually benign and has a low mortality rate unless complications ensue. Pneumonia (especially in infants), otitis media, and other bacterial infections are common. Patients with measles are highly susceptible to streptococcal infection. Measles causes transient suppression of delayed hypersensitivity, leading to a transient reversal of previously positive tuberculin and histoplasmin skin tests, and sometimes to worsening of active tuberculosis or reactivation of latent mycobacterial infection. An exacerbation of fever, change in blood count from leukopenia to leukocytosis, and development of malaise, pain, or prostration suggest a complicating bacterial infection.

Acute thrombocytopenic purpura, at times with severe hemorrhagic manifestations, may complicate the acute phase of measles.

Encephalitis occurs about once in 600 to 1000 cases. It usually occurs 2 days to 3 wk after onset of the exanthem, often beginning with high fever, convulsions, and coma. Although in most instances the CSF lymphocyte count is between 50 and 500/cu mm and the protein level is increased, a normal CSF at the time of initial symptoms does not rule out encephalitis. The course may be brief, with recovery in about a week, or may be prolonged and terminate in serious CNS impairment or death.

TABLE 1-4. DIFFERENTIAL DIAGNOSIS OF

Condition	Incubation (days)	Period of Communicability	Symptoms and Signs
Measles (Rubeola)	7–14	From 2 to 4 days before appearance of rash until 2 to 5 days after onset	Koplik's spots; fever, coryza, cough, conjunctivitis, photophobia, usually mild pruritus
Rubella (German measles)	14–21	Shortly before onset of symptoms until rash disappears; infected newborns are usually infective for many months	Malaise, fever, headache, rhinitis; postauricular & suboccipital lymphadenopathy, with tender nodes
Roseola infantum (Exanthem subitum)	Probably 4–7	Unknown	Infants & preschool children affected. Characteristic disappearance of high fever & simultaneous appearance of rash
Chickenpox (Varicella)	14–21	From a few days before onset of symptoms until all crops of vesicles have crusted over	Moderate fever, headache, malaise, occasional sore throat
Smallpox (Variola)	10–14	Usually from 24 to 48 h before onset of symptoms until all crusts have disappeared	Abrupt onset with chills, fever, rapid pulse & respiration; frequently nausea & vomiting. Also severe headache, backache, muscular pains
Infectious mononucleosis	5–15	Undetermined	Malaise, headache, fever, sore throat, splenomegaly, generalized lymphadenopathy
Scarlet fever (Scarlatina)	3–5 (Occasionally slightly shorter or longer)	Usually from 24 h before onset of symptoms until 2 to 3 wk thereafter, or even longer if complications occur (e.g., sinusitis, otitis media)	Sore throat, chills, fever, headache, vomiting; strawberry tongue; cervical lymphadenopathy; circumoral pallor, rapid pulse
Drug rash	History of use of drug	None	Variable, including fever, malaise, arthralgia, nausea, photophobia, pruritis

THE MORE COMMON EXANTHEMS

Eruption			Laboratory Findings
Site	Character	Onset; Duration	
Starts around ears, on face, neck, spreading over trunk & limbs. Limbs escape in mild cases	Maculopapular; brownish-pink in color & irregularly confluent in severe cases or even petechial. Discrete in mild cases	3 to 5 days after onset of symptoms; lasts 4 to 7 days	Granulocytic leukopenia. Virus in blood & nasopharynx
Face, neck, & spreading to trunk & limbs	Fine pinkish macules which become confluent & often scarlatiniform or pinpoint on 2nd day	1 or 2 days after onset of symptoms; lasts 1 to 3 days	WBC count usually normal or slightly reduced. Virus in blood and nasopharynx
Chest & abdomen, with moderate involvement of face & extremities	Either diffuse macular or maculopapular	On about 4th day; rash appears as temperature drops suddenly to normal; lasts 1 to 2 days	Granulocytic leukopenia
Usually 1st on trunk, later on face, neck, extremities; infrequently on palms & soles	Lesions discrete; progress from macule to papule to vesicle to crusting; appear in crops, hence these various stages of development are present simultaneously	Shortly after onset of symptoms; lasts a few days to 2 wk	Presence of virus in vesicle fluid
First face, neck, upper chest, hands. Most on exposed surfaces; may involve palms, soles, pharynx	Shot-like papules changing to vesicles & finally to umbilicated pustules, which become confluent as they enlarge. Usually only 1 crop of lesions, in contradistinction to chickenpox	On 3rd or 4th day; lasts 2 to 5 wk	Initially, leukopenia; later, during pustular phase, leukocytosis. Virus can be detected in skin lesions
Most prominent over trunk	Occurs in about 15% of cases, as a morbilliform, scarlatiniform, or vesicular rash	Appears 5 to 14 days after onset of illness; lasts 3 to 7 days	Positive heterophil antibody test; leukocytosis with atypical enlarged lymphocytes ("mononucleosis"); appearance of antibodies to Epstein-Barr virus
Face, neck, chest, abdomen, spreading to extremities. Entire body surface may be involved	Diffuse pinkish-red punctate flush of skin, blanching on pressure & with Schultz-Charlton blanching reaction	On 2nd day; lasts 4 to 10 days	Granulocytosis; throat culture positive for β-hemolytic streptococcus, erythrogenic-toxin producing
Generalized; sometimes restricted to exposed surfaces	May be morbilliform, scarlatiniform, erythematous, acneform, vesicular, bullous, purpuric, or exfoliating	Variable	Agranulocytosis may be present; test urine for drug

Measles virus is also associated with **subacute sclerosing panencephalitis (SSPE),** a previously unexplained chronic brain disease of children and adolescents, which occurs months to years (usually years) after an attack of measles, causes intellectual deterioration, convulsive seizures, and motor abnormalities, and is usually fatal. Measles virus has been identified in brain tissue by electron microscopy, by demonstration of measles antigen through fluorescent antibody technics, and by isolation of the agent from brain biopsies.

Diagnosis

Measles may be suspected in a child with coryza, photophobia, and evidence of bronchitis, but before the rash appears a definite diagnosis can be made only by identifying Koplik's spots. These, followed by high fever, malaise, and the rash with its characteristic cephalocaudal progression, establish the diagnosis in most cases. The virus can be grown in tissue culture, and serologic tests are available, of which the CF test is the most widely used.

Differential diagnosis includes rubella, scarlet fever, drug rashes, serum sickness, roseola infantum, infectious mononucleosis, and echo- and coxsackievirus infections. Distinguishing features of rubella include its mild course with few or no constitutional symptoms, enlarged (and usually tender) postauricular and suboccipital lymph nodes, low fever, normal blood count, usual absence of a recognizable prodrome, and short duration. Scarlet fever may be suggested at first by the pharyngitis and fever, but the leukocytosis of scarlet fever is absent. Koplik's spots, the severe cough, and the characteristic rash of measles clarify what might be a difficult diagnosis. Drug rashes (e.g., from phenobarbital or sulfonamides) resemble the measles eruption, but the typical prodrome, cough, and cephalocaudal progression of the rash are absent and the palms and soles are more likely to be prominently involved. Here, even more than usual, the history is important. Roseola infantum produces a skin rash similar to that of measles, but is seldom seen in children over age 3. It can usually be differentiated by its high initial temperature, the absence of Koplik's spots and malaise, and the appearance of the rash simultaneously with defervescence.

Prophylaxis

Several live attenuated virus vaccines are available, all capable of providing the same permanent immunity as natural measles. The vaccines produce mild, or inapparent, noncommunicable infection and an antibody response near that of natural measles. Fever over 38 C (101 F) occurs 5 to 12 days after inoculation in < 5% of vaccinees, often followed by a rash. CNS reactions are exceedingly rare, and with the Schwartz and more attenuated Enders' Edmonston strains, simultaneous administration of measles immune globulin **(MIG)** or immune serum globulin with the vaccine is unnecessary and contraindicated.

Contraindications to the use of any live measles virus vaccine include generalized malignancies (e.g., leukemia, lymphoma), immunologic deficiency diseases, and therapy with corticosteroids, irradiation, alkylating agents, or antimetabolites. Reasons to defer vaccination include pregnancy, any acute febrile illness, active untreated tuberculosis, or administration of antibody (as whole blood, plasma, or any immune globulin) within the past 8 wk.

For **routine immunization,** see ROUTINE IMMUNIZATION PROCEDURES in §22.

Exposed susceptibles may be protected if the live vaccine is given within 2 days of exposure. Alternatively (e.g., in pregnant patients, children under 3 yr of age, or patients with tuberculosis or an acute febrile illness), MIG or immune serum globulin 0.25 ml/kg body wt IM is given immediately, followed by a live vaccine 8 wk later or as soon after that as health permits. An exposed susceptible patient with a condition which contraindicates the use of *any* live measles virus vaccine (leukemia, immunosuppression, combined immunodeficiency, etc.) is given MIG or immune serum globulin 20 to 30 ml IM.

Treatment

Confinement to bed during fever is advisable to prevent complications. Patients should be protected from exposure to streptococcal infections. Treatment is symptomatic. Itching may be relieved by applying phenolated calamine lotion several times/day.

Secondary bacterial complications require appropriate antibacterials. Immune serum globulin is ineffective in encephalitis; symptomatic care is the only available treatment.

RUBELLA
(German Measles; Three-Day Measles)

A contagious exanthematous disease with usually mild constitutional symptoms, but which may result in abortion, stillbirth, or congenital defects in infants born to mothers infected during the early months of pregnancy. Congenital rubella is discussed under NEONATAL INFECTIONS in §10, Ch. 2.

Etiology and Epidemiology

The disease is caused by an RNA virus of uncertain classification (probably a togavirus) spread by airborne droplet nuclei or by close contact. A patient can transmit the disease from 1 wk before onset of the rash until 1 wk after it fades. (Congenitally infected infants are potentially infectious for months after birth.) Rubella is apparently less contagious than measles, and many persons are not infected during childhood; as a result, 10 to 15% of young adult women are susceptible. Many cases are misdiagnosed or are so mild as to go unnoticed. Epidemics occur at irregular intervals during the spring; major epidemics occur at about 6- to 9-yr intervals. Immunity appears to be lifelong following natural infection.

Symptoms and Signs

After a 14- to 21-day incubation period, a 1- to 5-day prodrome, usually consisting of malaise and lymphadenopathy, occurs in children but may be minimal or absent in adolescents and adults. Tender swelling of the suboccipital, postauricular, and postcervical glands is characteristic, and, with the typical rash, suggests the diagnosis.

The rash is similar to that of measles but is less extensive and more evanescent. It begins on the face and neck and quickly spreads to the trunk and extremities. At the onset of the eruption, a flush simulating that of scarlet fever may appear, particularly on the face. A mild enanthem of discrete rose-colored spots is present on the palate, later coalescing into a red blush and extending over the fauces. There is a reddening of the pharynx at the onset, but no complaint of sore throat. The rash usually lasts about 3 days. On the 2nd day, it often becomes more scarlatiniform (pinpoint) with a reddish flush. The slight skin discoloration that remains as the rash fades may disappear in a day.

Constitutional symptoms in children are mild—slight malaise and occasional arthralgias. Adults characteristically complain of few or no constitutional symptoms, although fever, malaise, headache, stiff joints (occasionally with overt, transient arthritis), a slight feeling of lassitude, and mild rhinitis may be noted. They may become aware of the disease by noting the rash on the chest, arms, or forehead, or by discovering the characteristic postauricular lymphadenopathy while washing or on combing the hair. Encephalitis is an unusual but occasionally fatal complication that has occurred during extensive outbreaks of rubella among young adults in the armed services.

Diagnosis

Measles, scarlet fever, secondary syphilis, drug rashes, infectious mononucleosis, and echo-, coxsackie-, and adenovirus infections must be considered. Rubella is clinically differentiated from measles by the milder, more evanescent rash, and by the absence of Koplik's spots, coryza, photophobia, and cough. A patient with measles is sicker, and the illness lasts longer. With even mild scarlet fever, there are usually more constitutional symptoms than in rubella, including a severely red, sore throat. The WBC count is elevated in scarlet fever but normal in rubella. Observation for a day usually establishes the diagnosis in scarlet fever.

The eruption and adenopathy of rubella can be simulated by secondary syphilis, but the adenopathy of syphilis is not tender and the skin eruption is bronze-like. If there is doubt, a quantitative STS should be done and repeated observations made. Infectious mononucleosis may also cause a rubella-like adenopathy and skin rash but can be differentiated by the initial leukopenia followed by leukocytosis, the many typical mononuclear cells in the blood smear, the appearance of antibodies to the Epstein-Barr virus, and, in many cases, an increase in the heterophil antibody titer. In addition, the pharyngeal angina of infectious mononucleosis is usually prominent, and malaise is greater and lasts much longer than in rubella.

A clinical diagnosis of rubella is subject to error without laboratory confirmation, especially since enteroviral exanthems closely mimic rubella. Acute and convalescent serums should be obtained, if possible, for serologic testing; a 4-fold or greater rise in specific HI antibodies is confirmatory.

Prophylaxis (See also §22, Ch. 10, ROUTINE IMMUNIZATION PROCEDURES)

The purpose of rubella immunization programs is to prevent congenital rubella catastrophes. The most successful method is not yet known. The routine use of live rubella vaccine in all susceptible mothers immediately following delivery has been suggested, but routine vaccination of children between the ages of 15 mo and puberty is more common. The hope is that the latter procedure will eradicate the reservoir of infection in the early age group that is presumed responsible for most adult exposures. Another suggested procedure is to screen women of childbearing age for rubella HI antibodies (the history, whether positive or negative, being too unreliable a criterion of immunity) and selectively immunize those who are seronegative. Such immunization, however, cannot be undertaken unless conception is prevented for at least 2 mo afterward.

Live virus vaccines prepared in duck embryo, rabbit kidney, and human diploid fibroblast tissue cultures have been shown to be effective, with antibody production in about 95% of recipients. Transmission of vaccine virus from vacinees to susceptible contacts rarely, if ever, occurs and is not a contraindication to immunization. The attenuated-virus vaccine is not recommended. In children vaccinated with live virus vaccines, solid immunity lasts more than 9 yr, and may be permanent.

Fever, rash, lymphadenopathy, polyneuropathy, arthralgia, or overt arthritis are now rare with vaccination in children; joint pain and swelling still occasionally follow vaccination in adult women.

Vaccine should not be given to any person with a defective or altered immune mechanism (e.g., with leukemia, lymphoma, other malignancy, or a febrile illness, or during prolonged corticosteroid or x-ray treatment). Data suggest that the vaccines can infect a fetus during early pregnancy and their use is therefore **contraindicated** throughout pregnancy.

Treatment

Uncomplicated rubella requires little or no treatment. Otitis media, a rare complication, requires appropriate treatment. There is no specific therapy for encephalitis.

ROSEOLA INFANTUM
(Exanthem Subitum; Pseudorubella)

An acute disease of infants or very young children characterized by high fever, absence of localizing symptoms or signs, and appearance of a rubelliform eruption simultaneously with, or following, defervescence.

Etiology and Epidemiology

The cause and mode of spread are not known, but the disease is probably communicable and caused by a neurodermotropic virus. It occurs most often in the spring and fall. Minor local epidemics have been reported.

Symptoms and Signs

The incubation period is probably between 4 and 7 days. Fever of 39.5 to 40.5 C (103 to 105 F) begins abruptly and persists for 3 or 4 days without any evident cause. Convulsions are common during this period. Leukopenia with relative lymphocytosis is present, usually by the 3rd day. The spleen may be slightly enlarged.

The fever usually falls by crisis on the 4th day, and the macular or maculopapular eruption appears; it is profuse on the chest and abdomen and mild on the face and extremities. The temperature is normal at this stage, and the child feels and acts well. The evanescent rash may be unnoticed in mild cases.

Diagnosis

If roseola is known to be in the community, it should be suspected when a child aged 1 to 3 yr develops a persistently high temperature without apparent cause. A presumptive diagnosis usually can be made, to the relief of the parents, if pyelonephritis, otitis media, and central pneumonia can be ruled out.

Treatment

This is symptomatic and includes antipyretic measures to keep the child comfortable. For treatment of convulsions, see §14, Ch. 3. When the temperature falls to normal and the eruption appears, the patient is so nearly well that further treatment is unnecessary.

CHICKENPOX
(Varicella)

An acute viral disease, usually ushered in by mild constitutional symptoms that are followed shortly by an eruption appearing in crops and characterized by macules, papules, vesicles, and crusting.

Etiology and Epidemiology

That chickenpox and herpes zoster are caused by the same virus has been established by immunologic and antigenic analysis, chickenpox apparently being the acute invasive phase of the varicella-zoster virus, and zoster (shingles) being the reactivation of the latent phase of the virus. This viral identity is demonstrated by the occasional simultaneous occurrence of the two conditions in the same family or even in the same child, and by the cross-immunity which either infection may afford.

Chickenpox shares with measles the highest rate of communicability. Epidemics occur in winter and early spring in 3- to 4-yr cycles (the period required to develop a new group of susceptibles). Susceptibility is high from birth until the disease is contracted. Some infants may have partial immunity until age 6 mo, probably acquired transplacentally.

Chickenpox is believed to be spread by infected droplets from the nose and throat. The period of greatest communicability is during the short prodrome and early stages of the eruption. By the time the final lesions have crusted, the patient can no longer transmit the disease. Isolation for 6 days after the first vesicles appear is usually sufficient to control cross-infection. Indirect transmission (by third persons or objects) probably does not occur.

Symptoms and Signs

Mild headache, moderate fever, and malaise may be present during the 3rd wk after exposure, about 24 to 36 h before the first series of lesions appears. The prodrome is usually unrecognized in young children, is more likely to be present in children over age 10, and is usually severe in adults.

The initial rash, a morbilliform eruption, may be accompanied by an evanescent flush. Following the appearance of the characteristic itchy monolocular "teardrop" vesicles, containing clear fluid and standing out from their red areolas, diagnosis can usually be made. The typical chickenpox lesions progress from macule to papule to vesicle within 24 to 48 h. Lesions erupt in successive crops, some macules just appearing as earlier crops are beginning to crust. The eruption may be generalized in severe cases; otherwise, the face and extremities are partially spared. When only a few lesions are present, the upper trunk is the most frequent site. Lesions may also be present on the mucous membranes. In the mouth the vesicles rupture immediately, are indistinguishable from those of herpetic stomatitis, and often cause pain on swallowing. Laryngeal or tracheal vesicles may cause severe dyspnea. Lesions are frequently present on the scalp, resulting in tender, enlarged suboccipital and posterior cervical lymph nodes.

Chickenpox in childhood is usually benign. However, it may be severe or fatal in patients with leukemia or those receiving corticosteroids.

Complications

Secondary streptococcal infection of the vesicles may lead to erysipelas, sepsis, acute hemorrhagic nephritis, or, rarely, gangrene of the skin. Staphylococci may also infect the vesicles, resulting in bullous impetigo. Pneumonia may complicate severe chickenpox, which is encountered in adults and newborn infants but is unusual in young children. Myocarditis, transient arthritis, and hemorrhagic complications have also been reported.

Post-chickenpox encephalitis is unusual. Like that following measles, it tends to occur toward the end of the disease or 1 to 2 wk after its termination. One of the most common neurologic complications is acute cerebellar ataxia. Transverse myelitis, cranial nerve palsies, and multiple-sclerosis-like clinical manifestations have also occurred. Encephalitis may be fatal, but the prognosis for complete recovery from CNS complications is generally good and is far better than in measles encephalitis. Reye's syndrome is an unusual, but severe, complication that may begin 3 to 8 days after onset of the rash.

Diagnosis

Secondary syphilis, impetigo, infected eczema, insect bites and stings, drug rashes, contact dermatitis, and erythropoietic porphyria (hydroa aestivale) must be considered in the differential diagnosis. Under certain epidemiologic circumstances, smallpox must also be considered. In chickenpox, the monolocular, superficial lesions appear in 3 or 4 distinct crops about 1 day apart, so that after about a day the patient clearly has lesions in various stages of development. Smallpox lesions progress simultaneously and are usually multiloculated, umbilicated, and more deeply seated than those of chickenpox, and feel "shotty" when palpated. The distribution of smallpox lesions is typically centrifugal (head, extremities), whereas chickenpox lesions tend to be centripetal (most numerous over the head, neck, and trunk). Where diagnosis is important, as in distinguishing atypical chickenpox from modified or unusually mild smallpox, a smear may be made from the floor of the vesicle. Stained with Giemsa's stain, this shows giant epithelial cells in chickenpox (and in herpes zoster), but not in smallpox. The fluid from smallpox vesicles, but not from chickenpox vesicles, produces lesions on scarified rabbit cornea (as described under SMALLPOX, below) and on the chorioallantoic membrane of embryonated hens' eggs.

Prophylaxis

There is no vaccine for chickenpox at present. Zoster immune globulin (ZIG), prepared from the plasma of convalescent zoster patients with demonstrably high antibody content, provides passive protection against chickenpox in exposed susceptible children when injected in 2- to 5-ml doses IM within 72 h after exposure. It is available on a very limited basis from the Center for Disease Control, Atlanta, Ga. 30333, for susceptibles with leukemia, severe malnutrition, immune deficiency syndromes, or other debilitating illness, or those receiving corticosteroids, who have had a documented exposure within 72 h. Use of ZIG (or pooled immune globulin) should also be considered for neonates during the first 2 days postpartum if the mother has developed chickenpox lesions just prior to delivery.

Treatment

Mild cases require only symptomatic treatment. Wet compresses may be applied to control itching, which may be extreme and, from scratching, may lead to widespread infection and disfigurement. Local or systemic antihistamines may be used in severe cases. Because of the frequency of staphylococcal or streptococcal infection in the vesicles, the patient should be bathed often with soap and water and kept in clean underclothing; the hands should be kept clean and the nails clipped. Antiseptics should not be applied to individual lesions unless they become secondarily infected. An infected vesicle may be treated with neomycin-bacitracin ointment applied b.i.d.; widespread staphylococcal or β-hemolytic streptococcal infection is treated with appropriate systemic antibiotics.

HERPES ZOSTER
(Shingles; Zona; Acute Posterior Ganglionitis)

An acute CNS infection involving primarily the dorsal root ganglia, and characterized by vesicular eruption and neuralgic pain in the cutaneous areas supplied by peripheral sensory nerves arising in the affected root ganglia.

Etiology, Incidence, and Pathology

Herpes zoster is caused by the varicella-zoster virus, the same virus that causes chickenpox. It may be activated by local lesions involving the posterior root ganglia, by systemic disease, particularly Hodgkin's disease, or by immunosuppressive therapy. It may occur at any age but is most common after age 50. Inflammatory changes occur in the sensory root ganglia, the posterior horn of the gray matter, the meninges, and the dorsal and ventral roots.

Symptoms and Signs

Prodromal symptoms of chills and fever, malaise, and GI disturbances may be present for 3 or 4 days before distinctive features of the disease develop, with or without pain along the site of the future eruption. On about the 4th or 5th day,

4

characteristic crops of vesicles on an erythematous base appear, following the cutaneous distribution of one or more posterior root ganglia. The involved zone is usually hyperesthetic, and the associated pain may be severe. The eruptions occur most often in the thoracic region, and spread unilaterally. They begin to dry and scab about the 5th day after their appearance. Zoster may become generalized. If dissemination occurs or the lesions persist beyond 2 wk, an underlying malignancy or immunologic defect becomes more suspect.

One attack of herpes zoster usually confers immunity. Most patients recover without residua, except for scarring of the skin. However, postherpetic neuralgia may persist for months or years, most frequently in the elderly.

Geniculate zoster (Ramsay Hunt syndrome) results from involvement of the geniculate ganglion. There is pain in the ear and facial paralysis (rarely permanent) on the involved side. Vesicular eruptions are present in the external auditory canal and on the auricle, the soft palate, and the anterior pillar of the fauces. (See also HERPES ZOSTER OTICUS in §17, Ch. 4.)

Ophthalmic herpes zoster (see also in §19, Ch. 9) follows involvement of the gasserian ganglion. There is pain and a vesicular eruption in the distribution of the ophthalmic division of the 5th nerve. A 3rd nerve palsy may be present. Vesicles on the tip of the nose indicate that the nasociliary branch of the 5th nerve and the cornea are involved, with probable corneal ulcerations and opacities.

Diagnosis

Though difficult in the pre-eruption stage, diagnosis is made readily after the vesicles appear in characteristic distribution. Pleurisy, trigeminal neuralgia, Bell's palsy, and, in children, chickenpox must be differentiated. The pain may resemble that of appendicitis, renal colic, cholelithiasis, or colitis, depending on the location of the involved nerve. Herpes simplex virus may produce nearly identical zosteriform lesions. Herpes simplex tends to recur, but herpes zoster rarely ever does. The viruses can be differentiated by culture and serologically.

Treatment

There is no specific therapy. However, a corticosteroid, if given early, may relieve pain in severe cases. The initial dose should be relatively large (e.g., prednisone 50 mg/day orally for an adult), and duration should not exceed 3 wk; all the precautions associated with prescribing corticosteroids should be observed. Locally applied wet compresses are soothing. Aspirin 600 mg, alone or with codeine 15 to 60 mg, orally q 4 to 6 h, may relieve pain.

For ophthalmic herpes zoster, see §19, Ch. 9. (CAUTION: *Before using corticosteroids one must be certain that the disease is not acute ocular herpes simplex, in which corticosteroids are* **contraindicated;** *close supervision and follow-up of the patient are required).*

HERPES SIMPLEX
(Fever Blister; Cold Sore)

A recurrent viral infection characterized by the appearance on the skin or mucous membranes of single or multiple clusters of small vesicles, filled with clear fluid, on slightly raised inflammatory bases.

Etiology

The infecting agent is the relatively large herpes simplex virus (herpesvirus hominis, **HVH**). There are 2 HVH strains. Type 1 commonly causes herpes labialis and keratitis; Type 2 is usually genital and is ordinarily transmitted venereally. The time of initial HVH infection is usually obscure except in the primary systemic infection that is occasionally seen in infants and is characterized by generalized or localized cutaneous and mucosal lesions accompanied by severe constitutional symptoms. Localized infections ordinarily occur more frequently in childhood, but may be delayed until adult life. Presumably, the virus remains dormant in the skin or nerve ganglia, and recurrent herpetic eruptions can be precipitated by overexposure to sunlight, febrile illnesses, physical or emotional stress, or certain foods and drugs. The trigger mechanism is unknown in many instances.

Symptoms and Signs

The lesions may appear anywhere on the skin or mucosa, but are most frequent about the mouth, on the lips, on the conjunctiva and cornea, and on the genitalia. Following a short prodromal period of tingling discomfort or itching, small tense vesicles appear on an erythematous base. Single clusters vary in size from 0.5 to 1.5 cm, but several groups may coalesce. Herpes simplex on skin tensely attached to underlying structures (e.g., the nose, ears, or fingers) may be painful. The vesicles persist for a few days, then begin to dry, forming a thin yellowish crust. Healing usually begins 7 to 10 days after onset and is complete by 21 days. Healing may be slower, with secondary inflammation, in moist body areas. Individual herpetic lesions usually heal completely, but recurrent lesions at the same site may cause atrophy and scarring.

Variations and Complications

Genital herpes is discussed in §21, Ch. 1; herpes simplex keratitis in §19, Ch. 9; and primary and recurrent herpetic stomatitis and herpes labialis in §18, Ch. 14. Gingivostomatitis and vulvovaginitis may occur as a result of herpes infection in infants or young children. Symptoms include irritability, anorexia, fever, gingival inflammation, and painful ulcers of the mouth and occasionally of the vulva and vagina. In infants and sometimes in older children, primary infections may cause extensive organ involvement and fatal viremia. Women with Type 2 HVH infection late in pregnancy may transmit the infection to the fetus, with the development of severe viremia. Herpes simplex may also cause fatal encephalitis. **Kaposi's varicelliform eruption (eczema herpeticum)** is a potentially fatal complication of infantile or adult atopic eczema; patients with extensive atopic dermatitis should therefore **avoid** exposure to persons with active herpes simplex. Herpes simplex may be followed by typical erythema multiforme, but the relationship is uncertain since a variety of other infectious agents and drugs can also induce an identical syndrome.

Diagnosis

Herpes simplex may be confused with herpes zoster, but the latter is rarely recurrent and usually causes more severe pain and larger groups of lesions distributed along the course of a sensory nerve. Differential diagnosis also includes varicella, genital ulcers or gingivostomatitis due to other causes, and vesicular dermatoses, particularly dermatitis herpetiformis and drug eruptions.

When herpes simplex is suspected, cultures for the virus, a progressive increase in serum neutralizing or CF antibodies, and biopsy findings readily confirm the diagnosis.

Prophylaxis

Smallpox vaccinations are probably psychotherapeutic only, and may be dangerous. Patients who find sunlight a precipitating factor should avoid overexposure and apply a topical sunscreen preparation (e.g., 3.5% digalloyl trioleate or 10% sulisobenzone lotion). There is no vaccine available at present.

Treatment

No local or systemic chemotherapeutic agent is effective, with the possible exception of topical idoxuridine **(IDU)** in superficial herpetic keratitis. Reports on this compound in cutaneous herpes are conflicting.

Gentle cleansing with soap and water is recommended, but keeping lesions moist may aggravate the inflammation and delay healing. Drying lotions or liquids (e.g., camphor spirit or 70% alcohol) may be applied to oozing skin lesions. In secondary infections, topical antibiotics (e.g., neomycin-bacitracin ointment) or, if severe, appropriate systemic antibiotics, are indicated. Topical treatment with neutral red dye and phototherapy (photoinactivation), and with topical ether or alcohol, has been suggested, but their efficacy and potential dangers have not yet been established. (CAUTION: *Corticosteroids, either topical or systemic,* **should not be used** *in ocular herpes simplex because the lesions may progress to hypopyon or corneal perforation.*)

In herpes simplex with systemic manifestations, vigorous supportive therapy (control of electrolyte balance, parenteral fluid, blood transfusions, and systemic antibiotics) may be necessary. Systemic treatment with potentially toxic agents, such as IDU, cytarabine, or vidarabine (adenine arabinoside), has been attempted in serious infections such as encephalitis or disseminated neonatal disease, but their efficacy remains questionable.

SMALLPOX
(Variola)

An acute, highly contagious viral disease, initiated by sudden severe constitutional symptoms and characterized by a progressive cutaneous eruption often resulting in permanent pits and scars.

Etiology and Epidemiology

Smallpox is caused by a virus closely related to the vaccinia and other variola viruses. It is present through all stages of the disease—in the vesicle, pustule, crust, nasopharyngeal secretion, and excreta—and can be recovered from the blood during the first 2 days of clinical illness but seldom thereafter except in fatal cases. The virus resists drying and may be transmitted in the dried scales of the lesions, or it may be airborne in the droplet nuclei from nasopharyngeal secretions. The disease may be transmitted directly from person to person or by contact with contaminated clothing or household articles. It is frequently transmitted by patients with unrecognized smallpox (e.g., the mild sporadic variety—possibly in persons vaccinated a long time previously—or the severe hemorrhagic type in which the patient dies before the rash appears). One attack confers permanent immunity. The disease is now endemic only in isolated areas of southern Asia and Africa, and it is hoped that complete eradication will be achieved by the 1980s or sooner.

Symptoms, Signs, and Course

After a 10- to 14-day incubation period, onset is abrupt, with chills, high fever, and great prostration—similar to severe influenza. Headache, backache, and muscular pains may occur. Persistent vomiting and convulsions are common in small children. This prodromal period may last up to 2 days and is accompanied by a morbilliform, scarlatiniform, or petechial rash that is not suggestive of smallpox.

The characteristic eruption appears on the 3rd day, accompanied by a drop in temperature and a decrease in symptoms. Pink-red macules, 1 to 2 mm in diameter, generally appear first on the forehead, temples, and about the mouth, then spread rapidly to the scalp, ears, neck, arms, and hands, reaching the trunk after 24 h. In severe cases, it becomes generalized and may be profuse on the palms and soles and in the axillas, sites usually spared by other eruptions. The individual lesions enlarge; they are deep in the skin (not on it) and feel "shotty" on palpation. By the 3rd day of the eruption, the lesions, all chronologically in the same phase of development, are umbilicated and multilocular, surrounded by a pinkish areola, and filled with clear serum. Lesions may become confluent. In the next 1 or 2 days, the lesions all become pustules simultaneously and fever returns with severe prostration. The characteristic umbilicated lesions may be seen on the mucous membranes of the mouth, pharynx, larynx, vagina, urethral meatus, and rectum.

By the 8th or 9th day of the eruption, most of the lesions have passed their peak, many have ruptured, and some are shrinking. The skin shows purulent material and crusting. There may be extensive cutaneous desquamation and loss of hair, eyebrows, and nails. Healing is slow and may continue for another 2 wk, with the deeper or coalesced lesions leaving permanent pockmarks and deep pits.

The fulminant ("sledgehammer") form begins with high fever, severe prostration, bone marrow depression, hemorrhagic skin lesions, and bleeding, progressing to death in 3 to 4 days with typical focal skin lesions.

Leukopenia is characteristic in the early stages. Leukocytosis is noted with the onset of the suppurative phase (usually on the 5th or 6th day of the eruption). In severe hemorrhagic smallpox, prothrombin time is prolonged and fibrinogen decreased.

Clinical Variants

Smallpox in previously vaccinated persons is likely to be mild and is often designated as **varioloid. Alastrim (variola minor),** another mild form that occurred predominantly in South America, showed the manifestations of smallpox, but was mild and lacked complications. The virus of alastrim is indistinguishable by laboratory methods from that of severe smallpox, but it reproduces true to form and continues to cause mild disease even after several passages through susceptible persons.

Prognosis and Complications

The mortality rate of virgin variola is high in the very young or very old. In others, the fatality rate increases from 5% when the rash remains discrete, to about 60 or 80% in the fulminant confluent and hemorrhagic types. Fatal smallpox is usually accompanied by hemorrhage into coalesced areas of the eruption. Gangrene of the skin and damage to the eyes and ears from local lesions may occur. CNS or heart lesions are uncommon.

Diagnosis

This is based clinically on the history, prodromal symptoms, and characteristic eruption. Features that distinguish the eruption of chickenpox are described under that disease. Virus isolation, direct electron microscopy of the vesicle fluid or crust extracts, and agar gel precipitin tests are valuable diagnostic methods. Sometimes used in diagnosis are a CF test using material from the crusts and vesicles, and the demonstration of Guarnieri bodies (rounded clumps of virus lying close to the cell nucleus). These bodies are produced within a few hours after inoculating a rabbit's cornea with material from early-stage vesicles, and are demonstrated by scraping the scarified area and staining with methylene blue and eosin.

Prophylaxis

The efficacy of smallpox vaccination is unquestioned. Successful vaccination provides relative immunity within 8 days, a high level of protection for at least 3 yr, substantial but waning immunity for 10 yr or more, and, apparently, protection against death from the disease for an even longer period. Revaccination every 3 yr is required to maintain adequate immunity.

Routine pediatric immunization is no longer recommended in the USA. Vaccination is necessary for travelers to endemic or infected areas, and vaccination every 3 yr is strongly recommended for hospital and other health personnel who would be at high risk if importation of infection occurs.

Following known or suspected **exposure to smallpox,** those whose vaccination is over 3 yr old should be revaccinated immediately. Vaccination of household contacts within 7 days after contact has been shown to provide significant protection against the disease. Previously unvaccinated contacts should also be vaccinated immediately, and should be kept under observation for 3 wk. Isolation is mandatory if fever develops during observation. Vaccinia immune globulin will prevent or modify the disease if given within 24 h after exposure but is no longer available in the USA.

Contraindications: Persons who are ill, immunodeficient, or immunosuppressed, or who have a malignant disease, should not be vaccinated. Unless there are compelling reasons for vaccination, pregnancy may be considered a contraindication, since fatal vaccinia infection of the fetus has been reported. Individuals with extensive skin eruptions, particularly infants or children with eczema or impetigo, should not be vaccinated nor be allowed near recently vaccinated persons, since they are likely to develop **eczema vaccinatum (Kaposi's varicelliform eruption),** which may be generalized and fatal. Infants under 1 yr old are more likely to have vaccination complications—postvaccinal encephalitis, disseminated vaccinia, vaccinia necrosum, and accidental secondary inoculation of the eye or other sites.

The well-known technic of smallpox vaccination will not be described since information is enclosed with each batch of vaccine. The best site at all ages is on the arm (preferably the less-used arm), at the dimple over the deltoid insertion.

Currently, only two classifications of **results** are accepted by WHO: (1) **"Major reaction"** indicates a successful immunization. A small pink-red papule appears in 3 to 5 days, serous vesicles form, surrounded by a red areola, and the lesion reaches maximum width in 8 to 14 days. The vesicle becomes pustular, gradually flattens, and forms a crust which, if unmolested, sloughs in 3 wk. A glistening red scar remains for a considerable time, but within 1 or 2 yr becomes white and pitted ("vaccination mark"). If there is partial immunity, the reaction may be **accelerated,** with maximum lesion size 5 to 8 days after immunization. In either case, a typical vesicle in some stage of development should be présent 7 days after the vaccination. (2) **"Equivocal reaction"** includes any reaction other than a major reaction. It may represent partial immunity or only an allergic reaction to the inactive vaccine components. *If there is no evidence of a vesicle or crust* 6 to 8 days post-vaccination, it is classified as equivocal and revaccination should be done with a different lot of vaccine.

Treatment

Therapy is largely symptomatic (provision for caloric, fluid, and electrolyte needs), but penicillin or broad-spectrum antibiotics are given when secondary bacterial invasion in the vesicular and pustular stages is suspected. The eyes require nursing care if swelling and inflammation are pronounced. They may be irrigated several times a day with 2% sodium bicarbonate or 0.5% methylcellulose solution. If conjunctival inflammation is severe, 10% sulfacetamide ophthalmic ointment may be used 2 or 3 times/day to control the inflammation and protect the cornea from infection and vascularization.

Isolation: In most countries, public health laws require strict quarantine of smallpox cases (and suspected cases pending diagnosis) until the disease is over and all scabs and crusts have disappeared. Bed linen, clothing, and other items used by smallpox patients can harbor the virus and must be sterilized.

RESPIRATORY VIRAL DISEASES

THE COMMON COLD
(Upper Respiratory Infection; URI; Acute Coryza)

An acute, usually afebrile, catarrhal respiratory tract infection, with major involvement in any or all airways, including the nose, paranasal passages, throat, larynx, and often the trachea and bronchi.

Etiology
Many respiratory viruses may be causative, including rhino- and adenoviruses, influenza and parainfluenza viruses, respiratory syncytial virus, and certain echo- and coxsackieviruses. More than 95 rhinovirus serotypes have been established and several more are as yet untyped. Serologic tests and virus isolation are necessary to establish the specific etiologic agent of each illness.

Predisposing factors have not been clearly identified. Chilling of the body surface will not by itself induce colds and susceptibility is not affected either by the person's health and nutrition or by upper respiratory tract abnormalities (e.g., enlarged tonsils or adenoids). Infection may be facilitated by excessive fatigue, allergic nasopharyngeal disorders, or inhalation of noxious fumes, and during the midphase of the menstrual cycle.

Pathogenic bacteria that normally inhabit the nasopharynx are the cause of infrequent purulent complications such as otitis media and sinusitis. Bronchitis may be of viral etiology, but secondary bacterial infection is the more likely cause if the sputum becomes purulent.

Symptoms and Signs
Onset is characteristically abrupt after an 18- to 48-h incubation period. Illness generally begins with a scratchy sensation in the throat, followed by sneezing, rhinorrhea, and varying degrees of malaise. Though it is characteristically an afebrile infection, fever of 38 to 39 C (100 to 102 F) is common in infants and small children. The disease may be limited to part of the upper respiratory tract or may also involve the accessory nasal sinuses. Purulent sinusitis or otitis media are bacterial complications, although the secretions thicken in the natural course of uncomplicated infection. Hacking cough may be present, together with a moderate laryngitis or a tracheitis manifested by substernal tightness and burning discomfort. Severe tracheobronchial involvement with purulent sputum suggests primary or secondary bacterial or mycoplasmal invasion.

Symptoms normally resolve in 4 to 10 days, but complications such as sinusitis, adenoiditis, tonsillitis, eustachitis, laryngitis, tracheitis, and bronchitis may last longer.

Diagnosis
Clinical symptoms and signs do not permit early specific etiologic diagnosis. Many serious disorders (including measles, diphtheria, streptococcal pharyngitis,

meningitis, and whooping cough) also cause catarrhal upper respiratory tract symptoms at onset and may therefore be confused with primary coryza. Differentiation depends on characteristics that develop later. Many cases of influenza are similar to the common cold. The presence of fever and more severe symptoms usually differentiates influenza. Hay fever and other allergies may also be mistaken for coryza; differentiation usually depends on persistence of the allergy. Leukocytosis indicates a disorder other than an uncomplicated common cold.

Prophylaxis

Immunity is type-specific. Effective experimental vaccines have been prepared for single types of rhinoviruses, but the many types and strains of causative viruses preclude production of a useful viral vaccine. Many other measures to prevent acquisition and spread of common colds have been tried, including polyvalent bacterial vaccines, alkalis, citrus fruits, vitamins, ultraviolet light, and glycol aerosols, but none have been unequivocally effective. In controlled trials, large (as much as 2 Gm/day) prophylactic oral doses of vitamin C have not altered the frequency of acquisition of common rhinovirus colds or the amount of virus shedding, but some studies have shown a reduced duration of disability among persons who took as much as 8 Gm/day on the first day of disease. Such persons might be transmitters of the infection since the person's sense of well-being is enhanced while virus shedding is not reduced.

Large doses of exogenous human interferon have shown a protective and beneficial effect, and prophylactic administration of a chemical interferon inducer, N,N-dioctadecyl-N′N′-bis(2-hydroxyethyl) propanediamine, was also found to be effective in decreasing infection, reducing virus shedding, and accelerating interferon production, which diminishes illness.

Treatment

Bed rest is indicated for infants, preadolescents, and all febrile patients; it is usually impossible to enforce and of little importance in afebrile adults. Though antipyretics and analgesics are commonly used in the early stage, aspirin has been found to increase virus shedding while producing only slight symptomatic improvement in persons with afebrile rhinovirus infections. Thus, aspirin is not recommended unless symptoms are severe enough to keep the patient at home in relative isolation.

Other measures used in the early stage are anticholinergic preparations such as atropine 0.25 mg orally t.i.d. or belladonna tincture 0.3 to 1 ml orally t.i.d. to dry the nasal mucosa, and oral phenylpropanolamine 15 to 50 mg, 0.5% phenylephrine or ephedrine nose drops or spray, or a nasal inhaler (not more often than q 3 or 4 h) to provide temporary nasal decongestion. Steam inhalations will relieve chest tightness. If necessary, cough syrups (especially those containing codeine; e.g., terpin hydrate and codeine 5 to 10 ml orally q 3 to 4 h) can be used to control coughing; an expectorant (e.g., iodinated glycerol 60 mg orally q.i.d. or potassium iodide saturated solution 300 to 600 mg [0.3 to 0.6 ml] orally q 2 h) may help. Antihistamines may reduce rhinorrhea in allergic patients. Antibiotics do not affect the common cold and are *not recommended* unless a specific bacterial complication develops.

RESPIRATORY SYNCYTIAL VIRUS (RSV)

RSV is one of the most important causes of lower respiratory illness (including bronchiolitis and pneumonia) in infants and young children, and can be fatal. The sudden death of a baby with respiratory disease is often believed to be due to RSV infection. In adults, RSV causes mild upper respiratory illness and is also a very important cause of primary bronchopneumonia, secondary bacterial pneumonia, and exacerbations of chronic bronchitis.

Etiology

RSV is an RNA virus, classified as a paramyxovirus. It biologically and behaviorally resembles influenza and parainfluenza viruses more than other taxonomic virus groups, but is serologically and, in several ways (e.g., by its failure to grow in eggs or produce hemagglutinin), biologically distinct from them. Only one clinically important type has been recognized.

Epidemiology

RSV is associated with a sharp annual outbreak of acute respiratory disease occurring in late autumn or in winter. Like influenza, it causes increased morbidity and mortality from bronchitis and pneumonia, and also frequently milder disease in adults. The annual recurrence of a single RSV serotype indicates that reinfection, with illness, occurs. Thus, although about 70% of persons have serum antibody against RSV by age 5, infections continue to occur in persons of all ages. The poorly protective effect of serum antibody against infection, and, perhaps, the immunologic enhancement of disease are indicated by the increased severity of infection seen in some infants under 6 mo old, who have maternal antibody but develop severe lower respiratory tract disease, which causes an appreciable number of deaths.

Symptoms and Signs

The clinical manifestations of RSV infection are of little help in identifying the specific cause of the infection. Dyspnea, cough, and wheezing are the most prominent symptoms; fever and bronchiolitis are the most frequent findings. Crepitant rales are characteristic; bronchopneumonia is often apparent in chest x-rays. The leukocyte count is usually normal, but granulocytes may be moderately elevated. In adults, infection may be inapparent or only an afebrile URI (the common cold), although bronchopneumonia may result, and RSV infections account for about 15% of hospital admissions for acute exacerbations of chronic bronchitis. Secondary bacterial pneumonia (most commonly pneumococcal) may be a more common complication than is thought.

Diagnosis

RSV can be isolated from respiratory secretions on tissue cultures of a human epithelial cell strain. Since the virus only poorly tolerates freezing and thawing unless protected by special media, it may be difficult to store or ship specimens. RSV infection is usually confirmed serologically. A rise in serum antibody can be detected by CF with a standard antigen. However, serologic findings may be difficult to evaluate. Very young infants often have maternal antibody, children may show acquired antibody in the early-phase serum, an antibody rise may not be demonstrable in young children, and mild disease in adults causes no increase in titer.

Prophylaxis

Since serum antibody does not prevent and may worsen disease, inactivated parenteral vaccine would be valueless and contraindicated. Attempts to develop an attenuated live virus vaccine for respiratory tract administration have not yet been successful.

Treatment

Mild and inapparent infections are probably quite frequent and resolve without special attention. Severe disease in infants and children requires hospitalization and careful observation to ensure adequate respiration. Adults with bronchopneumonia and acute bronchitis may also require respiratory support.

INFLUENZA
(Grippe; Grip; "Flu")

A specific acute viral respiratory disease characterized by fever, coryza, cough, headache, malaise, and inflamed respiratory mucous membranes. It usually occurs as an epidemic in the winter, affecting several members of a family and many persons in a locale. Prostration, hemorrhagic bronchitis, pneumonia, and sometimes death occur in severe cases.

Etiology

Influenza is caused by myxoviruses. These are RNA viruses 80 to 120 nm in size with a core of helical nucleic acid and a soluble nucleoprotein (NP or S) antigen. On the basis of the reaction of this antigen with specific antibody in a CF test, influenza viruses are classified into Types A, B, and C. The virion has a limiting membrane and is enveloped in a coat composed principally of two glycoproteins, one having hemagglutinating activity (HA) and one having enzymatic activity as a neuraminidase (NA), that appear as spikes extending from the capsid of the virus and represent the strain-specific antigens. Myxoviruses require a specific glycoprotein receptor site on the cell surface for attachment by the hemagglutinin. The virus is then engulfed, its envelope fuses with the vacuolar membrane, and the viral genetic material enters the cell. After intracellular replication of the viral components, the virus is assembled at the cell surface and is released from the cell by a budding process in which the viral NA participates.

Different serotypes of Type A influenza viruses are numbered H_0N_1, H_1N_1, H_2N_2, and H_3N_2 according to the major human antigenic types recognized since the virus was first isolated in 1933. Only the most recent serotype (H_3N_2) causes epidemics. Earlier strains disappear with the appearance of new types. Influenza B viruses show some marked strain-specific variations, but the cross-relationships among strains are much greater than with influenza A. Specific numbers are not assigned to the Type B surface antigens. Influenza C is not a prevalent virus and serotypes, if they occur, are not defined.

Epidemiology

Influenza A virus is the most frequent cause of clinical influenza. Spread is by person-to-person contact and airborne droplet spray. Infection produces sporadic respiratory illness every year. Acute epidemics usually occur about every 3 yr, generally nationwide during late fall or early winter. A major shift in the prevalent antigenic type of influenza A virus occurs about once in a decade and results in an acute major pandemic. Persons of all ages are afflicted, but prevalence is highest in school children, and severity is greatest in the very young, aged, or infirm. Epidemic illness often occurs in two waves—the first in students and active family members, the second mostly in shut-ins and persons in semi-closed institutions.

Influenza B causes epidemics about every 5 yr and is much less often associated with pandemics. Influenza C is an endemic virus which sporadically causes mild respiratory disease.

Symptoms and Signs

The incubation period is about 48 h. Transient viremia may occur before infection localizes in the lower respiratory tract. Influenza A or B is sudden in onset, with chilliness and fever up to 39 to 39.5 C (102 to 103 F) developing over 24 h. Prostration and generalized aches and pains (most pronounced in the back and legs) appear early. Headache is prominent, often with photophobia and retrobulbar aching. Respiratory tract symptoms may be mild at first, with sore throat, substernal burning, nonproductive cough, and sometimes coryza, but later become dominant. Cough may become severe and productive. The skin, especially on the face, is warm and flushed. The soft palate, posterior hard palate, tonsillar pillars, and posterior pharyngeal wall may be reddened, but there is no exudate. The eyes water easily and the conjunctiva may be mildly inflamed. Usually, after 2 to 3 days acute symptoms subside rapidly and fever ends, though fever lasting up to 5 days may occur without complications. Weakness, sweating, and fatigue may persist for several days or occasionally for weeks.

In severe cases, hemorrhagic bronchitis and pneumonia may develop within hours or days. Fulminant fatal viral pneumonia occasionally occurs; dyspnea, cyanosis, hemoptysis, pulmonary edema, and death may proceed as soon as 48 h after onset of the influenza. Such severe disease is most likely to occur during a pandemic caused by a new influenza A serotype. Persons at **high risk** of developing severe disease are those with chronic pulmonary diseases; those with valvular heart disease with or without preceding congestive heart failure, or other heart disease with pulmonary edema; pregnant women in the third trimester; and persons who are aged, very young, or confined to bed. Influenza B, but not influenza C, has infrequently caused equally severe disease.

Complications

Secondary bacterial infection of the bronchi and sometimes pneumonia are suggested by persistence of fever, cough, and other respiratory symptoms for more than 5 days. Pneumonia should be suspected if dyspnea, cyanosis, hemoptysis, rales, a secondary rise in temperature, or a relapse develops. With pneumonia, cough increases and·purulent or bloody sputum is produced. Crepitant or subcrepitant rales may be detected over the involved pulmonary segments. The bacterial etiology of this secondary pneumonia is related to age and environment. Pneumococci, streptococci, and *Haemophilus influenzae* are common causes, especially in ambulatory nonhospitalized or young patients. Pneumococci, staphylococci, and *Klebsiella pneumoniae* are the most common causes in older, infirm, or hospitalized patients.

Encephalitis, myocarditis, and myoglobinuria may also occur as complications of influenza, usually during convalescence. The virus is rarely recovered from affected organs and the specific relationship and pathogenesis of these diseases cannot be positively established. However, an increase in such diseases regularly follows influenza A pandemics. Reye's syndrome has been prominently associated with epidemics of influenza B.

Diagnosis

An etiologic diagnosis of influenza cannot be made clinically except during epidemics. In the early stages of infection or in uncomplicated cases, chest examination is usually normal. In mild cases, the symptoms are those of a febrile or afebrile common cold. Pulmonary symptoms may simulate those of mycoplasmal or atypical pneumonia, especially during epidemics. In distinguishing influenza from other respiratory tract infections, one should consider the season and whether an influenza epidemic is in progress; the mode of onset and severity of symptoms; and the presence or absence of a tonsillar or pharyngeal exudate, other signs of localized infection, or evidence of suppurative disease. The leukocyte count is low in uncomplicated cases; sometimes a leukopenia with a relative lymphocytosis may be present. Fever and severe constitutional symptoms differentiate influenza from the common cold. An exudate or a membrane is often present over the tonsils and pharyngeal wall in hemolytic streptococcal tonsillitis but not in influenza.

A specific diagnosis of influenza can be made by virus isolation or serologic tests. During the early stages of the disease, the virus can be recovered from respiratory tract secretions. The specimen can be collected as sputum, but more often throat washings are obtained by gargling a buffered saline solution, usually with a small amount of protein such as albumin or gelatin; if necessary, diluted skim milk can be used. The recently prevalent strains of influenza virus have not been difficult to isolate either in tissue cultures or embryonated eggs. During epidemics, it is important to isolate and identify influenza viruses early. For this purpose, State Health Laboratories and, through them, the National Center for Disease Control and International Influenza Reference Centers assist in strain identification.

Serologic tests used are predominantly CF and HI tests. Serial serum specimens are best, the first collected at the onset of illness and another a week or more later. The 2 specimens are tested simultaneously to demonstrate a rise in the specific antibody titer. If only a single serum specimen is available after the disease is already well developed, a high CF antibody titer may indicate recent infection; the HI titer may reflect previous infection or vaccination.

Leukocytosis, with young granulocytes in the blood smear, is a valuable diagnostic sign of complicating bacterial pneumonia. Purulent sputum should be smeared, gram-stained, and examined for leukocytes and bacteria. Appropriate sputum and blood cultures and other examinations should be made to identify the specific bacterial species and to determine the extent of secondary infection.

Prognosis

Recovery is the rule in uncomplicated influenza. However, viral pneumonia and other virus-related complications may cause death in some patients, especially those identified above as being at high risk. Chemotherapy decreases the fatality rate of severe secondary bacterial pneumonia.

Prophylaxis

Vaccines that include the prevalent strains of influenza viruses effectively reduce the incidence of infection among vaccinees for 1 or 2 yr after vaccination. The immunity is less when appreciable antigenic drift occurs in the virus, and when a major antigenic mutation occurs no significant protection is afforded unless the new strain is incorporated into the vaccine. Vaccine is prepared as inactivated whole virus or as subunits of the virus, either semi-purified viral hemagglutinin or disrupted virion components. Both types of vaccine are equally protective.

Vaccination is especially important for the aged and for patients with cardiac, pulmonary, or other chronic diseases. Pregnant women expected to deliver during the winter months should be vaccinated also. Immunization, preferably in the fall, usually consists of 1 dose of vaccine, but when new strains arise primary immunization should consist of 2 or 3 injections of vaccine containing the new strains, given at monthly intervals. About 2 wk is required for immunity to develop after vaccination. Because immunity from vaccination lasts only 1 or 2 yr, an annual booster dose early in the fall is required for optimal protection. Primary or booster doses are 0.5 to 1 ml s.c. or IM. The intradermal route is *not recommended.* With the presently available purified vaccines, local or constitutional reactions are uncommon or minor. Nevertheless, a history of sensitivity to eggs should be sought and epinephrine should be at hand if a person with such a history is vaccinated.

Under development are new attenuated live virus vaccines given intranasally. They have the advantage of eliciting specific secretory antibody at the portal of virus entry. Also under investigation are recombinant vaccines of influenza A viruses which are the progeny of a genetic crossing in the laboratory of an old and a new strain of virus.

Amantadine 100 mg q 12 h orally (for adults) can be used prophylactically against influenza A. During influenza A epidemics, it should be given to family members and other close contacts of patients, to persons at high risk, and, optimally, to all unvaccinated persons, in order to augment antibody immunity and to protect against variant strains. Vaccine should be given, after which amantadine may be discontinued in 3 wk. If vaccine cannot be given, amantadine must be continued for the duration of the epidemic, usually 6 or 8 wk. It is ineffective against influenza B.

Influenza renders the patient temporarily immune to reinfection with the same virus serotype, and incompletely immune to variants from antigenic drift; it has no effect on other strains of influenza virus.

Treatment

Treatment is symptomatic. The patient should remain in bed or rest adequately and avoid exertion during the acute stage and for 24 to 48 h after the temperature becomes normal. If constitutional symptoms of acute uncomplicated influenza are severe, antipyretics and analgesics (e.g., aspirin 600 mg, alone or with codeine 15 to 30 mg, orally q 4 h) are helpful. To relieve nasal obstruction, 1 or 2 drops of 0.25% phenylephrine may be instilled into the nose periodically. Gargles of warm isotonic saline are useful for sore throat. Steam inhalation may alleviate respiratory symptoms somewhat and also prevent drying of secretions. Treatment of respiratory symptoms may be unnecessary in less severe cases. A codeine cough mixture (e.g., terpin hydrate and codeine 5 to 10 ml orally q 3 to 4 h) may be indicated during some stages of the disease.

No therapeutic agent of proved value is available for control of pulmonary infection due to the influenza virus, but amantadine has a slight effect if given early in uncomplicated influenza A. It has shown no benefit when used for pneumonia. Complicating bacterial infections require appropriate antibiotics.

PARAINFLUENZA VIRUSES

A group of viruses causing a number of respiratory illnesses varying from the common cold to influenza-like pneumonia, with febrile croup as their most common manifestation.

Etiology

The parainfluenza viruses are RNA paramyxoviruses and consist of 4 serologically distinct agents categorized as Types 1, 2, 3, and 4. Early human isolates of parainfluenza Types 1 and 3 were called "hemadsorption (HA) viruses." The initial Type 2 isolates were designated "croup-associated (CA) viruses." Though the 4 types tend to cause diseases of different severity, they share common antigens, as evidenced by cross-reactive antibody responses, and are similar structurally and biologically. Type 4 has antigenic cross-reactivity with mumps. Though each type of parainfluenza virus has a corresponding serotype that causes specific diseases in animals, cross-infection of animals to man or vice versa either does not occur or the transfer is very inefficient. The corresponding strains of animal origin for Types 1, 2, and 3 are Sendai virus (mice), Simian virus 5 (SV-5), and shipping fever virus of cattle (SF-4).

Epidemiology

Infections with Types 1 and 3 are common in early childhood; sharp localized outbreaks occur in nurseries, schools, pediatric wards, and orphanages. Widespread community epidemics are prevented by almost universal immunity in adults. Infection with each type produces different epidemiologic patterns. Parainfluenzal infections, unlike influenza, occur in all seasons, but epidemic disease in the fall is more likely to be due to Type 1 and in the summer to Type 3. Type 1 disease occurs more cyclically; Type 3 disease is highly endemic and contagious.

Type 3 can cause explosive outbreaks that seldom last longer than 7 to 10 days; sporadic infections continue to occur throughout the year. Type 1 epidemics are usually less explosive, with milder disease. The incubation period is usually 24 to 48 h with Type 3, and 4 to 5 days with Type 1. Type 2 infection is not as endemic as infection with Types 1 and 3. It is more sporadic and causes modest epidemics of infantile croup (acute laryngotracheobronchitis). The parainfluenza viruses are considered to be a chief cause of this condition. Type 4 causes mild respiratory illness, but only rarely.

Second and even third infections with the same strains of virus, particularly with Types 1 and 3, are not uncommon, though the partial immunity developed during previous episodes may reduce the spread and severity of subsequent infections.

Symptoms and Signs

The most common illness produced in children is an acute febrile respiratory infection that is clinically indistinguishable from influenza or other respiratory virus infection occurring in the same age group. Type 3 causes the most severe disease; Type 4, the mildest. Onset is marked by fever and moderate coryza. The degree of malaise is directly related to the height of the fever. In many cases, the temperature does not exceed 38 or 39 C (101 or 102 F); in others, it may peak several times to 40 C (104 F). Moderate sore throat and a dry cough usually develop early in the disease. Hoarseness and croup are prominent symptoms in many cases, especially with Type 1 or 2 infections. This **acute laryngotracheobronchitis** (see CROUP in §10, Ch. 4) is the most severe and dangerous manifestation of parainfluenza virus infections.

Fever may subside promptly or continue for 2 or 3 days. In some patients, particularly those who develop lower respiratory tract involvement, fever lasting a week or more may recur one or more times.

Bronchitis and "walking" pneumonia often develop during or after the initial acute episode in children and sometimes adults infected with Type 3. Pneumonia is detected by auscultation that reveals moist rales in one or more lung areas, or by chest x-ray. Bacterial complications are not common.

Diagnosis

A firm diagnosis of parainfluenzal infection cannot be made clinically. Virus isolation and identification require tissue culture inoculation. CF, HI, and hemadsorption-neutralization tests with acute and convalescent serums will confirm a parainfluenzal infection but serologic cross-reactions can make it difficult to identify the specific parainfluenza virus without a viral isolate.

Prognosis

Except for infantile croup, illnesses due to the parainfluenza viruses, although frequent, are usually mild, self-limited, and of brief duration. The bronchitis and pneumonia associated with Type 3 infections seldom cause serious disability and are rarely, if ever, fatal.

Prophylaxis

Experimental tissue culture vaccines have been given preliminary trials but they are not highly antigenic and, because reinfection occurs in the presence of serum antibody, it may be necessary to develop preparations that are given directly into the respiratory tract in order to elicit specific local secretory antibody. Attenuated live virus vaccines are a possibility, but safe and effective strains must still be established.

Treatment

There is no specific therapy. Nonexertion and a comfortable environment are the best remedies. Aspirin is not recommended unless the fever is high or the symptoms prevent sleep. If necessary, antitussives (e.g., codeine 1 to 1.5 mg/kg/day orally in 6 divided doses) will suppress cough. For treatment of croup, see that discussion in §10, Ch. 4.

ADENOVIRUSES

A group of viruses causing various acute febrile disorders characterized by inflammation of the respiratory and ocular mucous membranes and hyperplasia of submucous and regional lymphoid tissue.

Etiology

Adenoviruses are DNA viruses 60 to 90 nm in size. The virion is shaped like an icosahedron. Three major antigens can be directly related to the capsid structures. Most important is the hexon, a 6-sided capsomere comprising 240 of the 252 capsomeres. It reacts with specific antiserums in a non–type-specific CF reaction and thus serves as a group antigen to identify all types of adenoviruses. However, virus-neutralizing antibody is type-specific. The 2nd major antigen is associated with a penton, a 5-sided capsomere located at the 12 common vertices of the 20 triangles that form the icosahedron. It is a type-specific antigen that can be differentiated in neutralization or HI tests. The 3rd antigen is a fiber antigen related to the thread-like structure extending from the apices of the virion. Not infrequently, adenoviruses have another smaller DNA virus associated with them, called **adenoassociated virus (AAV)**. It is a defective virus that requires complementation by adenovirus in order to replicate. The importance of AAV in adenovirus infections is not known.

Epidemiology

About 4 to 5% of clinically recognized respiratory illnesses in civilian populations are caused by adenoviruses. Of the 33 known serotypes, only a few have been adequately observed in relation to human disease to determine their prevalence and ability to produce illness (see TABLE 1-5). Different serotypes have quite different epidemiologies. Types 1, 2, and 5 cause sharp, limited outbreaks of respiratory or enteric illness during the first few months or years of life. Type 2 has been relatively more common in some of these episodes. In older children and adults, Type 3 causes a characteristic syndrome of acute pharyngoconjunctival fever **(APC)**, especially among patrons of summer camps and swimming pools. Acute respiratory disease **(ARD)** occurs in military camps and is caused by Types 4, 7, 14, and 21. In some countries, ARD epidemics have also been apparent among civilian populations, but not in the USA. Epidemic keratoconjunctivitis **(EKC)** is caused by Type 8 and is seen largely in industrial plants and eye clinics.

Adenoviruses also infect the intestinal tract, usually without causing symptoms, although enteritis, mesenteric adenitis, and intussusception can occur. Following infection with Types 1, 2, and 5, the virus may remain latent in the tonsils and adenoids; about 80% of excised tonsils yield such virus.

The ratio of manifest disease to infection rates varies with the different syndromes and serotypes and according to the season when infected. In winter, infection of military recruits with adenovirus Types 4 or 7 causes recognizable illness in most cases and about 25% require hospitalization for fever and lower respiratory tract disease. APC occurs in a high proportion of Type 3 infections in the summer. The ratio of illness to infection is lower with Types 1, 2, 5, and some of the less studied, higher numbered adenoviruses.

TABLE 1-5. SYNDROMES CAUSED BY ADENOVIRUSES

Disease	Serotypes Implicated		Comments
	Common	Less Common	
Respiratory only: Acute febrile respiratory disease of children	1, 2, 3, 5, 6	Other types	Probably the most frequent manifestation of adenoviruses; Types 1, 2, & 5 endemic; Type 3 occasionally epidemic; more prevalent during cold months
Acute respiratory disease (ARD)	4, 7	14, 21	Epidemic in military recruits; sporadic in adult civilians; Types 4 & 7 infections rare in children
Viral pneumonia: Infants	7	1, 3	Rare; occurs in hospital nurseries; may be fatal; similar to Goodpasture's inclusion body pneumonitis
Adults	4, 7	3	Predominantly associated with acute respiratory disease; cold agglutinins not developed
Ocular only: Acute follicular conjunctivitis	3, 7	2, 6, 9, 10, 21	Sporadic; adults chiefly affected; in children, usually associated with respiratory & systemic effects
Epidemic keratoconjunctivitis (EKC)	8 (classic)	3, 7 (mild)	Epidemic; adults mainly affected; widespread in Japan, rare in USA
Combined respiratory & ocular: Acute pharyngoconjunctival fever (APC)	3, 7	1, 2, 5, 6, 14, 21	Epidemic in children; sporadic in adults; summer epidemics frequently associated with swimming in pools or lakes

Pathology

Adenoviral infections are rarely fatal and have few, if any, recognizable long-term pathologic effects. Some deaths have occurred in infants with giant-cell pneumonia associated with adenovirus Types 3 or 7. Autopsies have disclosed microscopically an extensive and unique inclusion body pneumonia, the intranuclear inclusions appearing to be similar to those considered characteristic of adenoviral cellular invasions in tissue cultures. Biopsies of superficial lesions produced by adenoviruses in conjunctival and pharyngeal mucosa show capillary dilation, occasional submucous hemorrhage, and mononuclear leukocyte infiltration, but no intranuclear inclusions. The conjunctivitis caused by the common respiratory types of adenoviruses is benign, but keratoconjunctivitis caused by Type 8 can produce corneal opacities and impaired vision.

Symptoms and Signs

Acute febrile respiratory disease is the usual manifestation of known adenoviral infection in children. Adenoviruses Types 1, 2, 3, 5, and 6 have been isolated most commonly, though infection with these types is often not directly associated with any specific illness. Infection is airborne or waterborne (by swimming), or acquired by direct contact. The incubation period is 2 to 5 days. In a typical outbreak confined to a household or nursery, some affected children have fever only, without localizing signs; others have fever and pharyngitis; others have fever with pharyngitis, tracheitis, and bronchitis, a moderately persistent nonproductive cough, and, rarely, pneumonia. Cough with adenoviral pneumonia has been confused with pertussis in children. Pharyngeal lymphoid hypertrophy sometimes persists and leads to eustachian tube obstruction and possibly otitis media. Regional lymph nodes are frequently enlarged and sometimes tender, but they never suppurate. Laboratory findings are generally within normal limits, though some children may show a lymphocytosis.

Acute respiratory disease (ARD) is observed almost exclusively in military recruits. Adenovirus Types 4 and 7 have been reported in most outbreaks in the USA, but Types 14 and 21 have also been incriminated. ARD is marked by malaise, fever, chills, and headache. Respiratory manifestations include nasopharyngitis, hoarseness, and dry cough. The disease may resemble streptococcal pharyngitis with exudate on the faucial pillars and posterior pharyngeal wall. Cervical adenopathy is present, but the nodes are not as tender as in streptococcal pharyngitis. Viremia and viruria may occur and there may be a fine erythematous macular rash on the body, but the viruria occurring with these respiratory strains of adenoviruses does not produce symptoms like the epidemic hemorrhagic cystitis which occurs as a primary disease with Type 11. Physical signs are minimal except in about 10% of patients, who develop rales and x-ray evidence of pneumonia. Fever usually subsides within 2 to 4 days; convalescence, while uneventful, may require another 10 to 14 days.

Viral pneumonia of infants, due chiefly to Type 7, is a rare but specific clinicopathologic entity. Small outbreaks have occurred in France, the USA, and Japan, with fatalities due to extensive pneumonia. Onset is sudden, affecting infants in the first few days or weeks of life with high fever and rapid upper and lower respiratory tract involvement. The pneumonia is lobular but may be so extensive as to suggest lobar pneumonia. Several fatal cases developed a maculopapular rash and encephalitis, with focal necrosis apparent in the brain, skin, and lungs.

Acute pharyngoconjunctival fever (APC) classically produces the clinical triad of fever, pharyngitis, and conjunctivitis. Infection is sometimes waterborne. The incubation period is 5 to 8 days. Adenovirus Types 3 and 7 have been reported in nearly all outbreaks. In a typical outbreak, 50% or more of the patients have all three components, while others may have only one or two. The acute conjunctivitis is initially unilateral and sometimes painful. Involvement of the lower respiratory tract may occur in addition to pharyngitis. The illness usually subsides within a week, but follicular conjunctivitis may persist for another week.

Conjunctivitis without constitutional symptoms appears to be a rather common manifestation of infection with several different adenovirus serotypes. It occurs most often in young adults, chiefly parents of children with APC, and is self-limited and benign. Onset is sudden and usually unilateral. Symptoms and signs include a foreign-body sensation in the eye, lacrimation, and focal erythema of the palpebral and bulbar conjunctiva. The discharge is mucoid but not purulent. The other eye is subsequently involved in about half the patients, usually less severely. Persistent follicular enlargement of submucous lymphoid tissue under the palpebral conjunctiva, even resembling early trachoma, may be seen about 2 to 4 days after onset. Preauricular and posterior cervical lymphadenopathy, more prominent on the same side as the more involved eye, is usual. A mild sore throat occasionally develops, often on the same side as the affected eye. The course is usually mild, though focal conjunctival hemorrhages and extensive periorbital edema occasionally occur.

Epidemic keratoconjunctivitis (EKC) is a specific, severe, epidemic disease caused almost exclusively by adenovirus Type 8. Observed for many years in Japan, it became epidemic in the USA during World War II, chiefly among shipyard workers on both coasts. It has occurred only sporadically in this country since then, but widespread epidemics have occurred in Europe and Asia. Onset is sudden, one eye showing redness and chemosis followed by periorbital swelling, preauricular lymphadenopathy, and superficial corneal opacities. Unlike herpetic keratitis, it does not result in corneal ulceration; local pain like that from foreign-body irritation is usual, however. The other eye may become involved within a week. Systemic symptoms and signs are mild or absent. The illness usually lasts 3 to 4 wk, though opacities may persist much longer and vision has sometimes been permanently impaired.

Mild, transient corneal involvement has been observed in eye infections (e.g., APC) with other adenoviruses (Types 3 and 7), but the opacities are seldom noticeable except to an ophthalmologist.

Diagnosis

Clinical identification of adenoviral infection is only presumptive except in typical APC, EKC, and ARD in military recruits, in which conditions the clinical or epidemiologic characteristics, or both, are unique. During the acute stages of adenoviral illnesses, the virus can be isolated from respiratory and ocular secretions, and frequently from feces and urine. Several serologic procedures (CF, HI, and neutralization tests) can be performed on acute and convalescent serums. A 4-fold rise in the serum antibody titer indicates recent adenoviral infection. The CF test is group-specific for any adenovirus serotype. HI and neutralization tests are type-specific. Commercial antigen is available for the CF test but not for the latter two tests.

Prognosis

Adenoviral infections are generally benign and of relatively short duration. Except for rare cases of fulminating primary pneumonia in young infants, even severe adenoviral pneumonia is not fatal.

Prophylaxis

Live Type 4 and 7 adenovirus vaccine, given orally in an enteric-coated capsule, has caused a marked reduction in ARD in military populations. Though spread of the vaccine virus to family members can occur, it either does not occur or is of no importance under the conditions of military use. The live oral vaccine is neither recommended nor available for civilian use. Vaccines for other serotypes have not been developed.

Treatment

Treatment is symptomatic and supportive. Bed rest at home or infirmary care may be required during the acute febrile period. Aspirin is not recommended unless headache and malaise are distressing; analgesics such as codeine are rarely necessary. Severe pneumonia in infants and EKC require early hospitalization and close supervision to prevent death in the former and permanently impaired vision in the latter. Topical corticosteroids relieve symptoms and shorten the course of EKC and adenoviral conjunctivitis. Such therapy is dangerous in ulcerative corneal conditions, however, and should always be supervised by an ophthalmologist.

ENTEROVIRAL DISEASES

A group of diseases caused by the enteroviruses (polio-, coxsackie-, or echoviruses).

Etiology and Epidemiology

Because of similar biologic, chemical, and physical properties, the **enteroviruses** (**polio-, coxsackie-,** and **echoviruses**) and the rhinoviruses are placed together taxonomically as subgroups of the family **picornaviruses** (*pico,* small; *rna,* their characteristic nucleic acid component). For a discussion of the polioviruses and the symptoms they produce, see POLIOMYELITIS, below. For rhinoviruses, see THE COMMON COLD.

The **coxsackieviruses** are an antigenically heterogeneous group divided into Groups A (24 types) and B (6 types). They resemble the polioviruses in their size, resistance to physical and chemical agents, prevalence during summer and fall,

TABLE 1-6. SYNDROMES CAUSED BY ENTEROVIRUSES

Disease	Serotypes Most Often Implicated	Comments
Herpangina	Coxsackievirus A 2, 4–6, 8, 10; probably 3 and others	Most common in infants and children; characteristic pharyngeal lesions
Hand, foot, and mouth disease	Coxsackievirus A 16	Most common in young children; vesicular exanthem usually brief and benign
Epidemic pleurodynia (Bornholm disease)	Coxsackievirus B 1–6	Most common in children, but any age group may be affected
Aseptic meningitis	Coxsackievirus A 2, 4, 7, 9, 23 and others, B 1–6 Poliovirus 1–3 Echovirus 4, 6; others less commonly	Most common in infants and children; course usually benign
Paralytic disease	Poliovirus 1–3 Coxsackievirus A 7 and others Echovirus 4, 6, and others	See POLIOMYELITIS
Myocarditis Pericarditis	Coxsackievirus B 2–5 Coxsackievirus A 23, B 1–5 Echovirus 1, 6, 8, 16	May occur at any age; myocarditis neonatorum has high mortality
Exanthems: With fever alone	Coxsackievirus A 23, B 2, 3, 5; A 4–6, 9, 16 also implicated Echovirus 4; 2, 6, 11, 14, 16, 18, 30 also implicated	Course generally benign
With aseptic meningitis	Coxsackievirus A 16, 23; B 4 Echovirus 4, 16	Course generally benign
Respiratory disease	Echovirus 4, 8, 20, and others Coxsackievirus A 21, B 1, 3, 4, 5 Poliovirus 1–3	Most common in infants and children; course generally mild
Gastroenteritis	Echovirus 6, 14, and 18 proved cause in newborns; many other enteroviruses suspected in all age groups	Probably most important in newborn or premature nursery

and largely person-to-person spread. They have been isolated from oral secretions, stools, blood, and CSF.

The **echoviruses** (enteric cytopathogenic human orphan), like the coxsackieviruses, are small, heterogeneous, most prevalent in summer and fall, and widely distributed geographically; 31 serotypes are recognized. These viruses have been isolated from the pharynx, feces, blood, CSF, and CNS tissues.

RECOGNIZED DISEASE ENTITIES

Herpangina

Any of the 24 Group A coxsackieviruses, and occasionally other enteroviruses, may cause herpangina. It tends to occur in epidemic form, most commonly in infants and children, and is characterized by sudden onset of fever with sore throat, headache, anorexia, and, frequently, pains in the neck, abdomen, and extremities. Vomiting and convulsions may occur in infants. Within 2 days after onset, a few (rarely > 12) characteristic small (1 to 2 mm in diameter) grayish papulovesicular lesions with erythematous areolas appear, most frequently on the tonsillar pillars, but also on the soft palate, tonsils, uvula, or tongue. During the next 24 h, the lesions become shallow ulcers, seldom > 5 mm in diameter, which heal in 1 to 5 days. Complications are unusual and the patient is generally asymptomatic by the 4th day. Permanent immunity to the infecting strain follows infection, but repeated episodes, caused by other Group A viruses, are possible.

Diagnosis is based on the symptoms and characteristic oral lesions. It is best confirmed by isolating the virus from the lesions or by demonstrating a rise in specific antibody titer. Differential diagnosis includes herpetic stomatitis, which occurs during any season and shows larger, more persistent ulcers; and recurrent aphthae and Bednar's aphthae, which rarely occur in the pharynx and generally are not associated with systemic symptoms. **Treatment** is entirely symptomatic.

Hand, Foot, and Mouth Disease

This is usually associated with coxsackievirus A 16 and occurs particularly among young children. The course is similar to that of herpangina, but with a vesicular exanthem distributed over the buccal mucosa and palate, and with similar lesions on the hands and feet and occasionally in the diaper area. **Treatment** is also symptomatic.

Epidemic Pleurodynia (Bornholm Disease)

This disease may occur at any age but is most common in children. It may be caused by any of the 6 Group B coxsackieviruses, and is characterized by sudden onset of severe, frequently intermittent, pain in the epigastrium or lower anterior chest, with fever and often headache, sore throat, and malaise. Local tenderness, hyperesthesia, muscle swelling, and myalgias of the trunk and extremities may occur. The disease usually subsides in 2 to 4 days, but relapse may develop within a few days and symptoms may recur for several weeks. In some cases, symptoms are continuous for a few weeks. Complications include orchitis, fibrinous pleuritis, pericarditis, and, rarely, aseptic meningitis.

Diagnosis is obvious during an epidemic. However, in sporadic cases or in the early stages of an epidemic, the disease may be mistaken for poliomyelitis, myocardial infarction, spontaneous pneumothorax, acute appendicitis, pancreatitis, a perforated viscus, or an influenza-like respiratory infection. Laboratory diagnosis consists of isolating the virus from throat washings or stool, or demonstrating a rise in specific neutralizing antibody titers.

Prognosis is good in uncomplicated cases, although a few deaths have been reported. Repeated infections with other Group B coxsackieviruses are possible. **Treatment** is entirely symptomatic.

Aseptic Meningitis

Aseptic meningitis in infants and young children is frequently caused by a poliovirus, a Group A or B coxsackievirus, or an echovirus. Viruses other than enteroviruses are frequently responsible in older children and adults (see ARBOVIRUS ENCEPHALITIDES, below; and ACUTE VIRAL ENCEPHALITIS AND ASEPTIC MENINGITIS in §14, Ch. 7). Headache, pain and stiffness in the neck and back, and muscular aches may be abrupt in onset or preceded by prodromal symptoms of fever, malaise, anorexia, and vomiting. Kernig's and Brudzinski's signs are usually positive. Symptoms generally subside by the end of a week, but fatigue and irritability may persist for months. CSF findings consist of a normal or slightly elevated protein level, a normal glucose level, and a cell count usually < 500/cu mm; neutrophils may predominate in the early stages, but lymphocytes are more common later. Encephalitic signs occasionally develop and may be severe.

Meningitis due to coxsackie- or echovirus is usually impossible to differentiate clinically from other viral meningitides during the acute stages. **Diagnosis** is made by isolating the virus from throat washings, stool specimens, or, occasionally, the CSF, or by demonstrating a rise in neutralizing antibody titer.

Prognosis is generally good, but death may occur in the newborn. **Treatment** should follow that for nonparalytic poliomyelitis (see POLIOMYELITIS, below) since the two diseases are clinically indistinguishable in the acute stages.

Paralytic Disease

Certain Group A and B coxsackieviruses (especially A 7) and several echoviruses may produce muscle weakness or paralysis that is clinically indistinguishable from paralytic poliomyelitis. The causative virus can be identified by laboratory technics; **treatment** is the same as for paralytic poliomyelitis.

Myocarditis; Pericarditis

Myocarditis neonatorum, caused by Group B coxsackieviruses and some echoviruses, occurs in newborns infected after birth (rarely, in utero). It is characterized by sudden onset of fever, feeding difficulties, pharyngitis, tachycardia, cyanosis, and tachypnea, frequently associated with cardiac murmurs and hepatomegaly. The ECG may show signs of myocarditis. CNS, hepatic, pancreatic, or adrenal lesions may be present concomitantly. Recovery may occur within a few weeks, but death due to circulatory collapse is not unusual.

Myocarditis or pericarditis in older children or adults also may be due to a Group B coxsackievirus, and, in a few instances, to a Group A coxsackievirus or an echovirus. Symptoms and signs are usually localized only to the myocardium or pericardium, and complete recovery is usual.

Diagnosis is made, as in other coxsackievirus infections, by virus isolation or antibody titer studies. **Treatment** is symptomatic, including strict bed rest and control of heart failure and arrhythmias. The value of corticosteroids has not been established; their use is best reserved for severe cases of myocarditis with associated cardiac failure.

Exanthems With or Without Aseptic Meningitis

Certain echo- and coxsackieviruses may cause a rubelliform rash, which is generally discrete, nonpruritic, nondesquamative, and usually confined to the face, neck, and chest. The rash is sometimes maculopapular or morbilliform, occasionally hemorrhagic or vesicular. Fever is common. Aseptic meningitis may develop. The disease is usually epidemic, with exanthems predominating among infants and children, but sporadic cases occur. The course is generally benign.

Respiratory Disease

Enteroviruses have been implicated in some infants' and children's respiratory illnesses characterized by fever, coryza, and pharyngitis, sometimes with diarrhea and vomiting. Bronchitis and interstitial pneumonia have occasionally occurred in infants. **Treatment** is symptomatic (see THE COMMON COLD, above).

Diarrhea; Gastroenteritis

Enteroviruses, particularly echoviruses 6, 14, and 18, have occasionally been isolated from the stools of newborn infants with acute diarrheal disease. A large variety of enteroviruses and a few adenoviruses have been isolated from the stools of older infants and young children with acute gastroenteritis, but their importance in the etiology of this disease is questionable. Other enteric viruses, called "epidemic gastroenteritis viruses," have been demonstrated by oral inoculation of volunteers with stool filtrates, and by electron microscopy of the feces in acute cases, particularly in infants and young children. The identity of these viruses has not yet been clearly established, but the majority appear not to be enteroviruses. **Treatment** of the enteric infections is symptomatic (see ACUTE INFECTIOUS GASTROENTERITIS in §10, Ch. 4).

CENTRAL NERVOUS SYSTEM VIRAL DISEASES
(See also §14, Ch. 7)

POLIOMYELITIS
(Infantile Paralysis; Acute Anterior Poliomyelitis)

An acute viral infection in which only a small percentage of those infected develop clinical signs—fever, headache, stiff neck and back, and sometimes flaccid paralysis of various muscle groups.

Etiology

Poliovirus, the causative agent, is one of the enteroviruses, a subgroup of the picornaviruses. It is a small (28 nm), ether-resistant RNA virus, stable for months at 4 C and for years at −20 C or lower. Electron micrographs show the virus particles aggregated in crystalline array in the cytoplasm of infected cells. Polioviruses exist in 3 immunologic types; Type I is the most paralytogenic and is responsible for most epidemics. Man, chimpanzees, and monkeys are susceptible; some strains (particularly of Type II) can be adapted to mice and other small rodents. All strains grow in primary outgrowth tissue cultures of primate cells and in a variety of continuous cell lines originating from primate hosts.

Epidemiology

Infections with wild polioviruses are common in unimmunized populations, but overt disease is relatively rare except in epidemics; even then the ratio of inapparent infections to clinical cases probably exceeds 100:1. Poliomyelitis vaccines have had a marked impact on disease incidence in those parts of the world where they have been extensively used. In the USA, the number of cases has fallen from an average of 21,000/yr in the 5-yr period before introduction of vaccine in 1955, to 7 in 1974. Similar successful control has been achieved in other large geographic areas, but first epidemics are still appearing in some countries, particularly in the tropics where vaccination programs are often inadequate. The few recent cases in the USA have chiefly been in unimmunized individuals. Epidemics localized to pockets of unvaccinated children have occurred without spread of the disease to the well-immunized surrounding community.

Polioviruses are spread primarily by human association; the healthy carrier is as infectious as the frank case. During active infection the virus is present in the throat and in intestinal excreta. Transmission probably occurs by the fecal-oropharyngeal route and, particularly during epidemics, by spread from the pharynx of one person to the oropharynx of another. The period of communicability, not accurately known, is probably greatest during the few days before and after onset of illness. Young children are the most susceptible in any population and are also the most effective virus spreaders. There is a marked seasonal incidence of poliomyelitis in temperate climates, with sharp increases in summer and fall; cases tend to occur year round in tropical areas.

Poliomyelitis occurs in all parts of the world. The shift from an endemic to an epidemic disease, which occurred in the late 19th century in Scandinavia and the USA, has been correlated with changes in the sanitary environment. The viruses are widely disseminated in populations with poor sanitation and hygiene. Under these circumstances, infection and immunity are acquired in the first few years of life, epidemics do not occur, and sporadic cases are confined largely to children under age 5 yr. With economic development and improved sanitation and hygiene, exposure and infection are delayed and the number of susceptibles builds up. An epidemic may result when a virulent strain is introduced unless prophylactic vaccination has been carried out.

Pathogenesis and Pathology

The virus enters the body by the oropharynx and is implanted in the walls of the pharynx and the intestinal tract, where primary multiplication occurs. Virus is present in the throat, blood, and feces 3 to 4 days after exposure, which corresponds to the period of the "minor illness." Viremia precedes the onset of the CNS phase, lasts several days, and disappears as antibodies develop. Virus can be recovered from the throat for 10 to 14 days, and is excreted in the feces for 3 to 6 wk or longer. CNS invasion is apparently via the bloodstream, though experiments in monkeys indicate that poliovirus can travel along neural pathways; such spread may possibly occur in the natural infection under certain circumstances. What determines whether circulating virus lodges in the CNS and produces neuronal damage is not known, but factors predisposing to serious neurologic involvement include increasing age, recent tonsillectomy, recent inoculations (most often DTP), pregnancy, and physical exertion concurrent with onset of the CNS phase of the disease.

The characteristic lesions of poliomyelitis are found in the gray matter of the spinal cord, the medulla, the precentral gyrus of the cerebral cortex, and the deep nuclei of the cerebellum. Neuronal necrosis, chromatolysis, neuronophagia, and loss ("outfall") of cells occur. Focal and diffuse leukocytic infiltration and perivascular cuffing are found in areas of neuronal damage. Lymph node hyperplasia is often observed, and, occasionally, myocarditis.

Symptoms and Signs

Clinical forms are extremely varied, but two basic response patterns are recognized: the "minor illness," or abortive type, and the "major illness." The **minor illness** (first phase), accounting for 80 to 90% of clinical infections, may be so mild as to go unnoticed. After a 3- to 5-day incubation period, slight fever, malaise, headache, sore throat, and sometimes vomiting develop. Examination discloses no evidence of CNS involvement and the CSF is normal. Recovery occurs within 24 to 72 h. This is usually the entire course of the disease and, because of its nonspecific character, it cannot be diagnosed clinically as poliomyelitis. In a few patients, symptoms recur after several days of well-being (the biphasic course) and the major illness, with CNS signs, appears.

The **major illness** (second phase) more commonly begins without previous minor illness, particularly in older children and adults. The incubation period is commonly 7 to 14 days, but may be as long as 35 days. Fever, severe headache, stiff neck and back, deep muscle pain, and sometimes hyperesthesias and paresthesias are present. Asymmetric weakness of various muscles and loss of superficial and deep reflexes occur in paralytic cases. The site of paralysis depends on the location of lesions in the spinal cord or medulla. The cranial nerve nuclei are involved in the bulbar form, resulting in paralysis of the pharyngeal, laryngeal, facial, or other muscle groups innervated by the cranial nerves. Dysphagia, nasal regurgitation, and nasal voice are early signs of bulbar involvement. Encephalitic signs occasionally predominate. During the major illness, the CSF usually shows a slightly increased protein content and an increased cell count of 20 to 300 cells/cu mm (largely lymphocytes), although the cell count is occasionally normal even in the presence of paralysis. The peripheral blood usually shows either moderate leukocytosis or a normal WBC count.

Diagnosis and Differential Diagnosis

Flaccid limb paralyses or bulbar palsies without sensory loss occurring during the course of an acute febrile illness in a child or young adult almost always indicate poliomyelitis, though, rarely, certain coxsackie- and echoviruses produce the same clinical picture. In the Guillain-Barré syndrome, which is often confused with paralytic poliomyelitis, the course is afebrile, muscle weakness is symmetric, sensory findings are characteristic, and the CSF protein is elevated in the presence of a normal cell count. CNS involvement due to mumps or herpes viruses, tuberculous meningitis, or brain abscess should also be considered. Encephalitis due to arboviruses may be confused with poliomyelitis in certain geographic areas.

Nonparalytic poliomyelitis (i.e., aseptic meningitis due to poliovirus) cannot be clinically distinguished from aseptic meningitis due to a variety of agents, including other enteroviruses (coxsackie- and echo-); arboviruses; mumps, lymphocytic choriomeningitis (LCM), and herpes viruses; and leptospires. An etiologic diagnosis can be made only on such laboratory evidence as virus isolation or antibody titer rise.

Prognosis

In the abortive and nonparalytic forms, recovery is complete. In paralytic poliomyelitis, fewer than 25% of patients suffer severe permanent disability, about 25% have mild disabilities, and over 50% recover with no residual paralyses. Mortality is 1 to 4% but may increase to 10% in adults and with the bulbar type.

Prophylaxis

Active immunization is recommended for all infants and children. Two kinds of vaccine have been used: the formalin-inactivated **Salk** type **(IPV)** given parenterally, and the oral **Sabin** live attenuated virus vaccine **(OPV)**. OPV has gradually replaced IPV because of its immunogenic superiority and logistic simplicity, and trivalent OPV is now the preparation used routinely in the USA. OPV induces an inapparent infection that simulates the natural one. Not only circulating antibodies are induced, but also a state of resistance in the alimentary tract associated with local secretory (IgA) antibody production. This serves to block virus implantation and multiplication, thus protecting the individual and providing a barrier to dissemination of the virus in the community. The vaccine is easily given and immunity is rapidly achieved (7 to 10 days), making it an effective means of halting an epidemic. Very rarely, the trivalent vaccine has been associated with paralytic poliomyelitis in recipients and in contacts of vaccinees, the rates per million doses being 0.06 for recipients and 0.2 for contacts.

Schedules for routine immunization of infants and children are given in Routine Immunization Procedures, in §22. Because the current incidence of poliomyelitis in the USA is extremely low, the likelihood of exposure of adults is virtually nil; oral vaccine is recommended for unimmunized adults only for travel to areas where the disease is endemic, or during an epidemic. Hospital personnel might also be considered at special risk, especially if cases are occurring in the community.

Passive immunization with immune serum globulin is not recommended.

Treatment

No specific therapy is known. Patients with abortive or mild nonparalytic poliomyelitis need only bed rest for several days. In more severe cases during the early febrile stage of the major illness, symptomatic treatment is similar to that for other acute infectious diseases. Fluid and electrolyte balance should be maintained; mild analgesics, such as aspirin 600 mg, alone or with codeine 30 to 60 mg, orally q 4 to 6 h, are given for headache, pain, and discomfort. (N.B.: These are adult doses and should be proportionately reduced for children.) Sedatives should be used with caution because of the danger of depressing respiration.

During **active myelitis,** emphasis should be on rest with avoidance of strain, unnecessary movement, or exertion. Relief of muscle spasm and pain is best accomplished by several 20-min applications/day of hot, moist packs. In patients with paralysis of the legs, urine retention is a frequent complication; it often responds to a parasympathomimetic such as bethanechol 5 to 30 mg orally or 2.5 to 5 mg s.c. 3 or 4 times/day. Catheterization should be avoided if possible because of the hazard of urinary tract infection. Antimicrobial therapy should be instituted early if infection occurs.

Respiratory failure in poliomyelitis may be due to (1) paralysis of the muscles of respiration, (2) involvement of the respiratory centers in the medulla, (3) airway obstruction from weakness of the pharyngeal muscles and larynx, and (4) pulmonary edema.

Respiratory failure from involvement of vital medullary centers occurs in bulbar poliomyelitis. It is usually associated with obstruction due to paralysis of the pharyngeal muscles, inability to cough, and pooling of bronchotracheal secretions. Continuous O_2 inhalation, postural drainage, and suction removal of secretions generally suffice in mild uncomplicated cases. A high tracheostomy is indicated if these measures fail to keep the airway clear. Adequately humidified O_2 can then be given through the tracheostomy tube. Concentrations of 40 to 60% are used, though emergencies may necessitate 100% for brief periods.

Positive pressure respiration through a cuffed tracheostomy tube may be instituted in patients needing artificial respiration because of paralysis of the muscles of respiration. Further details regarding respiratory intensive care can be found in §5, Ch. 3.

In patients with respiratory failure, pulmonary atelectasis frequently occurs and may require repeated bronchoscopy and aspiration. Antimicrobial prophylaxis has not proved effective in lessening the incidence of pulmonary infection, but once infection occurs, an appropriate antibiotic should be given.

Physical therapy is the principal treatment of paralytic poliomyelitis during convalescence. The greatest return of muscle function occurs in the first 6 mo, but improvement may continue for 2 yr. An important aspect of general care is management of the emotional problems that often arise in patients suddenly faced with severe physical disabilities.

RABIES
(Hydrophobia)

An acute infectious disease of mammals, especially carnivores, characterized by CNS irritation followed by paralysis and death.

Etiology and Epidemiology

The etiologic agent is a neurotropic virus often present in the saliva of rabid animals which bite animals or humans and thus transmit the infection. Rabies may also be acquired by exposure of a mucous membrane or fresh skin abrasion to infected saliva. Three cases of apparently respiratory infection have been reported, one following laboratory exposure and two from the poorly ventilated atmosphere of a cave infested by millions of guano bats. Worldwide, rabid dogs still present the highest risk to man. In the USA, vaccination has largely controlled canine rabies, and bites of infected wild animals have caused most cases of human rabies since 1960. Infected wildlife continues to be the major source of human exposure in the USA. The most commonly infected wild animals are skunks, foxes, bats, and raccoons.

Infected dogs may have either **furious rabies**, characterized by agitation and viciousness, followed by paralysis and death; or **dumb rabies**, in which paralytic symptoms predominate. Rabid wild animals may show "furious" behavior, but less obvious behavior changes (diurnal activity of normally nocturnal bats, skunks, and foxes; lack of normal fear of humans) are more likely.

Pathology

The virus has an affinity for nervous tissue. It travels from the site of entry via peripheral nerves to the spinal cord and the brain where it multiplies, subsequently continuing through efferent nerves to the salivary glands and into the saliva. Postmortem examination shows vessel engorgement and associated punctate hemorrhages in the meninges and brain; microscopic examination shows perivascular collections of lymphocytes but little destruction of nerve cells. The presence of intracytoplasmic inclusion bodies (Negri bodies), usually found in the cornu Ammonis, is pathognomonic of rabies, but these are not always found.

Symptoms and Signs

In man, the incubation period varies from 10 days to > 1 yr (average, 30 to 50 days). It is usually shortest in patients with extensive bites or bites about the head or trunk. The disease commonly begins with a short period of mental depression, restlessness, malaise, and fever. Restlessness increases to uncontrollable excitement, with excessive salivation and excruciatingly painful spasms of the laryngeal and pharyngeal muscles. The spasms, which result from reflex irritability of the deglutition and respiration centers, are easily precipitated—e.g., by a slight breeze or an attempt to drink water. As a result, the patient is unable to drink, though his thirst is great (hence, "hydrophobia"). Death from asphyxia, exhaustion, or general paralysis usually occurs within 3 to 10 days.

Diagnosis

The fluorescent antibody test and virus isolation have replaced examination of the animal's brain for Negri bodies as the preferred method of diagnosis. A dog or cat that bites a human but is otherwise asymptomatic should, when practicable, be confined and observed by a veterinarian for 10 days. If the animal remains healthy, it can be safely concluded that it was not infectious at the time of the bite. When the biting animal was apparently rabid or was a wild animal (i.e., whenever a biting animal must be proved uninfected to avoid human treatment), it should be immediately killed and the brain submitted to a diagnostic laboratory for fluorescent antibody testing.

In patients, diagnosis is made from a history of a compatible animal bite once the characteristic clinical symptoms appear. Hysteria due to fright may follow a bite and give the impression of rabies, but the symptoms should subside promptly once the patient is assured that he is in no immediate danger and can be protected from rabies.

Control

The prevention and control of rabies requires impoundment of stray dogs, and restraint of other dogs by their owners. Immunization of 70% or more of the canine population has been effective in restricting transmission of the disease even in areas where rabies is endemic among wildlife.

Control of rabies in wildlife reservoirs is more difficult. Rabies usually becomes a problem when the wildlife host population is high. Locally, it becomes self-limiting because it decimates susceptible hosts until epidemic disease can no longer be propagated. If conducted on an adequate scale, systematic reduction of host species will bring about the same result and effectively prevent spread. However, because of the difficulty and expense, such control efforts are best limited to locales where human contact with wildlife is high (e.g., campgrounds, farm areas).

Prophylaxis

Postexposure: Rabies rarely occurs in man if proper local and systemic prophylaxis is carried out immediately after exposure. **Local wound treatment** may be the most valuable measure in preventing rabies. The contaminated area should be immediately and thoroughly cleansed with a 20% solution of medicinal soft soap. Deep puncture wounds should be flushed with soap through catheters. Cauterizing or suturing the wound is not advised.

Systemic postexposure prophylaxis (see TABLE 1-7) should be started immediately (1) if the animal is rabid or develops rabies during confinement; or (2) if the animal is not available for observation or examination, *and* if it was behaving in an atypical manner or if the bite was unprovoked, *and* if there is rabies in the area. The state health department may be consulted on the last point. Skunks, raccoons, foxes, and bats are particularly suspect among wild animals and, unless the animal is proved uninfected by examination, their bites generally necessitate rabies treatment. Rabbits and rodents (including squirrels, chipmunks, rats, and mice) are very rarely infected and their bites seldom justify rabies treatment.

TABLE 1-7. POSTEXPOSURE ANTIRABIES GUIDE

The following guide should be used in conjunction with knowledge of the animal species involved, circumstances of the bite or other exposure, vaccination status of the animal, and presence of rabies in the region.

Animal and Its Condition		Systemic Treatment	
Species	Condition at Time of Attack	Kind of Exposure	
		Bite	Non-Bite*
Wild Skunk, Fox Raccoon, Bat	Regard as rabid	S + V†	S + V†
Domestic Dog, Cat	Healthy	None‡	None‡
	Escaped (unknown)	S + V	V§
	Rabid	S + V†	S + V†
Other	Consider individually: Bites of rodents seldom require prophylaxis		

S = Antirabies serum or human rabies immune globulin; V = Rabies vaccine.

* Scratches, abrasions, or open wounds.

† Discontinue vaccine if fluorescent antibody tests of animal killed at time of attack are negative.

‡ Begin S + V at first sign of rabies in biting dog or cat during holding period (10 days).

§ 14 doses of duck embryo vaccine.

Adapted from USPHS Advisory Committee on Immunization Practices (ACIP) Recommendations, *Morbidity and Mortality Weekly Report* Vol. 21, No. 25 Supplement, June 24, 1972.

The administration of antirabies serum followed by vaccine gives the best specific postexposure prophylaxis and is indicated when the likelihood of rabies exposure is high. Less suspect exposures may be treated with vaccine alone.

The importance of prompt postexposure prophylaxis cannot be stressed too highly. For **passive immunization**, human rabies immune globulin 20 IU/kg body wt is given. Up to ½ the total dose is inoculated directly into the wound; the remainder is given IM. If equine origin antirabies serum must be used, 40 u./kg is given in the same manner. **Active immunization** with a course of 14 to 21 daily subcutaneous injections of duck embryo vaccine (in the manufacturer's recommended dose) should also begin immediately. If antirabies immune globulin or serum is administered, 21 doses of vaccine are given, plus 2 booster doses, given 10 days and 20 days after the completion of the initial vaccine course. Local reactions at the vaccine injection site are usual, but generalized systemic allergic reactions are uncommon and rarely serious.

More highly immunogenic tissue culture vaccines now being tested give promise of less vigorous vaccine regimens, with minimal allergic reactions and a superior immune response.

Pre-exposure: Because of the relative safety of the duck embryo vaccine, prophylactic vaccination of persons with a high occupational risk of exposure to rabid animals is well justified. Two alternative regimens are recommended: either two 1-ml doses of duck embryo vaccine 1 mo apart with a third inoculation 6 mo later, or (for more rapid immunization) three 1-ml doses 1 wk apart with a fourth inoculation 3 mo later. Serologic confirmation of antibody response should be obtained 3 to 4 wk after the last injection, and booster doses given, if needed, until antibody is detected. Persons with continuing exposure should have booster doses (1 ml) every 2 to 3 yr. If a previously immunized person (antibody response confirmed) is bitten by a rabid animal, he should receive 5 daily doses of duck embryo vaccine and a booster dose 20 days later; for a nonbite exposure, a single dose of the vaccine is sufficient.

Treatment

If rabies develops, treatment is symptomatic. Vigorous supportive treatment is **recommended.** Death from rabies had been considered inevitable if symptoms developed, but recovery has occurred following aggressive, vigorous, supportive treatment to control respiratory, circulatory, and CNS symptoms.

ARBOVIRUS AND ARENAVIRUS DISEASES

Arboviruses: *Viruses that are maintained in nature through transmission between vertebrate hosts and hematophagous arthropods; they multiply in both the vertebrates and the arthropods.* **Arenaviruses:** *Lymphocytic choriomeningitis and morphologically related viruses that are transmitted by rodents and can show man-to-man transmission.*

ARBOVIRUS ENCEPHALITIDES

The arboviruses (**arthropod-bo**rne viruses) number > 250; at least 80 immunologically distinct arboviruses cause disease in humans. Arboviruses are transmitted among vertebrates by biting insects, chiefly mosquitoes and ticks. Birds are often important sources of infection for mosquitoes, which then transmit the infection to horses, other domestic animals, and humans. Man is a "dead-end" host

TABLE 1-8. IMPORTANT ARBOVIRUS AND ARENAVIRUS DISEASES IN MAN:
            CLINICAL AND EPIDEMIOLOGIC FEATURES

Major Clinical Syndrome	Viral Agent	Group Classification	Vector	Major Distribution
Fever, malaise, headaches, myalgia	Venezuelan equine encephalitis (VEE)	Group A	Mosquito	Fla., Tex., La., Mexico, Central America, Northern S. America
	Naples Sicilian	Phlebotomus fever	Sandfly	Italy, India, Egypt, Iran, Pakistan
	Punta Toro Chagres	Phlebotomus fever	Sandfly	Panama
	Candiru	Phlebotomus fever	Sandfly	Brazil
	Colorado tick fever	Ungrouped	Tick	Western USA
	Rift Valley fever	Ungrouped	Mosquito	E. Africa
Fever, malaise, headaches, myalgia, arthralgia, rash	Chikungunya	Group A	Mosquito	S. Africa, India, S.E. Asia
	O'nyong-nyong	Group A	Mosquito	E. Africa
Fever, malaise, headaches, myalgia, rash, lymphadenopathy	Dengue 1–4	Group B	Mosquito	Worldwide (includes Caribbean, Hawaii)
	West Nile	Group B	Mosquito	S. & W. Africa, Middle East, India, Malaysia
Fever with CNS involvement	Eastern equine encephalitis (EEE)	Group A	Mosquito	Eastern Canada & USA, Caribbean, Eastern S. America
	Western equine encephalitis (WEE)	Group A	Mosquito	Canada, USA, Mexico, Brazil, Argentina
	Japanese encephalitis	Group B	Mosquito	Japan, China, S.E. Asia, Malaysia, Australia, New Zealand
	Kyasanur Forest disease	Group B	Tick	India
	Murray Valley encephalitis	Group B	Mosquito	Australia, New Guinea
	Powassan	Group B	Tick	Canada, USA
	St. Louis encephalitis	Group B	Mosquito	USA, Caribbean, Panama, Brazil, Argentina
	California encephalitis	California Group	Mosquito	USA
	Lymphocytic choriomeningitis	Arenavirus	Rodent	Worldwide (includes USA)

(Continued)

TABLE 1-8.   IMPORTANT ARBOVIRUS AND ARENAVIRUS DISEASES IN MAN:
CLINICAL AND EPIDEMIOLOGIC FEATURES *(Cont'd)*

Major Clinical Syndrome	Viral Agent	Group Classification	Vector	Major Distribution
Fever, malaise, headaches, myalgia, hemorrhagic signs	Chikungunya	Group A	Mosquito	S.E. Asia, Malaysia, India
	Dengue 1–4	Group B	Mosquito	S.E. Asia, Malaysia, India, Philippines
	Omsk hemorrhagic fever	Group B	Tick	USSR
	Yellow fever	Group B	Mosquito	Africa, Central & S. America
	Crimean-Congo hemorrhagic fever	Ungrouped	Tick	S. USSR, Central Africa, W. Pakistan, Bulgaria
	Junin (Argentinian hemorrhagic fever)	Arenavirus (Tacaribe group)	Rodent	Argentina
	Machupo (Bolivian hemorrhagic fever)	Arenavirus (Tacaribe group)	Rodent	E. Bolivia
	Lassa	Arenavirus	Rodent Man-to-Man	Central W. Africa
	Far Eastern or Korean hemorrhagic fever	?Arenavirus	?Rodent ?Mite	E. USSR, Manchuria, China, Korea

(i.e., incidental to the natural cycle and ineffective in virus perpetuation) for most of the agents, but is a definitive host (i.e., part of the natural cycle and necessary for transmitting the infection) in urban yellow fever, phlebotomus fever, and dengue. The agents are widely distributed throughout the world, depending on the availability of lower vertebrate hosts and appropriate vectors.

The arboviruses are classified by antigenic structure into 24 groups and 1 supergroup with 11 subgroups; there is also an ungrouped category for agents showing no serologic relationships. Many of the important disease-producing agents are in Group A (Eastern, Western, and Venezuelan equine encephalitis viruses) or Group B (the viruses of yellow fever; dengue; West Nile fever; St. Louis, Murray Valley, and Japanese encephalitis; and Kyasanur Forest disease).

In the USA, Western equine encephalitis **(WEE)** occurs throughout the country in all age groups, but a disproportionate number of cases occur in children under 1 yr old. Eastern equine encephalitis **(EEE)** occurs in the eastern USA, mainly in young children and persons over age 55, and has a higher mortality rate than WEE. In children under 1 yr old, WEE and EEE tend to be severe, with permanent sequelae. Epidemics of both WEE and EEE are associated with epizootics in horses. Urban and rural outbreaks of St. Louis encephalitis have occurred throughout the USA; morbidity and mortality are greatest in older age groups. The California encephalitis virus group is widely distributed throughout the USA, and mainly affects children in rural or suburban areas.

Symptoms, Signs, and Treatment

Arboviruses may cause CNS syndromes (including aseptic meningitis and encephalitis), minor nonspecific febrile illnesses, and, most commonly, inapparent infection. Except in epidemics, the clinical findings in meningitis and encephalitis rarely permit specific identification. Headache, drowsiness, fever, vomiting, and stiff neck are the usual presenting symptoms. Tremors, mental confusion, convulsions, and coma may develop rapidly. Paralysis of the extremities occasionally occurs. Treatment is supportive, as in other viral encephalitides (see in §14, Ch. 7).

YELLOW FEVER

An acute arbovirus infection of variable severity, characterized by sudden onset, fever, a relatively slow pulse, and headache. Intense albuminuria, jaundice, and hemorrhage, especially hematemesis, are characteristic but occur only in the proportionately few severe cases.

Etiology and Epidemiology

The virus of **urban yellow fever** is transmitted by the bite of an *Aëdes aegypti* mosquito infected 2 wk previously by feeding on a viremic patient. **Jungle (sylvatic) yellow fever** is transmitted by *Haemagogus* and other forest canopy mosquitoes which acquire the virus from wild primates. Yellow fever is endemic in central Africa and areas of South and Central America.

Symptoms and Signs

(1) Period of incubation: *3 to 6 days.* Prodromal symptoms are usually absent. **(2) Period of invasion:** *2 to 5 days.* Onset is sudden with fever of 39 to 40 C (102 to 104 F). The pulse, usually rapid initially, by the 2nd day becomes slow for the degree of fever present **(Faget's sign).** The face is flushed and the eyes are injected; the tongue margins are red and the center is "furred." Nausea, vomiting, constipation, epigastric distress, headache, muscle pains (especially in the neck, back, and legs), severe prostration, restlessness, and irritability are common symptoms. If mild, the illness ends at this stage after 1 to 3 days. **(3) Period of remission:** In moderate or severe illness, the fever falls by crisis 2 to 5 days after onset and a remission of several hours or days ensues. **(4) Period of intoxication:** *3 to 9 days.* The fever recurs but the pulse remains slow. Jaundice, extreme albuminuria, and hematemesis ("black vomit"), the three characteristic clinical features, appear. Oliguria or anuria may occur, and petechiae and mucosal hemorrhages are common. The patient is dull, confused, and apathetic. Delirium, convulsions, and coma occur terminally. **(5) Period of convalescence:** This is usually short except in the most severe cases. There are no known sequelae.

Diagnosis and Laboratory Findings

Albuminuria occurs in 90% of patients, usually on the 3rd day, and may reach 20 Gm/L in severe cases. The WBC count is usually low and drops to 1500 to 2500 by the 5th day; leukocytosis may occur terminally. Experimental evidence suggests that disseminated intravascular coagulation may occur. Serum bilirubin is mildly elevated.

The clinical features are nonspecific during the period of invasion, but the diagnosis is suggested by Faget's sign. During the period of intoxication, the characteristic triad of intense albuminuria, jaundice, and hematemesis should suggest the diagnosis. Diagnosis is confirmed by isolation of the virus from the blood, by a rising antibody titer, or at autopsy by the characteristic midzonal liver cell necrosis. Needle biopsy of the liver during illness is **contraindicated** by the risk of hemorrhage.

Prognosis

Up to 10% of clinically diagnosed cases end fatally, but overall mortality is actually lower since many mild or inapparent infections are undiagnosed.

Prophylaxis

Active immunization with the 17D strain of live attenuated yellow fever virus vaccine (0.5 ml s.c. every 10 yr) effectively prevents outbreaks and sporadic cases. In the USA, the vaccine is given only at USPHS-authorized Yellow Fever Vaccination Centers. Countries vary in their vaccination requirements; current information and addresses of vaccination centers can be obtained from state and local health departments.

To prevent further mosquito transmission, patients should be isolated in well-screened rooms sprayed with residual insecticides. Since transmission of infection can occur through laboratory accidents, hospital and laboratory personnel should be careful to avoid self-inoculation with patients' blood.

Eradication of urban yellow fever requires widespread mosquito control and mass immunization. During sylvatic outbreaks, work in the area should be discontinued pending immunization and mosquito control.

Treatment

Management is supportive and directed toward alleviating major symptoms. Complete bed rest and nursing care are important. Correction of fluid and electrolyte imbalance is imperative (see §11, Ch. 6).

Hemorrhagic tendencies should be combated with calcium gluconate 1 Gm IV once or twice/day, or with phytonadione (see VITAMIN K DEFICIENCY, Treatment, in §11, Ch. 3). Transfusion may be necessary. Heparin may be given if there is evidence of disseminated intravascular coagulation (low fibrinogen levels, prolonged thrombin time, thrombocytopenia, and elevation of fibrin split products in full-blown cases; in less acute forms some of these laboratory findings may not occur). Typical heparin dosage is 50 to 100 u./kg body wt initially, then 10 to 15 u./kg/hour, given by IV infusion.

Nausea and vomiting may be alleviated with dimenhydrinate 50 to 100 mg orally or rectally, or 50 mg IM, q 4 to 6 h; or with prochlorperazine 5 to 10 mg orally, parenterally, or rectally q 4 to 6 h. Fever may be reduced with tepid-water sponge baths. Headaches may require codeine 15 to 60 mg orally or s.c. q 4 to 6 h, or meperidine 50 to 100 mg orally or IM q 4 to 6 h.

DENGUE
(Breakbone or Dandy Fever)

An acute febrile disease characterized by sudden onset, with headache, fever, prostration, joint and muscle pain, lymphadenopathy, and a rash that appears simultaneously with a second temperature rise following an afebrile period. A hemorrhagic fever syndrome associated with dengue occurs in children (see below).

Dengue is endemic throughout the tropics and subtropics. The causative agent, a Group B arbovirus with 4 distinct serogroups, is transmitted by the bite of *Aëdes* mosquitoes.

Clinical Course

Following an incubation period of 3 to 15 (usually 5 to 8) days, onset is abrupt, with chills or chilly sensations, headache, postorbital pain on moving the eyes, lumbar backache, and severe prostration. Extreme aching in the legs and joints occurs during the first hours of illness. The temperature rises rapidly to as high as 40 C (104 F), with a relative bradycardia and hypotension. The bulbar and palpebral conjunctivas are injected, and a transient flushing or pale pink macular rash (particularly of the face) usually appears. The spleen may be soft and slightly enlarged. Cervical, epitrochlear, and inguinal lymph nodes are usually enlarged.

Fever and other symptoms persist for 48 to 96 h, followed by rapid defervescence with profuse sweating. This ushers in an afebrile period, with a sense of well-being, which lasts about 24 h. A second rapid temperature rise follows, usually with a lower peak than the first, producing a "saddle-back" temperature curve. A characteristic maculopapular eruption simultaneously appears, usually spreading from the extremities to cover the entire body except the face, or distributed patchily over the trunk and extremities. The palms and soles may be bright red and edematous. The fever, rash, and headache and other pains constitute the "dengue triad." Cases have occurred without the second febrile period.

Mortality is nil in typical dengue. Convalescence is often prolonged, lasting several weeks, and accompanied by asthenia. An attack produces immunity for a year or more.

Diagnosis and Laboratory Findings

Leukopenia is present by the 2nd day of fever; by the 4th or 5th day, the WBC count has dropped to 2000 to 4000 with only 20 to 40% granulocytes. Moderate albuminuria and a few casts may be found.

Dengue may be confused with Colorado tick fever, typhus, yellow fever, or other hemorrhagic fevers. Serologic diagnosis may be made by HI and CF tests using paired serums, but is complicated by cross-reactions with other Group B arbovirus antibodies.

Prophylaxis and Treatment

Prevention requires control or eradication of the mosquito vector. To prevent transmission to mosquitoes, patients in endemic areas should be kept under mosquito netting until the second fever has abated. **Treatment** is symptomatic. Complete bed rest is important. Aspirin 600 mg and codeine 15 to 60 mg may be given orally q 4 h for severe headache and myalgia.

DENGUE HEMORRHAGIC FEVER SHOCK SYNDROME
(DHFS; Philippine, Thai, or Southeast Asian Hemorrhagic Fever)

An acute disease occurring in children living where dengue is endemic, and characterized by an abrupt febrile onset followed by hemorrhagic manifestations and circulatory collapse. It is prevalent in Southeast Asia and India. Virtually all patients are under age 10.

Symptoms and Signs

Onset is abrupt, with fever, headache, nausea, vomiting, abdominal pain, cough, pharyngitis, and dyspnea. Shock occurs 2 to 6 days after onset, with sudden collapse or prostration, cool clammy extremities (the trunk is often warm), weak thready pulse, and circumoral cyanosis. Bleeding tendencies occur, usually as purpura, petechiae, or ecchymoses at injection sites; sometimes as hematemesis, melena, or epistaxis; and occasionally as subarachnoid hemorrhage.

Hepatomegaly is common, as is bronchopneumonia with or without bilateral pleural effusions. Myocarditis may be present. Mortality ranges from 6 to 30%; most deaths occur in infants under 1 yr old.

Laboratory Findings and Diagnosis

Hemoconcentration (Hct > 50%) is present during shock; the WBC count is elevated in $\frac{1}{3}$ of the patients. Thrombocytopenia (< 100,000/cu mm), a positive tourniquet test, and a prolonged prothrombin time are characteristic and indicative of the coagulation abnormalities. Minimal proteinuria may be present. SGOT levels may be moderately increased. Serologic tests usually show high CF antibody titers against Group B arboviruses, suggestive of a secondary immune response.

Presumptive diagnosis is based on abrupt onset of fever followed by sudden shock or collapse 2 or more days later, and bleeding abnormalities, including thrombocytopenia without manifest bleeding.

Treatment

The degree of hemoconcentration, dehydration, and electrolyte imbalance must be immediately evaluated and closely monitored for the first few days, since shock may occur or recur precipitously. Cyanotic patients should be given O_2. Vascular collapse and hemoconcentration require immediate and vigorous fluid replacement, preferably with a crystalloid solution such as Ringer's lactate (overhydration must be avoided). Plasma or human serum albumin should also be given if there is no response in the first hour. Fresh blood or platelet tranfusions may control bleeding. Agitated patients may be given paraldehyde or chloral hydrate. Hydrocortisone, pressor amines, α-adrenergic blocking agents, and vitamins C and K are of doubtful value.

LYMPHOCYTIC CHORIOMENINGITIS (LCM)

An acute viral infection caused by an RNA virus now classified as an arenavirus, usually appearing as an influenza-like illness or aseptic meningitis, rarely as encephalitis, orchitis, parotitis, or hemorrhagic fever.

LCM infection is endemic in rodents. Human infection is most commonly from exposure to dust or food contaminated by the gray house mouse or hamsters, which harbor the virus for life and excrete it in urine, feces, semen, and nasal secretions. When transmitted by mice the disease occurs primarily in adults, in the winter.

LCM virus is an uncommon cause of aseptic meningitis. As in aseptic meningitis from other causes, fever, headache, stiff neck, and lymphocytic CSF pleocytosis (usually 100 to 500/cu mm, but occasionally 1000 or more) are characteristic. The course may be biphasic, with an influenza-like syndrome followed by remission and then a CNS phase, or may end before meningeal involvement. The course is usually benign, with complete recovery in 10 to 14 days, although fatal encephalomyelitis or systemic infection has been reported.

During the acute stage, the virus can be recovered from blood, urine, and CSF by inoculation of suckling mice or guinea pigs. CF antibodies appear in the serum 7 to 21 days after onset; neutralizing antibodies may not appear for 5 to 8 wk. **Therapy** is supportive.

OTHER SYSTEMIC VIRAL DISEASES

MUMPS
(Epidemic Parotitis)

An acute, contagious, generalized viral disease, usually causing painful enlargement of the salivary glands, most commonly the parotids.

Etiology and Incidence

The causative agent, a paramyxovirus, is spread by droplet infection or direct contact with materials contaminated with infected saliva. The virus probably enters through the mouth. It may be found in the saliva for 1 to 6 days before the salivary glands swell and for the duration of glandular enlargement. It has been isolated from patients' blood and urine, and from the CSF in patients with CNS involvement.

Mumps is endemic in heavily populated areas, but may occur in epidemics when large numbers of susceptible individuals are together under crowded conditions. Communicability is less than in measles and chickenpox. The peak incidence is in late winter and early spring. Although the disease may occur at any age, most cases are in children aged 5 to 15, the disease is unusual in children under 2, and infants up to 1 yr are ordinarily immune. One attack usually confers permanent immunity even though only one parotid may have been enlarged. About 25 to 30% of cases are clinically inapparent.

Symptoms, Signs, and Course

After a 14- to 24-day incubation period, onset occurs with chilly sensations, headache, anorexia, malaise, and a low to moderate fever which may last 12 to 24 h before salivary gland involvement is noted. These prodromal symptoms may be absent in mild cases. Pain on chewing or swallowing, especially on swallowing acidic liquids such as vinegar or lemon juice, is the earliest symptom of parotitis. There is marked sensitivity to pressure over the angle of the jaw. With development of parotitis, the temperature frequently rises to 39.5 or 40 C (103 or 104 F). Swelling of the gland reaches maximum about the 2nd day and is associated with swelling of the area in front of and below the ear, from tissue edema extending beyond the parotid.

Both parotid glands are involved in most cases. Occasionally, the submaxillary and sublingual glands also swell; more rarely, these are the only glands affected. Swelling of the neck beneath the jaw occurs in such cases, or, with submaxillary gland involvement, suprasternal edema. The oral duct openings of the involved glands are "pouting" and slightly inflamed. The skin over the glands may become tense and shiny. Involved glands are acutely tender during the 24- to 72-h febrile period. The WBC count may be normal, though a slight leukopenia with a reduction in granulocytes is usual.

Prognosis is excellent in uncomplicated mumps, although rarely a relapse occurs after about 2 wk.

Complications

Particularly in postpuberal patients, the disease may involve organs other than the salivary glands. Symptoms may precede, accompany, or follow salivary gland involvement, and may also occur without primary sialadenitis.

Orchitis occurs in about 20% of postpuberal male patients. Testicular atrophy may ensue. Sterility is unusual, but can follow bilateral postorchitic atrophy; hormonal function is not lost. Gonadal involvement in females (**oophoritis**) is less commonly recognized and far less painful.

Meningoencephalitis: CSF pleocytosis is common in mumps, emphasizing the reason for headache, one of the major symptoms of mumps. CSF glucose levels are occasionally low, between 20 and 40 mg/100 ml, mimicking bacterial meningitis. More severe encephalitic signs occur in about 5 or 10%, with drowsiness or even coma or convulsions that may be abrupt in onset. About 30% of CNS mumps infections occur without associated parotitis. The prognosis is favorable in most cases with CNS involvement, and is considerably better than in measles encephalitis, although permanent sequelae, such as unilateral (rarely bilateral) nerve deafness or facial paralysis, may result. As in other viral diseases, a para- or post-infectious form of encephalitis may rarely occur. Other rare CNS manifestations include acute cerebellar ataxia, transverse myelitis, and polyneuritis.

Pancreatitis: Toward the end of the first week, a few patients may have sudden severe nausea and vomiting, with abdominal pain that is most severe in the epigastrium, suggesting pancreatitis. These symptoms disappear in about a week and the patient completely recovers.

Miscellaneous: Prostatitis, nephritis, myocarditis, mastitis, polyarthritis, and lacrimal gland involvement are seen occasionally. Inflammation of the thyroid and thymus glands may cause edema and swelling over the sternum, as seen with submaxillary gland involvement.

Diagnosis

Diagnosis of typical cases during an epidemic is easy, but sporadic cases are more difficult. Swelling of the parotid or other salivary glands due to mumps virus must be distinguished from (1) bacterial parotid involvement in streptococcal throat infections, diphtheria, or debilitated patients with poor oral hygiene, typhoid, or typhus fever; (2) Mikulicz's syndrome, a chronic, usually painless parotid and lacrimal gland swelling of unknown etiology that occurs with TB, sarcoidosis, SLE, leukemia, and lymphosarcoma; (3) malignant and benign salivary gland tumors; (4) drug-related parotid enlargement (e.g., from iodides or guanethidine); and (5) obstruction produced by a calculus in Stensen's duct. Enlarged lymph nodes along the mandible may be mistaken for swollen salivary glands. Mumps meningoencephalitis, sometimes the only clinical manifestation, must be differentiated from other viral meningitides.

Paired acute and convalescent serums permit diagnosis by means of the CF test, preferably with both soluble (S) and viral (V) antigens. S antibodies increase in the first week of infection and drop rather rapidly, often disappearing after 6 to 8 mo; V antibodies usually rise later than S antibodies but drop slowly to a plateau. Thus, a single serum specimen may occasionally be diagnostic if both CF antigens are used. An elevated serum amylase level may also aid in diagnosis.

Prophylaxis

The patient should remain in isolation until glandular swelling subsides. Susceptible contacts should be followed up closely from the 14th to the 28th day after exposure. Mumps immune globulin 1.5 to 3 ml IM may provide some protection for postpuberal susceptibles if given during the first few days after exposure, but this has not been proved.

Live mumps virus vaccine is the agent of choice for active immunization (see ROUTINE IMMUNIZATION PROCEDURES in §22). A mumps neutralization antibody titer of 1:2 or greater is protective. This vaccine produces no significant local or systemic reaction and requires only one injection. It is not yet clear whether revaccination is required to maintain lifelong immunity. Postexposure vaccination does not protect against mumps from that exposure, but if mumps does not develop, the vaccination will give future protection.

Treatment

Treatment is symptomatic. Postpuberal patients should remain in bed until they are afebrile. A soft diet reduces pain caused by chewing. Analgesics (e.g., aspirin in a dosage appropriate for the patient's age) may be used for headache and general malaise, and a barbiturate (e.g., phenobarbital 15 mg orally t.i.d. or q.i.d.) for sedation as necessary.

Complications are also treated symptomatically. Patients with orchitis require bed rest. Supporting the scrotum in cotton on an adhesive-tape bridge between the thighs to minimize tension, or applying ice packs, often help to relieve pain. Codeine 30 mg and aspirin 600 mg orally q 4 h may relieve discomfort. Rarely, surgical incision of the tunica vaginalis may be necessary to relieve severe scrotal pain and swelling, and to shorten the period of disability.

If nausea and vomiting of pancreatitis are severe, oral feedings should be withheld and fluid balance restored by IV dextrose and saline solutions.

Neither corticosteroids nor mumps immune globulin has proved effective in any form of mumps infection.

INFECTIOUS MONONUCLEOSIS

An acute disease characterized clinically by high fever, sore throat, and generalized lymphadenopathy; pathologically by diffuse hyperplasia of lymphatic tissue; hematologically by an increase in lymphocytes, many of which are atypical; and serologically by development of transient heterophil antibodies to sheep, horse, and beef erythrocytes, and of persistent antibodies to the Epstein-Barr virus.

Etiology

That infectious mononucleosis is caused by the Epstein-Barr virus **(EBV)**, one of the herpes viruses, was established by the following: The disease occurs only in persons with no prior EBV antibodies. EBV-specific antibodies can be demonstrated early after onset. Antibody titers decline during convalescence, but remain detectable for life, correlating with immunity to the disease. The virus is regularly present in the oropharyngeal secretions of patients with infectious mononucleosis and often for months afterwards. As with other herpes-group viruses, a persistent carrier state follows primary EBV infection. The presence of the virus is demonstrated by its ability to transform cord-blood lymphocytes in vitro into continuously growing lymphoblasts which all show an EBV-determined nuclear antigen that is detectable by an anti-complement immunofluorescence technic. The transformation of lymphocytes is a biologic property of the virus. Lymphoid cells, taken from the blood during the acute phase, or from the lymph nodes or blood of viral carriers, all yield EBV-positive lymphoblast lines in culture, whereas lymphocytes from susceptible persons, who lack EBV antibodies, generally do not survive in culture.

Epidemiology

Despite the fact that oropharyngeal EBV excretion may persist for months, infectious mononucleosis is not very contagious; for example, the annual incidence among susceptible college students is below 15%. The disease is spread through close contact, mainly by the oral–respiratory route. In areas of poor sanitation and hygiene, primary EBV infections usually occur in early childhood and are often silent or too mild to be diagnosed. In higher socioeconomic groups, primary exposure to EBV is often delayed until adolescence or later, when infections usually lead to typical infectious mononucleosis. Though a vaccine would be desirable to protect high-risk susceptibles, such as high school and college students, none is yet in prospect.

EBV replication, yielding a largely defective viral progeny, is restricted to lymphocytic cells. The fact that EBV transforms lymphocytes indicates that it may be oncogenic. There is strong evidence that it is involved in the etiology of Burkitt's lymphoma, nasopharyngeal carcinoma, and possibly other malignancies. If so, additional factors (immunologic defects, genetic predisposition, environmental co-carcinogens, other infectious agents such as malaria or another virus) must contribute to tumor development.

Symptoms, Signs, and Complications

After a 4- to 7-wk incubation period (possibly shorter in children), vague grippe-like malaise, fatigue, headache, and chilliness develop, typically followed by an acute phase of high fever, sore throat, and generalized lymphadenopathy. Symptoms and signs may be confusing since almost any organ of the body may be affected. Splenomegaly is present in 50% of the patients; rarely, rupture of the spleen may occur spontaneously or following careless palpation. Liver function tests are abnormal in almost all patients; hepatomegaly is present in about 20%, and jaundice in fewer than 5%. Pericarditis and myocarditis occasionally occur. Chest pains, dyspnea, and cough indicate pneumonitis. Signs of CNS involvement such as meningoencephalitis, the Guillain-Barré syndrome, or Bell's palsy may occur during or after the acute phase or may occasionally be the only clinical manifestation. Renal involvement is rare and may mainly be due to antigen-antibody complexes. Eyelid and orbital edema is often present. A transitory maculopapular rash is seen occasionally, often precipitated by ampicillin therapy. Punctate petechiae may be present on the borders of the soft and hard palates. Hemolytic anemia and thrombocytopenic purpura are infrequent complications.

The **typhoidal** form of the disease occurs in 10% of the cases and is characterized by minimal or absent sore throat, prolonged fever, and delayed development of hematologic and serologic changes.

Diagnosis

Blood smear examination and serologic tests are the cornerstones of diagnosis.

Hemogram: By the 2nd or 3rd wk, the total WBC count is usually elevated to 10,000 to 15,000 with a relative and absolute lymphocytosis. Atypical lymphocytes are increased in number (i.e., > 20%) and frequently show cytoplasmic vacuolization; oval, kidney-shaped, or slightly lobulated nuclei, usually without nucleoli; and great cell-to-cell variation in size and staining characteristics. Their increased number is considered pathognomonic of infectious mononucleosis, although occasionally also found in viral hepatitis, measles, rubella, and serum sickness.

Heterophil antibody test (Paul-Bunnell-Davidsohn test): The heterophil test is described under SEROLOGY, in §24, Ch. 2. Reagents for highly specific, rapid slide tests are commercially available for use in general practice.

In adolescent and adult patients, heterophil antibodies are usually detectable within the first 2 wk of illness but may not develop until later. They generally disappear 3 to 6 mo after onset. Heterophil antibody tests are consistently negative in about 10% of adult patients, in a larger number of younger patients, and in nearly all children under 3 yr of age, so that the diagnosis is often missed in young children.

The heterophil antibodies are of the IgM class. Other IgM antibodies, including cold and anti-i agglutinins, are often elevated; total serum IgM levels may increase, therefore, by as much as 100% (and IgG levels by 50%). Tests for syphilis and rheumatoid factor may be transiently positive. Why primary EBV infections evoke these as well as heterophil antibody responses is unknown.

Liver function tests should be performed since hepatic involvement is common. Most indicative are tests for elevated alkaline phosphatase, SGPT, and SGOT.

EBV-specific serodiagnostic tests are now available in a few laboratories. All are based on titration of serums by immunofluorescence technics and use lymphoblasts from selected cultures which per se or after certain treatments reveal given EBV-determined antigens. These sophisticated tests are unnecessary if the clinical and hematologic features are characteristic and a heterophil antibody response is detected. However, they are essential for accurate diagnosis when characteristic clinical signs or heterophil antibodies do not develop, or when clinical manifestations are unusual.

Most significant is the demonstration of specific IgM antibodies to EB viral capsid antigens **(VCA)** in acute-phase serum and their subsequent decline. VCA-specific IgG antibodies are found at high titers by the time symptoms appear, but titers persist and these antibodies are therefore not diagnostically significant per se unless titers are very high, or increase at least 4-fold, or subsequently decline. A diagnostic increase in titer occurs in < 20% of patients. A second group of antigens are the EBV-induced early antigens **(EA)**, which are subdivided into diffuse **(D)** and restricted **(R)** components on the basis of immunofluorescent staining patterns. Diagnostically significant transitory anti-D responses occur in 70 to 80% of patients. Antibodies to the EBV-associated nuclear antigen **(EBNA)**, which is present in every EBV-transformed cell, usually develop late after onset of disease. The absence of anti-EBNA antibodies in serum that is anti-VCA–positive in the early acute phase is therefore of diagnostic significance, and the subsequent appearance of anti-EBNA antibodies provides further proof of a primary EBV infection. The differential use of these various procedures permits the serodiagnosis of current or recent primary EBV infections in about 95% of cases.

Differential Diagnosis

The disease must be differentiated from other acute infections associated with fever, sore throat, and lymphadenopathy due to bacteria (streptococcus, diphtheria, Vincent's angina), other viruses (rubella, adenoviruses, hepatitis A and B), and other agents (*Toxoplasma gondii*). Cytomegalovirus **(CMV)** causes a mononucleosis-like disease, but patients are usually older; moreover, while splenomegaly, hepatomegaly, and atypical lymphocytes are commonly present, sore throat, cervical lymphadenopathy, and heterophil antibody responses are usually absent. The post-perfusion syndrome (see CYTOMEGALOVIRUS INFECTIONS, below) is usually caused by CMV but occasionally by EBV. On occasion, lymphoproliferative disorders (leukemia, Hodgkin's disease, lymphomas) must also be excluded. In cases with CNS involvement, various other causes must be excluded.

Prognosis

Infectious mononucleosis usually spends itself in 1 to 4 wk but may linger for 2 to 3 mo. Sequelae are unusual and the ultimate outlook is excellent. Rarely, death may follow splenic rupture, acute pericarditis or myocarditis, CNS involvement, or airway obstruction. Because the oropharynx may excrete EBV for months, exacerbation of latent infection and the existence of chronic or recurrent disease is conceivable, but as yet unproved.

Treatment

Therapy is symptomatic. Bed rest should be enforced during the acute phase of fever and malaise, and prolonged in cases with hepatic involvement. Strenuous exercise must be avoided while the spleen is enlarged. Aspirin or other analgesics usually control headache; these and saline gargles relieve sore throat and other oropharyngeal symptoms. Corticosteroids should be given only to patients with severe complications such as airway obstruction, neurologic involvement, hemolytic anemia, thrombocytopenic purpura, myocarditis, or pericarditis. Rupture of the spleen requires immediate splenectomy and massive blood transfusions.

Isolation of patients is unwarranted. Antibiotics are of no value unless secondary bacterial infection is present.

CYTOMEGALOVIRUS (CMV) INFECTION
(Cytomegalic Inclusion Disease)

A virus infection occurring congenitally, postnatally, or later in life, and ranging in severity from a silent infection without consequences, through disease manifested by fever, hepatitis, and (in neonates) severe brain damage, to stillbirth or perinatal death. The restrictive appellation "cytomegalic inclusion disease" refers to the intranuclear inclusion bodies found in enlarged infected cells.

Etiology and Epidemiology

The human cytomegaloviruses ("salivary gland viruses") are members of the herpes group of viruses, all of which have a propensity for remaining latent in man. Antigenic dissimilarity between cytomegalovirus (CMV) isolates indicates that they are a subgroup of closely related agents. Cytomegaloviruses are highly host-specific and cannot be propagated in laboratory animals or in most non-human cell cultures.

The cytomegaloviruses are ubiquitous. Infected individuals may excrete virus in the urine or saliva for months; virus may be demonstrable in human cervical secretions, semen, and milk; fresh blood from asymptomatic infected donors may produce disease in susceptible recipients. Infection may be acquired transplacentally, during birth, or by contact with infected secretions or excretions at any time thereafter. Serologic surveys indicate that the incidence of infection gradually increases with age; 60 to 90% of adults have experienced infection. High infection rates may occur at an early age in closed populations such as orphanages. CMV disease in an immunologically impaired adult may be a newly acquired infection or an activation of a latent process.

Symptoms and Signs

Congenital infection: The extent of the pathologic process is highly variable. Most commonly, infection is manifested only by cytomegaloviruria in an otherwise apparently normal infant. At the other clinical extreme, CMV infection may cause abortion or stillbirth, or postnatal death from hemorrhage, anemia, or extensive hepatic or CNS damage. Infants born with severe nonfatal disease typically have a low birth weight and perinatally develop fever, hepatitis with jaundice, and hemorrhagic manifestations such as purpura. Hepatosplenomegaly, thrombocytopenia, chorioretinitis, microcephaly, and periventricular cerebral calcification may be present. Prognosis must be guarded in overt cases because psychomotor retardation, spastic diplegia, blindness, deafness, or seizures may develop. Infants with inapparent infections may later manifest hearing defects.

Acquired infection: Infections acquired postnatally or later in life are often asymptomatic. An acute febrile illness, termed **cytomegalovirus mononucleosis** or **cytomegalovirus hepatitis,** may result from iatrogenic or spontaneous contact with CMV. **Post-perfusion syndrome** develops 2 to 4 wk after tranfusion with fresh blood containing CMV and is characterized by fever lasting 2 to 3 wk, hepatitis of variable degree and with or without jaundice, a characteristic atypical lymphocytosis resembling that of infectious mononucleosis, and occasionally a rash. CMV infection in patients with malignancy or receiving immunosuppressive therapy may cause pulmonary, gastrointestinal, or renal involvement.

Diagnosis

CMV may be isolated from urine or other body fluids by inoculation of human fibroblastic cell cultures. However, CMV may be excreted for months or years after infection and cytomegaloviruria must be interpreted accordingly. The appearance of specific CF antibodies during illness provides supportive evidence. Morphologic demonstration of infected cells in urine is of limited value.

Congenital infection must be differentiated from bacterial, viral (e.g., rubella), and protozoan (e.g., toxoplasmosis) infections. Acquired infection must be differentiated from viral hepatitis and infectious mononucleosis. The absence of pharyngitis or lymphadenopathy, and a negative heterophil antibody test, are helpful in ruling out infectious mononucleosis.

Treatment

There is no specific therapy. Trials of drugs that interfere with viral DNA synthesis (floxuridine, cytarabine, and others) have not yielded clear-cut clinical results.

3. RICKETTSIAL DISEASES

A group of diseases characterized by sudden onset, a febrile course of one to several weeks, peripheral vasculitis, and, in most cases, a skin eruption, caused by various rickettsia species, and transmitted to man by animals, particularly arthropods.

Members of the order Rickettsiales are, with some exceptions, obligate intracellular organisms resembling both viruses and bacteria. Like bacteria, they possess metabolic enzymes, have cell walls, utilize O_2, and are susceptible to antibiotics; like viruses, they require living cells for growth. Most are pleomorphic coccobacilli characteristically staining with a Castaneda or Giménez stain; and most induce serum agglutinins against specific *Proteus* strains **(Weil-Felix reaction)** in convalescent and recovered patients. Since many of the Rickettsiales have a typical geographic distribution, the area where the patient lives or has recently been traveling often helps in diagnosis.

Rickettsias multiply in the endothelial cells of small blood vessels. The consequent endothelial proliferation, perivascular infiltration, and thrombosis cause the typical rash and headache, and may lead to gangrene. Initial rickettsial multiplication at the site of an arthropod bite results in a local lesion (eschar) in a number of rickettsioses.

The rickettsioses fall into 4 categories: (1) the typhus group—epidemic typhus, Brill-Zinsser disease, murine (endemic) typhus, and scrub typhus; (2) the spotted fever group—Rocky Mountain spotted fever, Eastern tick-borne rickettsioses, and rickettsialpox; (3) Q fever; and (4) trench fever.

EPIDEMIC TYPHUS
(European, Classic, or Louse-Borne Typhus; Jail Fever)

An acute, often severe, febrile disease characterized by prolonged high fever, intractable headache, and a maculopapular rash, caused by Rickettsia prowazekii, *and transmitted by lice.*

Etiology and Epidemiology

The causative organism, *Rickettsia prowazekii,* is found worldwide. It is transmitted to man in the feces of the human body louse, *Pediculus humanus,* when scratching the irritated bite puncture contaminates it with the infective material. Dried louse feces may also infect via the mucous membranes when rubbed into the eyes or inhaled. Infection is spread when an infected louse abandons a febrile patient or a corpse for an uninfected host.

Symptoms and Signs

Rapid onset of fever and headache follows a 10- to 14-day incubation period. Fever slowly rises to about 40 C (104 F) where it remains until recovery begins, about 13 to 16 days after onset. Headache is intense and difficult to treat. On the 4th to 7th day pink macules appear, usually on the upper trunk, and rapidly cover the body except for the face, soles, and palms. The lesions become dark and maculopapular; in severe cases, the rash is petechial or hemorrhagic. The spleen may be palpable. Hypotension may occur and potentially fatal renal insufficiency or vascular collapse may develop. Pneumonia and gangrene are also serious prognostic signs. Fatalities are rare in children under 10 yr, but mortality increases with age and may reach 60% in those over 50.

Diagnosis

Early symptoms are not sufficiently specific to differentiate the disease from other rickettsial infections, smallpox, relapsing fever, or typhoid fever. The characteristic appearance and course of the rash aid in diagnosis. Laboratory diagnosis may be made by isolation of the organism from the blood and by demonstration of IgM antibodies by CF or agglutination tests. *R. prowazekii* shares common soluble antigens with *R. typhi (mooseri)* but also has differentiating antigens. Nonspecific antibodies agglutinate *Proteus* OX-19 in the Weil-Felix reaction.

Prophylaxis

Immunization and louse control are highly effective. Live and killed vaccines are available. Lice may be eliminated by dusting infested persons with DDT, malathion, or lindane.

Treatment

Tetracyclines and chloramphenicol are highly effective if rickettsiostatic dosage is given sufficiently early. Since chloramphenicol is quickly absorbed from the gut, it may be preferable for oral therapy. An initial loading dose of 50 mg/kg body wt is given; then 50 mg/kg/day in 3 or 4 divided doses until fever begins to decline, followed by 25 mg/kg/day until the patient has been afebrile for 2 to 3 days. Tetracyclines are irregularly absorbed by the gut; 25 mg/kg/day is given orally in divided doses q 3 to 4 h.

Patients unable to take oral medication may be given tetracycline 1 Gm IV followed by 500 mg orally q 6 h, or chloramphenicol 1 Gm IV in glucose or saline solution, followed by 500 mg IV or orally q 4 to 6 h.

Nursing care is important to prevent hypostatic pneumonia and decubitus ulcers. Sponging with tepid saline may partially control high fever. Headache may be treated with aspirin or similar compounds.

BRILL-ZINSSER DISEASE

Recrudescence of prior epidemic typhus.

Etiology and Epidemiology

The causative agent is *R. prowazekii*. Patients previously have either had epidemic typhus or have lived in an endemic area, and may serve as a reservoir for epidemic typhus. It is postulated that epidemic typhus organisms are retained for long periods after the patient recovers, and that when host defenses are decreased the organisms are activated, giving rise to Brill-Zinsser disease. The disease is sporadic, occurring at any season and in the absence of infected lice.

Symptoms and Signs

Symptoms are similar to those of epidemic typhus except that the disease is milder, the duration shorter (7 to 11 days), the fever fluctuant, and the rash often evanescent or absent. Mortality is nil.

Diagnosis

A history of epidemic typhus or exposure to it is helpful. *R. prowazekii* may be recovered from lice fed on patients during the acute phase (xenodiagnosis). CF or agglutinating antibodies rise rapidly. Specific IgG antibodies develop early. The Weil-Felix reaction is often negative.

Treatment

Oral chloramphenicol or tetracycline is given as for epidemic typhus, but since the disease is mild, tetracycline is preferable. Body lice should be eradicated when cases occur in infested communities, since transmission of *R. prowazekii* to lice may result in epidemic typhus in other individuals.

ENDEMIC TYPHUS
(Murine, Rat, or Flea Typhus; Urban Typhus of Malaya)

A febrile disease clinically similar to, but milder than, epidemic typhus, caused by Rickettsia typhi *and transmitted by rat fleas.*

Etiology and Epidemiology

The causative agent, *R. typhi (mooseri)*, closely resembles *R. prowazekii* morphologically. The disease is prevalent in wild rats and mice and is transmitted to man by rat fleas *(Xenopsylla cheopis)*. It occurs worldwide; in the USA, foci of infection are found along the southern Atlantic and Gulf coasts.

Symptoms and Signs

Following a 6- to 14-day incubation period, fever develops, lasts 9 to 14 days, and terminates by rapid lysis. The rash and other symptoms are similar to those of epidemic typhus but are much less severe. Mortality is low; fatalities may occur in elderly patients.

Diagnosis

A history of contact with rats can often be elicited. It is not possible to differentiate this disease clinically from Brill-Zinsser disease or mild epidemic typhus. Agglutinins for *Proteus* OX-19 and specific CF and agglutinating IgM antibodies develop during the course of illness. Cross-reactions with *R. prowazekii* occur but specific differentiating antigens exist.

Prophylaxis and Treatment

Reduction of the rat and rat flea population is most important. Since rat fleas are more apt to bite humans when rats are scarce, flea populations are reduced first, by dusting rat runs, burrows, and harborages with DDT or another residual insecticide. A vaccine is available.

Treatment is as for epidemic typhus, with oral tetracycline rather than chloramphenicol since the disease is mild.

ROCKY MOUNTAIN SPOTTED FEVER
(Spotted Fever; Tick Fever; Tick Typhus)

An acute febrile disease caused by Rickettsia rickettsii *and transmitted by ixodid ticks.*

Etiology, Epidemiology, and Pathology

R. rickettsii is limited to the Western Hemisphere. Once thought to be restricted, in the USA, to some western states, it has now been found in many areas, especially on the Atlantic seaboard. The organisms are harbored by hard-shelled ticks (family Ixodidae), which can transmit *R. rickettsii* transovarially to their progeny, resulting in a reservoir independent of animal hosts. *Dermacentor andersoni* (the wood-tick) is the principal vector in the western USA; *D. variabilis* (dog tick) and *Amblyomma americanum* (lone-star tick), in the eastern and southern USA. The organism is also maintained in rabbits and other small mammals. The disease is seasonal, mainly occurring from May to September when adult ticks are active and when persons are most apt to be in areas infested by ticks. Though most cases occur in agricultural workers, incidence is high in children under age 15 and in others who frequent tick-infested areas for work or recreation.

Pathologically, small blood vessels are primarily involved. Endothelial cells are damaged and vessels may be blocked by thrombi. The skin, subcutaneous tissue, and CNS are the major sites affected, but the lungs, heart, liver, and spleen may also be involved.

Symptoms and Signs

The incubation period averages 7 days but may vary from 3 to 12 days; the shorter the incubation period, the more severe the infection. Onset is abrupt, with severe headache, chills, prostration, and muscular pains. Fever reaches 39.5 or 40 C (103 or 104 F) within 2 days and remains high (for 15 to 20 days in severe cases), though morning remissions may occur. An unproductive cough develops. About the 4th day of fever, a rash appears on the wrists, ankles, palms, soles, and forearms, then rapidly extends to the neck, face, axilla, buttocks, and trunk. Initially macular and pink, it becomes maculopapular and dark. In about 4 days, the lesions become petechial and may coalesce to form large, hemorrhagic areas that later ulcerate. Neurologic symptoms include headache, restlessness, insomnia, delirium, and coma. Hypotension develops in severe cases. Hepatomegaly may be present but jaundice is infrequent. Localized pneumonitis may occur. Untreated patients may develop such complications as pneumonia, tissue necrosis, and circulatory failure; and such sequelae as brain and heart damage.

Diagnosis

A history of working or vacationing in tick-infested areas or discovery of a tick bite or a feeding tick aids in diagnosis. Tularemia, Colorado tick fever, and Q fever are also transmitted by *D. andersoni* in certain areas, but the pathognomonic rash serves to differentiate spotted fever from these diseases, other rickettsial infections, typhoid fever, and meningococcemia.

R. rickettsii can be isolated from the blood during the 1st wk of illness. Specific CF antibodies (IgM) develop after the 2nd wk of illness; agglutinins against *Proteus* OX-2 and especially OX-19 are found during convalescence.

Prognosis

Antibiotic therapy has significantly reduced mortality, formerly about 20%, and higher in localized areas and in those over age 50. No sequelae result if therapy is instituted early.

Prophylaxis

A vaccine is available but is only recommended for persons who frequently encounter ticks during work or recreation. Tick repellents such as dimethyl phthalate should be used by all who live or work in tick-infested areas. Good personal hygiene should be practiced, with frequent body searches for ticks. Gradual traction with a small forceps will usually remove ticks from the body. Care must be taken when removing ticks from the body or from household animals since cases have occurred after handling crushed ticks. Tick populations may be reduced in limited areas by controlling small-animal populations; spraying the area with DDT, dieldrin, or chlordane is also helpful. However, no practical means exist to rid entire areas of ticks, and personal hygiene must therefore be emphasized.

Treatment

A tetracycline is given in an initial oral dose of 25 mg/kg, followed by 25 mg/kg/day in 3 or 4 divided doses. Alternatively, chloramphenicol may be given in an initial oral loading dose of 50 mg/kg, followed by 50 mg/kg/day in 3 or 4 divided doses. Either antibiotic is given until the patient has been afebrile for 24 h. Supportive therapy, especially for peripheral circulatory collapse, and good nursing care are imperative.

TICK-BORNE RICKETTSIOSES OF THE EASTERN HEMISPHERE

(North Asian Tick-Borne Rickettsiosis; Queensland Tick Typhus; African Tick Typhus [Fièvre Boutonneuse])

Febrile diseases transmitted by ixodid ticks and characterized by an initial lesion and an erythematous maculopapular rash.

Etiology and Epidemiology

Rickettsia sibirica is the etiologic agent of North Asian tick-borne rickettsiosis, *R. australis* of Queensland tick typhus, and *R. conorii* of fièvre boutonneuse. North Asian tick-borne rickettsiosis is found in Armenia, Central Asia, Siberia, and Mongolia; Queensland tick typhus in Australia. Fièvre boutonneuse is known by the area in which it occurs: Kenya, South African, and Indian tick typhus are self-evident; Marseilles fever is found in the Mediterranean littoral.

Animal hosts for tick typhus include dogs (fièvre boutonneuse), marsupials (Queensland tick typhus), and many small mammals. The tick vectors include the dog tick *(Rhipicephalus sanguineus)* in the Mediterranean area and India, *Haemaphysalis leachi* and *R. simus* in Africa, and other ixodid genera in South Africa and elsewhere. Transovarial transmission of rickettsias occurs in a variety of ticks.

Symptoms, Signs, and Prognosis

After a 5- to 7-day incubation period, fever, malaise, headache, and conjunctival injection develop. With the onset of fever a local lesion appears (termed **eschar**, or, in fièvre boutonneuse, **tache noire**), a small button-like ulcer 2 to 5 mm in diameter with a black center. About the 4th day of fever, a red maculopapular rash appears on the forearms and extends to most of the body, including the palms and soles. Fever lasts into the 2nd wk of illness. Regional lymph nodes are enlarged. Complications are rare. Death is rare except among aged or debilitated patients.

Diagnosis

The local lesions of tularemia and rickettsialpox must be differentiated; measles and meningococcal infections must also be ruled out. Laboratory diagnosis depends upon the presence of antibodies; agglutinins for *Proteus* OX-2 are usually higher than for OX-19; specific CF and agglutinating antibodies appear during convalescence. *R. sibirica, R. australis,* and *R. conorii* share a common antigen with *R. rickettsii* and *R. akari.* They may be differentiated from these and each other by cross-immunity tests in guinea pigs, and by CF and mouse-toxin neutralization tests.

Prophylaxis and Treatment

Tick control is prophylactically important (see Rocky Mountain Spotted Fever, above).

Treatment is with tetracycline in the same doses as for spotted fever. Patients become afebrile after 2 or 3 days of treatment.

SCRUB TYPHUS
(Tsutsugamushi Disease; Mite-Borne Typhus; Tropical Typhus)

A mite-borne infectious disease caused by Rickettsia tsutsugamushi *and characterized by fever, a primary lesion, a macular rash, and lymphadenopathy.*

Etiology and Epidemiology

Occurring in the Asiatic-Pacific area bounded by Japan, India, and Australia, *R. tsutsugamushi* is transmitted in nature by trombiculid mites (usually *Leptotrombidium* species) transovarially and by feeding on forest and rural rodents, including rats, voles, and field mice. Human infection follows a chigger (mite larva) bite.

Symptoms and Signs

Following an incubation period of 6 to 21 days (average 10 to 12 days), onset is sudden with fever, chilliness, headache, and generalized lymphadenopathy. With onset of fever, a local lesion (eschar) develops at the site of the chigger bite. It is seen in Caucasians but rarely in Asians, usually where skin surfaces meet. Beginning as a red indurated lesion about 1 cm in diameter, it eventually vesiculates, ruptures, and is covered with a black scab; regional lymph node enlargement occurs. Fever rises during the 1st wk, often to 40 to 40.5 C (104 to 105 F). A macular rash develops on the trunk during the 5th to 8th day of fever, often extends to the arms and legs, and may disappear rapidly or become maculopapular and intensely colored. Cough is present during the 1st wk of fever and pneumonitis may develop during the 2nd wk. In severe cases, pulse rate increases, blood pressure decreases, and delirium, stupor, and muscular twitching may develop. Splenomegaly may be present and myocarditis may occur. In untreated patients, high fever may persist for 2 wk or more and falls by lysis over several days. With specific therapy, defervescence usually begins within 36 h, and recovery is prompt and uneventful.

Diagnosis

In endemic areas, lymphadenopathy and an eschar in a febrile patient with a history of exposure to mites suggests scrub typhus. Other rickettsial infections, dengue, leptospirosis, malaria, and typhoid fever must be differentiated.

The organism can be isolated from blood or tissues. *R. tsutsugamushi* shows extreme antigenic variations according to its geographic area. CF antibodies are only active against specific strains, but all pathogenic strains produce agglutinins against *Proteus mirabilis* OX-K. The simplest method of serologic diagnosis is demonstration of these agglutinins; they appear by the 3rd wk and may disappear 2 to 3 wk later. CF tests may also help to establish the diagnosis; tests using soluble antigens are of no value.

Prophylaxis

Clearing the brush and spraying infested areas with residual insecticides eliminates or decreases the mite population. Mite repellents such as dimethyl phthalate or benzyl benzoate should be used by individuals likely to be exposed.

Treatment

Chloramphenicol 50 mg/kg/day or tetracycline 25 mg/kg/day is given orally until the patient has been afebrile for 24 h. Since relapses may occur, a single oral 3-Gm dose of either drug is given on the 7th and 14th day after intensive treatment ends.

RICKETTSIALPOX
(Vesicular Rickettsiosis)

A mild self-limited febrile disease with an initial local lesion and a generalized papulovesicular rash, caused by Rickettsia akari *and transmitted from its murine host by mites.*

First observed in New York City, rickettsialpox has also occurred in other US areas and in Russia, Korea, and Africa. The mite vector, *Allodermanyssus sanguineus*, is widely distributed. It infects the house mouse *(Mus musculus)* and some species of wild mice, and can transmit *R. akari* transovarially. Humans may be infected by either chigger or adult mite bites.

Symptoms and Signs

An eschar resembling the tache noire of fièvre boutonneuse appears about 1 wk before onset of fever. Initially a small papule, it develops into a small ulcer with a dark crust, and heals leaving a scar; regional lymphadenopathy is present. The fever is intermittent and lasts about a week, with chills, profuse sweating, headache, photophobia, and muscle pains. Early in the febrile course, a generalized maculopapular rash with intraepidermal vesicles appears, sparing the palms and soles. The disease is mild and no deaths have been observed.

Diagnosis

Chickenpox and smallpox must be ruled out. The presence of an eschar before onset of fever is characteristic.

R. akari shares a common antigen with other members of the spotted fever group, but may be differentiated from them by demonstration of a rising titer of specific CF antibodies. The Weil-Felix reaction is usually negative.

Prophylaxis and Treatment

Mouse harborages must be destroyed and the vector controlled by residual insecticides.

The disease may be so mild that no **treatment** is indicated. When needed, tetracycline 25 mg/kg/day is given orally for 3 to 4 days.

Q FEVER

An acute disease with fever, headache, and interstitial pneumonitis, caused by Coxiella burnetii (Rickettsia burnetii). *In contrast to other rickettsial diseases, no agglutinins are developed against* Proteus *strains, rash is absent, and transmission to man occurs by inhalation of infective aerosols.*

Etiology and Epidemiology

The route of infection is usually inhalation. The disease is essentially worldwide. It is maintained as an inapparent infection in domestic animals, with sheep, cattle, and goats the principal sources of human infection. The organisms persist in feces, urine, milk, and tissues (especially the placenta), so that fomites and infective aerosols are easily formed. Thus, many occupational cases occur among workers in close contact with domestic animals or their products. The disease can also be contracted by ingestion of infective raw milk. Person-to-person infection has occurred.

C. burnetii is also maintained in nature through an animal–tick cycle, and the disease in the USA was first recognized in persons bitten by *Dermacentor andersoni*. Various arthropods, rodents, other mammals, and birds are naturally infected and may play a role in human infection.

Symptoms and Signs

The incubation period varies from 9 to 28 days (average 18 to 21 days). Onset is abrupt, with fever, severe headache, chilliness, severe malaise, myalgia, and, often, chest pains. Fever may rise to 40 C (104 F) and persist for 1 to > 3 wk. Rash is absent. A nonproductive cough with x-ray evidence of pneumonitis often develops during the 2nd wk of illness. Mortality is less than 1% in untreated patients, and even lower with antibiotic therapy, but endocarditis or lobar pneumonia may cause death in aged or debilitated patients. Chronic Q fever with cardiovascular symptoms may occur. Q fever endocarditis is said to be uniformly fatal but fortunately is rare.

Diagnosis

Q fever should be considered in a febrile patient with a history of association with domestic animals, animal products, or ticks. Symptoms are not characteristic and during the early stages may resemble influenza. Differential diagnosis includes brucellosis, typhoid and paratyphoid fever, hepatitis, leptospirosis, and, when pneumonitis occurs, psittacosis, coccidioidomycosis, tularemia, and viral pneumonitis.

C. burnetii may be isolated from the blood. The Weil-Felix reaction is negative. Specific CF and agglutinating antibodies appear during convalescence. Agglutination tests are more sensitive than CF tests; fluorescent antibody tests are also available. C. burnetii exists in two phases; antibodies against Phase I organisms are rarely produced in infected human serum but when present indicate chronic Q fever.

Prophylaxis

Animal-to-man transmission must be prevented: milk should be pasteurized; dust control in pertinent industries is essential; and animal placentas, feces, and urine should be incinerated. The sputum and urine of Q fever patients should be autoclaved and the patient isolated. Effective vaccines are available but are still experimental.

Therapy

Tetracycline is preferable to chloramphenicol. It is given orally in a dose of 2 to 3 Gm/day, as 4 divided doses, until 5 days after the patient becomes afebrile. Fever usually disappears 36 to 48 h after initiation of therapy.

TRENCH FEVER
(Wolhynian Fever)

A louse-borne febrile disease observed in military populations during World Wars I and II, and now rarely seen.

Etiology and Epidemiology

The causative organism, *Rochalimaea (Rickettsia) quintana,* grows extracellularly, unlike other rickettsias, and multiplies in the gut lumen of the body louse. *R. quintana* is transmitted to man by the rubbing of infected louse feces into abraded skin or into the conjunctiva. Man is considered the reservoir since *R. quintana* persists in the blood for months after clinical recovery. The disease may be endemic in Mexico.

Symptoms and Signs

Following a 14- to 30-day incubation period, onset is sudden with fever, weakness, dizziness, headache, and severe back and leg pains. Fever may reach 40.5 C (105 F) and persist for 5 to 6 days. In about half the cases, fever recurs 1 to 8 times at 5- to 6-day intervals. A transient macular or papular rash and, occasionally, hepatomegaly and splenomegaly are present. Although recovery is usually complete in 1 to 2 mo and mortality is negligible, the illness may be prolonged and debilitating.

Diagnosis

The disease may be suspected in persons living where louse infestaton is heavy. Leptospirosis, typhus fever, relapsing fever, and malaria must be ruled out. The organism may be identified by xenodiagnosis: normal body lice excrete *R. quintana* about 1 wk after ingestion of the patient's blood. Antibodies can be demonstrated by fluorescence or CF tests during convalescence.

Prophylaxis and Treatment

Body lice must be controlled (see EPIDEMIC TYPHUS, above). Chloramphenicol and the tetracyclines should be effective treatment though reliable information is unavailable.

---

4. CHLAMYDIAL DISEASES

The organisms responsible for psittacosis, lymphogranuloma venereum (LGV), trachoma, inclusion conjunctivitis, and possibly cat-scratch fever are now classified in the genus *Chlamydia (Bedsonia, Miyagawanella)*, which is divided into two species. *C. psittaci* is the agent responsible for psittacosis; *C. trachomatis* strains cause LGV, trachoma, and inclusion conjunctivitis. (The latter are often referred to as the "TRIC agents.")

Chlamydia organisms are nonmotile, gram-negative, obligate intracellular parasites. Originally considered viruses because they multiply in the cytoplasm of host cells, the chlamydias have since been shown to be more closely related to bacteria and rickettsias, since they contain both DNA and RNA, have a cell wall that is chemically similar to that of gram-negative bacteria, possess ribosomes, grow well in the yolk-sac of embryonated eggs, and are susceptible to the tetracyclines.

Although the *Chlamydia* organisms have only recently found their appropriate classification and nomenclature, the diseases they cause were settled long ago into their preferred sites. Therefore, PSITTACOSIS is discussed under PNEUMONIA in §5; LGV, a venereal disease, is in §21; and the ophthalmic disorders TRACHOMA and INCLUSION CONJUNCTIVITIS are in §19, Ch. 8. Cat-scratch fever, though not yet established as a chlamydial disease, remains to be discussed here.

CAT-SCRATCH DISEASE
(Nonbacterial Lymphadenitis; Benign Lymphorecticulosis)

A febrile disorder characterized by lymphadenitis, thought to be transmitted by cats.

Etiology

Indirect evidence suggests that the etiologic agent belongs to the genus *Chlamydia*. Several animals have been held responsible, but most patients have had contact with young, healthy cats. No causative agent has been isolated from incriminated cats.

Symptoms and Signs

A few days after a minor scratch, a papule or pustule develops at the site. Regional lymphadenopathy develops within 2 wk, usually unilaterally and in relation to the scratch site (i.e., axillary, epitrochlear, submandibular, cervical, or inguinal). The nodes are initially firm and tender, but later become fluctuant and may drain with fistula formation. Pathologic examination of involved nodes shows, sequentially, hyperplasia, a granulomatous response, and then suppurative necrosis and micro-abscess formation. Fever, malaise, headache, and anorexia accompany the lymphadenopathy. Erythema nodosum, thrombocytopenic purpura, Parinaud's syndrome, and osteolytic lesions are uncommon. Encephalitis is a rare but severe complication, usually occurring one or more weeks after onset.

Diagnosis, Treatment, and Prognosis

Diagnostic criteria include regional lymphadenopathy, a history of cat contact, characteristic histopathology, negative studies for other common causes of lymphadenitis, and a positive intradermal skin test with cat-scratch antigen (not commercially available).

Tetracycline **therapy** may shorten the course. Spontaneous node regression usually occurs within 4 wk. Surgical excision may be necessary, especially if fistulas drain. **Prognosis** is excellent.

---

5. BACTERIAL DISEASES

CAUSED BY GRAM-POSITIVE COCCI

STAPHYLOCOCCAL INFECTIONS

Epidemiology

Pathogenic staphylococci are *normally* carried in the anterior nares of about 50%, and on the skin of about 20%, of healthy adults. Hospital patients or personnel have slightly higher rates of carriage. While penicillin-resistant strains are common in hospitals, they are not rare in the community. Dangerous staphylococci are ubiquitous.

Certain groups of patients are predisposed to staphylococcal infections: newborns, nursing mothers, and patients with influenza, chronic bronchopulmonary disorders (e.g., cystic fibrosis, pulmonary emphysema), leukemia, neoplasms, renal transplants, tracheostomies, burns, chronic skin disorders, surgical incisions, diabetes mellitus, and indwelling intravascular plastic catheters. Patients receiving adrenal steroids, irradiation, immunosuppressives, or antitumor chemotherapy are also at an increased risk. Such predisposed patients may acquire antibiotic-resistant staphylococci from other colonized areas of their own bodies, or from infected hospital personnel, who may be only asymptomatic carriers. Patient-to-patient transmission via the hands of personnel is the most important means of spread.

Unlike other staphylococcal diseases, **staphylococcal food poisoning** (see in §7, Ch. 12) is caused by ingestion of a preformed enterotoxin produced by staphylococci in contaminated food, and not by infection with the organism itself. Victims of staphylococcal food poisoning are usually otherwise healthy.

Symptoms, Signs, and Diagnosis

The site of the staphylococcal infection determines its clinical picture. Common presentations include furuncles, carbuncles, abscesses, pneumonia, bacteremia, endocarditis, osteomyelitis, enterocolitis, and gastroenteritis. These are discussed in further detail in other appropriate sections of THE MANUAL.

Staphylococcal abscesses and the "scalded skin syndrome" (for the latter, see §16, Ch. 4, and NEONATAL INFECTION in §10, Ch. 2): **Neonatal infections** usually appear within 6 wk after birth. Most commonly seen are pustular or bullous skin lesions generally located in the axillary, inguinal, or neck skin folds, but multiple subcutaneous abscesses, exfoliation, bacteremia, meningitis, or pneumonia may also occur. Microscopic examination of the pus discloses polymorphonuclear neutrophils and staphylococci, often within the leukocytes.

Nursing mothers who develop breast abscesses or mastitis 1 to 4 wk postpartum should be considered as having penicillin-resistant staphylococcal infections, most probably derived from the infant.

Postoperative infections ranging from "stitch abscesses" to extensive wound involvement are commonly due to staphylococci. Such infections may appear within a few days or not until several weeks after an operation, and are particularly likely if the patient received antibiotics at the time of surgery.

Furuncles and **carbuncles** are discussed in §16, Ch. 4.

Staphylococcal pneumonia (see in §5, Ch. 9) should be suspected in patients with influenza who develop dyspnea, cyanosis, or persistent or recurrent fever, and in patients hospitalized with chronic bronchopulmonary disease or other high-risk diseases who develop low-grade fever, tachypnea, cough, cyanosis, and leukocytosis. In neonates, staphylococcal pneumonia is characterized by abscess formation, rapid development of pneumatoceles, and, often, complicating empyema. Microscopic examination of patients' sputum discloses numerous large gram-positive cocci, occasionally within neutrophils.

Staphylococcal bacteremia may occur in association with any localized staphylococcal abscess. It is a common cause of death in severely burned patients, generally 2 to 4 wk after injury. Symptoms and signs are discussed under BACTEREMIA in §1, Ch. 1. Persistent fever is usual and may be associated with shock. Bacterial endocarditis may develop. Diagnosis is established by positive blood cultures.

Staphylococcal osteomyelitis (see also §13, Ch. 14): Acute hematogenous osteomyelitis occurs predominantly in children, causing chills, fever, and pain over the involved bone. Redness and swelling subsequently appear. Periarticular infection frequently results in effusion, suggesting septic arthritis rather than osteomyelitis. The WBC count is usually > 15,000 and blood cultures are often positive. X-ray changes are not apparent for 10 to 14 days; it may be longer before bone rarefaction and periosteal reaction are detected. Acute rheumatic fever is the most common misdiagnosis, but the differential diagnosis is usually not difficult if the delayed development of x-ray abnormalities is appreciated.

Staphylococcal enterocolitis (see §7, Ch. 16) is suggested when hospitalized patients develop fever, ileus, abdominal distention, hypotension, or diarrhea, especially if they have had recent abdominal surgery, broad-spectrum antibiotics, or antibiotics for preoperative bowel preparation. If microscopic examination of the stools discloses clumps of staphylococci, the diagnosis is confirmed.

Prophylaxis

Aseptic precautions (e.g., thorough hand washing between patient examinations, sterilization of equipment) are important. Infected patients and their bedding should be isolated from other vulnerable patients. Hospital personnel with active staphylococcal infections, even of a local nature (e.g., boils), should not be allowed in contact with patients or equipment until their infections have been cured. Asymptomatic nasal carriers need not be excluded from patient contact unless the strains are particularly dangerous and the individual is the suspected source of an outbreak.

Treatment

Management includes abscess drainage, antibacterial therapy (parenterally, in a seriously ill patient), and general supportive measures. The choice of an antibiotic agent depends on the site of the infection, the severity of the illness, and the sensitivity of the organism. Cultures should be obtained before instituting or altering antibacterial regimens. Hospital-acquired staphylococci, and many community-acquired strains, are usually resistant to penicillin G, ampicillin, carbenicillin, streptomycin, and the tetracyclines. These antibiotics should not be used unless the organisms have been proved to be susceptible.

Virtually all strains are susceptible to penicillinase-resistant penicillins (methicillin, oxacillin, nafcillin, cloxacillin, dicloxacillin), cephalosporins (cephalothin, cefazolin, cephalexin, cephradine), gentamicin, vancomycin, lincomycin, and clindamycin; hence, one of these is usually the agent of choice. Many strains are also sensitive to erythromycin, kanamycin, bacitracin, and chloramphenicol. Chloramphenicol and bacitracin, however, are seldom indicated because of their potential toxicity and the availability of alternative agents. In staphylococcal enterocolitis, a nonabsorbed antistaphylococcal agent such as vancomycin is given orally, in combination with systemic therapy.

STREPTOCOCCAL INFECTIONS

Classification

Streptococcal infections can be classified **microbially** according to characteristics of the streptococcus and **clinically** according to the type of infection.

When grown on sheep-blood agar, β-hemolytic streptococci produce zones of clear hemolysis around each colony; α-streptococci (commonly called *Streptococcus viridans*) are surrounded by green discoloration due to incomplete hemolysis; and γ-streptococci are nonhemolytic. An additional classification, based on carbohydrates present in the cell wall, divides streptococci into the Lancefield Groups A to O. The members of Group D are often called **enterococci.** Extracellular Group A streptococcal antigens evoking antibody responses play important roles in the diagnostic tests to be described later.

Clinically, streptococcal infections can be divided into 3 broad groups: (1) the **carrier state,** in which the patient harbors streptococci without apparent infection; (2) **acute illnesses,** often suppurative, caused by streptococcal invasion of tissues; and (3) **delayed, nonsuppurative complications.** The nonsuppurative complications are the inflammatory states of acute rheumatic fever, chorea (both discussed in this chapter), and glomerulonephritis (discussed in §6). They occur most commonly about 2 wk after a clinically overt streptococcal infection, but the infection may be asymptomatic and the interval may be under or over 2 wk.

Clinical Manifestations

The symptoms and signs of acute invasive streptococcal infections depend on the affected tissue, the organism, the state of the host, and the host's response.

A **carrier state** exists when streptococci can be identified in material taken from a site that shows no evidence of inflammation. Group D enterococci are normally found in the gut, γ-streptococci in the throat and respiratory tract. β-Hemolytic streptococci of Groups A, B, C, and G—the groups generally regarded as pathogenic for man—can be cultured regularly from normal-looking throats of asymptomatic patients, and the term "carrier state" is usually reserved for such pharyngeal discoveries. The carrier state has importance as a cause of misdiagnosis in many pharyngeal or respiratory illnesses since bacteriologic demonstration does not prove that a streptococcus is responsible for the associated clinical manifestations.

Acute streptococcal infections can be *primary,* invading normal tissue, or *secondary,* invading tissue compromised by trauma or other disease. The organism in primary invasions is usually the Group A β-hemolytic streptococcus and the site is usually the pharynx. Secondary invasions can be caused by γ-hemolytic streptococci, by enterococci, or by Group A organisms. Group A erysipelas can occur in previously normal skin, or a streptococcal cellulitis can be imposed on traumatized skin or in subcutaneous tissue predisposed by venous insufficiency. A viral pneumonia or degenerative lung disease may be followed by a streptococcal pneumonia; *S. viridans* or enterococci may create bacterial endocarditis; enterococci are frequently found in urinary infections; and the endometritis of a postpartum uterus is often due to enterococci or Group A organisms. The eyes, ears, joints, bone, and gut are other sites of secondary streptococcal invasion.

Primary or secondary infections can spread through the affected tissues and along lymphatic channels to regional lymph nodes, and can also produce bacteremia. The development of suppuration depends on the severity of infection and the susceptibility of tissue.

The most common type of streptococcal disease is **primary pharyngeal infection with the Group A β-hemolytic organism.** In its typical form, the infection is manifested by sore throat, fever, a beefy red pharynx, and tonsillar exudate. This form occurs in about 20% of Group A infections; the remainder are asymptomatic, have fever or sore throat alone, or have nonspecific symptoms such as headache, malaise, nausea, vomiting, or tachycardia. Convulsions may occur in children. The cervical and submaxillary nodes may enlarge and become tender. In children under 4, rhinorrhea is frequent and sometimes the sole manifestation. None of these symptoms (including sore throat) and none of the signs (including pharyngeal exudate or occasional palatal petechiae) are specific for streptococcal infection, and any or all of these clinical features can occur in viral infections, particularly with the adenoviruses and in infectious mononucleosis. Cough and stuffy nose are uncharacteristic of streptococcal infection, and their presence suggests that other etiologic agents coexist or have exclusive responsibility for the clinical ailment. Definitive diagnosis rests on the laboratory technics described later.

Though formerly a common ailment, **scarlet fever** is uncommon today, probably because antibiotic therapy prevents the opportunity for the streptococcus to progress in individual patients or to create massive epidemics. Scarlet fever is associated with Group A streptococcal strains that produce an erythrogenic toxin, leading to a diffuse pink-red cutaneous flush that blanches on pressure. The rash, an additional feature of an illness that otherwise resembles streptococcal pharyngitis, is seen best on the abdomen, on the lateral chest, and in cutaneous folds. Among the characteristic manifestations of the rash are **circumoral pallor** surrounded by a flushed face, a **"strawberry tongue"** (inflamed beefy red papillae protruding through a white coating), and **Pastia's lines** (dark red lines in the creases of skin folds). The upper layer of the previously reddened skin often desquamates after the fever subsides. The course and management of scarlet fever are essentially the same as for other clinically evident Group A infections.

Laboratory Diagnostic Tests

Acute streptococcal inflammation is regularly associated with an elevation both in ESR (usually > 50 in the Westergren test or uncorrected Wintrobe value) and in WBC count (about 12,000 to 20,000), with 75 to 90% neutrophils, many of which are young forms. The urine commonly shows no specific changes except those attributable to fever (e.g., proteinuria).

The presence of streptococci can be established directly and promptly in material taken from the inflammatory site and examined by bacteriologic technics:

overnight incubation on a sheep-blood agar plate or, for Group A organisms, immediate staining with fluorescent antibodies. The fluorescent method obviates the need, when organisms are grown in culture, for serologic testing to differentiate Group A organisms from other β-hemolytic streptococci, but the fluorescence may often produce false-positive reactions with hemolytic staphylococci.

These direct tests can show that streptococci are *present* but *proof of infection* is obtained indirectly from streptococcal antibodies in the serum. The ASO titer rises in only 75 to 80% of infections, and, for completeness, streptococcal antihyaluronidase, anti-deoxyribonuclease B, anti-diphosphopyridine nucleotidase, and anti-streptokinase can also be used.

A single value of one antibody titer is only a crude index of recent streptococcal infection. Confirmation requires comparison of sequential specimens for recent *changes* in titer, since a single value may be high as a result of slow "decay" of antibodies from a long antecedent infection. Conversely, a single value lower than the laboratory's upper limit of normal may represent an elevation for an individual patient. Serums need not be taken more often than every 2 wk and may be as far apart as 2 mo. A significant rise (or fall) in titer should span at least 2 tube dilutions since a 1-tube increment may be due to laboratory variation. For greatest accuracy, the serums under comparison should be saved and tested on the same day, with the same reagents, by the same technician.

Because of the time interval between serial specimens, serologic testing is not useful in management of acute invasive streptococcal infections, where diagnosis depends on clinical manifestations and the results of bacteriologic tests. The "serial run" antibody tests are particularly useful, however, in the diagnosis of poststreptococcal inflammatory states. Evidence of a recent Group A streptococcal infection is critical for the diagnosis of rheumatic fever, which can generally be ruled out if no change in titer is demonstrated in a properly performed "serial run" with measurement of other appropriate antibodies besides ASO.

Course and Treatment

The secondarily invasive streptococcal infections can be life-threatening, particularly for a debilitated patient. Septicemias, puerperal sepsis, endocarditis, and pneumonias due to streptococci were frequent causes of death in the pre-antibiotic era, and remain serious, especially with an enterococcal infection. Though Group A streptococci and *S. viridans* are almost always sensitive to penicillin, enterococci are often resistant and require supplemental treatment with streptomycin or other antibiotics.

The primary pharyngeal infections, including scarlet fever, ordinarily have a finite course; the fever will drop after several days and recovery is complete within 2 wk. Though antibiotics will hasten the disappearance of symptoms, their value is primarily to prevent local suppurative events such as peritonsillar abscess (quinsy), otitis media, sinusitis, and mastoiditis. Most important, they are used to thwart the nonsuppurative complications that may follow untreated Group A infections.

Penicillin is the best therapeutic agent for an established Group A streptococcal infection. A single injection of benzathine penicillin G, at a dose of 600,000 to 900,000 u. IM for small children and 1.2 million u. IM for adolescents or adults, will usually suffice. Since the injection is often painful, oral therapy may be preferred if the patient can be trusted to maintain the regimen. The minor differences of absorption among the diverse oral preparations of penicillin do not seem as important as an adequately high dosage and duration of the regimen. At least 200,000 u. (and perhaps 400,000 u.) should be taken q.i.d. for at least 10 days to achieve the effect of a single injection of benzathine penicillin G. The 10-day course *must be completed* even though the patient has become asymptomatic. An alternative plan for patients considered unreliable or unable to take oral medication is to give 3 injections of procaine penicillin (each usually less painful than the one large benzathine dose): 600,000 u. IM is given on the 1st, 4th, and 7th days.

When penicillin is contraindicated, erythromycin 2 Gm/day or lincomycin 1.8 Gm/day can be given orally for 10 days in divided doses. Sulfadiazine, which is bacteriostatic, should not be used to treat an established infection though it is highly useful in preventing streptococcal infections. Tetracycline is undesirable because a significant number of β-hemolytic streptococci are resistant to it; moreover, in the young it may discolor growing teeth.

Antistreptococcal therapy can often be withheld for 1 or 2 days until bacteriologic verification has been obtained. An effective plan is to begin oral penicillin when infection is suspected and specimens for laboratory tests have been obtained. The treatment is then stopped if laboratory tests fail to confirm the presence of streptococci. Otherwise, oral treatment is continued or replaced by an injected agent.

Other symptoms of streptococcal infection can be treated with agents such as aspirin for sore throat, headache, or fever. Bed rest is unnecessary unless the patient wants it. Isolation technics are no longer warranted. Among the infected patient's close associates in family or friends, those who are debilitated or have a history of poststreptococcal complications should be examined for streptococci, then appropriately protected with antibiotics.

RHEUMATIC FEVER

A nonsuppurative acute inflammatory complication of Group A streptococcal infections, characterized mainly by arthritis, chorea, or carditis appearing alone or in combination, with residual heart disease as a possible sequel of the carditis.

Etiology and Incidence

The mixture of manifestations arbitrarily diagnosed as acute rheumatic fever occurs as a nonsuppurative inflammatory complication of Group A streptococcal infection and can affect one or more of 5 major sites: the joints (arthritis), the brain (chorea), the heart (carditis), the subcutaneous tissues (nodules), and the skin (erythema marginatum). The attack rates of rheumatic fever range from 0.1% in untreated people with mild or asymptomatic streptococcal infections to 3% in those with febrile exudative pharyngitis. Though the Group A streptococcus has been indicted as the provocation for rheumatic fever, the role of the host's constitutional and environmental susceptibility has not yet been clarified. Environmentally, malnutrition and overcrowding seem to predispose to the infections and subsequent rheumatic episodes. Rheumatic fever occurs most often during school age, with first attacks rare before age 4 and uncommon after 18. Familial susceptibility is of significant but not paramount importance.

Exact incidence rates of acute rheumatic fever are difficult to determine because so many episodes, particularly those with only mild asymptomatic carditis, are not brought to the physician's attention. Though incidence rates seem to have declined in recent years, the contribution of antibiotics is difficult to separate from a reduction due to more specific diagnostic criteria, so that the "rheumatic" label is applied to fewer patients. The prevalence of rheumatic heart disease is also difficult to determine because diagnostic criteria are not standardized for the living and necropsy is not performed routinely. According to recent surveys, rheumatic heart disease is the most common cardiac abnormality of school children, being found in about 1 to 2%. It is responsible for about half of the rejections from military service for cardiovascular reasons and in 1972 caused 14,118 deaths in the USA, compared with 7006 deaths during the same interval attributed to syphilis, tuberculosis, and infectious enteritis.

Pathology

The clinical pathology of rheumatic fever is manifested in systemic and local indexes of acute inflammation. Systemically, the ESR is elevated, often to levels > 120 mm/h in the Westergren method and > 50 in the uncorrected Wintrobe test. The WBC count reaches values of 12,000 to 20,000 and may go higher with corticosteroid therapy. The serum C-reactive protein is abnormally high; since it rises and falls faster than the ESR, a negative test is useful for confirming the absence of inflammation in a patient whose ESR is elevated for some time after an acute rheumatic episode has subsided clinically.

The local indexes of inflammation are found in synovial fluid, though aspiration is seldom necessary for diagnosis or therapy. The fluid is usually clear and sterile, with normal mucin concentration, an elevated WBC count, and a ropy acetic acid precipitate.

Prolongation of the P-R interval is the most common abnormality in the ECG. This finding has *not* correlated well with prognosis or with other evidence of carditis, and it is now regarded as due to a nonspecific abnormality, unrelated to cardiac inflammation, that chemically causes delayed A-V electrical conductivity in about 30% of patients with poststreptococcal complications. Other ECG abnormalities, when present, are due to pericarditis, enlargement of ventricles or atria, or cardiac arrhythmias.

The histopathology of acute rheumatic fever is difficult to assess because few patients die during the acute attack. Aschoff lesions are often, but not consistently, found in the myocardium and other parts of the heart of patients with carditis. Biopsy of subcutaneous nodules shows certain features resembling Aschoff lesions, but no characteristics that can distinguish the nodules from those of rheumatoid arthritis. Biopsy of inflamed synovial membrane shows nonspecific edema and hyperemia. Erythema marginatum seldom lasts long enough for biopsy, and when examined microscopically, has shown no specific lesions. No distinctive findings, beyond hyperemia, have been found in the brains of the few patients who died during an acute episode of chorea or in examinations performed in choreic patients who died years later.

The most characteristic and potentially dangerous anatomic lesion of rheumatic inflammation is the gross effect on cardiac valves. The mitral valve is involved most commonly; the aortic valve, often; the tricuspid valve, infrequently; and the pulmonic valve, rarely. An acute interstitial valvulitis may cause edema, thickening, fusion, and retraction or other destruction of leaflets and cusps, leading to stenotic or regurgitant functional changes. Similar involvement can shorten, thicken, or fuse chordae tendineae, adding to the regurgitation of damaged valves or producing regurgitation for a valve that is itself unaffected. Dilation of valve rings may be a third mechanism causing regurgitation. Regurgitation and stenosis are the usual effects on the leaflets of mitral and tricuspid valves; the aortic valve generally becomes regurgitant initially and stenotic only later.

Fibrinous nonspecific pericarditis, sometimes with effusion, is seen only in the presence of endocardial inflammation and almost always subsides without permanent damage.

Symptoms and Signs

Because the following 5 diverse major manifestations can appear alone or in various combinations, rheumatic fever has many clinical patterns. The cutaneous and subcutaneous features are uncommon and almost never occur alone, usually developing in a patient who already has chorea, arthritis, or carditis.

Erythema marginatum, a serpiginous, flat, painless rash, is transient, sometimes lasting less than a day. Its appearance is often delayed after the inciting streptococcal infection, and its occurrence as, or after, other aspects of rheumatic inflammation subside should not be mistaken for a new attack.

Subcutaneous nodules, which occur most frequently on the extensor surfaces of large joints, usually coexist with evidence of carditis. Ordinarily, the nodules are painless, transitory, and responsive to whatever agent is used for the associated arthritic or carditic inflammation.

Chorea, a complication of poststreptococcal inflammation, can occur alone or in association with other rheumatic manifestations (see SYDENHAM'S CHOREA, below).

Arthritis is the most common clinical manifestation of rheumatic fever and gives the disease its name. The joints become painful and tender, and may also become red, hot, and swollen, sometimes with effusion. Tenosynovitis may develop at the site of muscle insertions. The involved joints are usually the ankles, knees, elbows, or wrists. The shoulders, hips, and small joints of hands and feet may also be involved but almost never alone. If vertebral joints are affected, other disease should be suspected. Rheumatic arthropathy can be mono- or polyarticular, and the typical pattern of migratory polyarthritis is now seen mainly when bed rest and anti-inflammatory therapy have not been instituted promptly.

Carditis has its own spectrum of manifestations, with the appearance, alone or in various combinations, of pericardial rub, significant murmurs, cardiac enlargement, or congestive heart failure. In first attacks of rheumatic fever, carditis is present in about 50% of patients with arthritis. In the absence of arthritis (or chorea), a patient with carditis will seek medical attention only if he is sufficiently febrile, if pericarditis is present and painful, or if cardiac decompensation produces respiratory, peripheral, or abdominal manifestations. In the absence of these provocations, a patient with symptomless murmurs or cardiac enlargement may not seek medical help during the acute rheumatic attack. The cardiac damage may then not be discovered until much later, when the patient is found to have "rheumatic heart disease without a history of rheumatic fever." In about ½ of adults with rheumatic hearts, the disease develops in this insidious manner, with the ailment initially undetectable because it did not receive medical examination.

Since murmurs are the most frequent manifestation of carditis, careful auscultatory technics and rigorous interpretative criteria are required to avoid errors during the acoustic assessment of the heart. The soft diastolic blow of aortic regurgitation (heard best along the lower left sternal border) and the presystolic murmur of mitral stenosis (heard focally above or medial to the apex) may be undetected when present. Normal 3rd heart sounds at the apex may be regarded fallaciously as mid-diastolic murmurs; apical split 1st sounds, as presystolic murmurs; and the physiologic systolic murmur that occurs in the pulmonary artery may be called aortic stenosis when heard at the base or mitral regurgitation when heard at the apex. Criteria for interpretation of roentgenograms are also needed, to avoid misconstruing normal variations in the posteroanterior cardiac silhouette caused by respiration or diastolic expansion. The barium esophagram may be indented not by an enlarged left atrium, but by swallowed air or a backward rotation of the left ventricle. A normal but prominent pulmonary conus may be mistaken for right ventricle enlargement.

Cardiac decompensation may be undiagnosed in acutely ill children because it may produce manifestations different from those expected in adults. Included are dyspnea without rales, nausea and vomiting (due to gastric hyperemia), a right upper quadrant or epigastric ache (due to distention of the hepatic capsule), and a hacking nonproductive cough (due to pulmonary congestion). Conversely, the tachypnea of salicylate toxicity and the hepatomegaly that sometimes occurs during prolonged corticosteroid therapy may be mistaken for congestive heart failure.

Other Manifestations

Abdominal pain can occur in rheumatic fever either via the hepatic mechanism just described under cardiac decompensation or via a concomitant mesenteric adenitis. Because of the elevated WBC count and abdominal guarding, the situation may resemble acute appendicitis, particularly when other rheumatic manifestations are absent. A prompt response to diuretic or anti-inflammatory agents may confirm the diagnosis.

The arthralgias (**"growing pains"**) often attributed to rheumatic fever in the past are not part of rheumatic inflammation and are generally due to nonspecific myalgia or tenodynia in the para-articular zone. These pains can be distinguished from rheumatic arthropathy by the absence of tenderness during passive movement of the allegedly involved joint. Isometric contraction of the neighboring muscles or tendons will often reproduce the pain.

The lethargy, malaise, or fatigue often ascribed in the past to rheumatic fever can be caused by congestive heart failure, but, in the absence of cardiac decompensation, these symptoms are psychogenic rather than rheumatic manifestations. "Rheumatic" pneumonia or pleurisy is no longer regarded as a specific entity in rheumatic fever. The manifestations may be caused by other diseases (such as RA or SLE), or by conventional types of pulmonary infection or infarction, occurring in association with decompensated rheumatic hearts.

Diagnosis

No single test or other evidence is pathognomonic of rheumatic fever, and diagnosis at present usually depends on the patient's fulfillment of the modified Jones criteria, which require the presence of at least 1, and preferably 2, of the 5 major manifestations cited earlier, together with evidence not only of recent Group A streptococcal infection, but also of such "minor" manifestations of acute inflammation as fever and an elevated ESR or WBC count.

Gout, sickle cell anemia, leukemia, SLE, and embolic bacterial endocarditis are other causes of acute arthropathy. Other causes of joint pain (e.g., serum sickness, drug reactions, traumatic arthritis, gonococcal arthritis) can usually be distinguished by history or specific laboratory tests. The main diagnostic source of arthrologic confusion is juvenile RA, which sometimes begins with a relatively abrupt onset, occasionally with rheumatoid cardiac involvement, and often without positive serologic tests for rheumatoid factor. The absence of an antecedent streptococcal infection and the long clinical course of an arthropathic episode will usually distinguish rheumatoid from rheumatic arthritis.

Congenital heart disease with murmurs, cardiomegaly, or congestive heart failure in children and adolescents is distinguished by its characteristic murmurs, and by cyanosis, when present; cardiac catheterization or angiography can be used to verify difficult diagnoses. Also, subendocardial fibroelastosis has been increasingly recognized as an uncommon mimic of rheumatic cardiac abnormalities, and can be suspected when there is no convincing evidence of rheumatic or congenital lesions.

Clinical Course

Except for carditis, all manifestations of rheumatic fever subside without residual effects. Joint pain and fever usually subside within 2 wk, often more rapidly, and seldom last longer than a month; the ESR usually returns to normal within 3 mo in the absence of carditis. Patients with carditis usually have at least overt acoustic evidence of it when first encountered medically; if no worsening occurs during the next 2 to 3 wk, new manifestations of carditis will seldom occur thereafter. Since murmurs often do not disappear, and since new cardiac phenomena are not common during clinical observation, inflammatory rather than cardiac manifestations are the best indexes of therapeutic response. The acute evidence of inflammation, including ESR, usually returns to normal within 5 mo in uncomplicated carditis.

About 5% of rheumatic patients have prolonged attacks with clinical and laboratory manifestations of inflammation for 8 mo or longer, appearing in spontaneously recurrent outbreaks unrelated to intervening streptococcal infection or to cessation of antecedent anti-inflammatory therapy. Such attacks are more likely to occur during recurrent rheumatic episodes with carditis.

Rheumatic fever does not seem to produce chronic "smoldering" cardiac inflammation. Scars left by acute valvular damage may contract and change, and secondary hemodynamic difficulties may develop in the myocardium without the persistence of acute inflammation.

The long-term outcome depends on the cardiac severity of the initial attack. Patients without carditis seldom develop valvular damage; they are less likely to have rheumatic recurrences than are patients with carditis; and they are unlikely to develop carditis in the recurrences. Patients who had severe carditis during the acute episode are usually left with residual heart disease that is often worsened by the rheumatic recurrences to which they are particularly susceptible. The organic murmurs eventually disappear in about half of the patients whose acute episode was manifested by mild carditis without major cardiac enlargement or decompensation. Susceptibility to recurrences in this group is intermediate (between the low risk of the "no carditis" and the high risk of the "severe carditis" patients), but the recurrences may create permanent or further cardiac damage.

Treatment

In patients with **arthritis** only, therapy is directed toward relief of pain. In mild cases, codeine, other analgesics, or relatively small doses of aspirin are adequate. In more severe situations, complete **salicylization** is necessary. Aspirin is given in an escalating pattern, resembling that of digitalization, until clinical effectiveness has been attained or toxicity supervenes. Measurements of blood or urinary levels of salicylate are unnecessary because the correlation with the clinical effects is inconsistent. The starting dose of aspirin for children and adolescents is 30 mg/lb body wt (about 60 mg/kg) divided into 4 daily doses. If not effective overnight, the dose is increased to 90 mg/kg the next day, 120 mg/kg on the following day, and 180 mg/kg on the day after. High doses can be divided into 5 or 6 portions rather than 4 daily installments. Aspirin should be abandoned in favor of a corticosteroid if a therapeutic effect has not been produced after the 4th day.

Enteric-coated, buffered, or complex salicylate molecules appear to have no advantages over ordinary aspirin. Local gastric reactions can be avoided (or treated, when they occur) by giving milk or antacids ½ h after ingestion of the aspirin. Systemic toxicity of salicylate is manifested by tinnitus, headache, or tachypnea and may not appear until after a week or more of fixed dosage. The toxicity is managed by reducing the dose if the drug appears therapeutically effective, or by abandoning it otherwise.

The goal with **carditis** is to suppress clinical inflammation while simultaneously avoiding the post-therapeutic rebound that often follows anti-inflammatory suppression. Salicylate is preferable to corticosteroid therapy as a first choice, because an 8-wk course of salicylate is seldom followed by such rebounds, and also because salicylate treatment can avoid the cutaneous striae and acne that often accompany prolonged, high-dosage corticosteroid therapy.

With severe carditis, particularly when congestive heart failure is present, the acute inflammation may be too great for suppression with salicylates. A **cortico-**

steroid program should be started promptly if a trial of salicylization fails. One useful regimen consists of prednisone, in a total daily oral dose of 40 to 80 mg, depending on the size of the patient. If inflammation is not suppressed after a 2-day trial at this dose, a total daily amount of 120 to 160 mg may be needed. The fully suppressive dose of corticosteroid should be maintained until the ESR has remained normal for at least 1 wk; the dosage is then halved for the next week. To prevent post-steroid rebounds, an overlap of full-scale salicylate therapy is begun simultaneously, maintained throughout the tapering of the corticosteroid, and continued until 2 wk after the corticosteroid has been stopped. The tapering of the corticosteroid may proceed at the rate of 5 mg every 2 days.

These procedures are intended only for acute rheumatic inflammation. Cardiac arrhythmias or decompensation should be treated with appropriate agents. A post-therapeutic rebound manifested only by fever or joint pain often subsides spontaneously without the need for resuming anti-inflammatory treatment that might be followed by a re-rebound, but congestive heart failure in a rebound, if uncontrollable by cardiotonic agents, requires resumption of anti-inflammatory therapy. In patients with the type of prolonged, spontaneously recurrent attacks described under Clinical Course, immunosuppressive agents—such as nitrogen mustard or mercaptopurine—may be effective.

Other Therapeutic Procedures

The acutely ill patient's choice of **physical activities** is usually as good as arbitrary medical decisions. Patients will usually limit themselves accordingly if symptomatic with arthritis, chorea, or congestive heart failure. In the absence of carditis, no restrictions are needed after the acute arthritis or chorea has disappeared. The most difficult medical decision about physical restrictions is for asymptomatic patients with carditis. Strict bed rest in such patients has no proved value, and its enforcement may create undesirable psychologic reactions.

Though the poststreptococcal inflammation is well developed by the time a rheumatic patient is medically detected, an eradicating course of **antibiotics** is useful to remove any lingering organisms. Appropriate regimens have been described under Course and Treatment of streptococcal infections.

No particular diet is necessary unless salt restriction is required for congestive heart failure unresponsive to other modes of management.

Subsequent Management

Antistreptococcal prophylaxis should be maintained continuously after an attack of acute rheumatic fever (or chorea) to prevent recurrent attacks. The most potent method is benzathine penicillin G in a monthly IM injection of 1.2 million u., but the injections have the disadvantages of pain and the need for monthly medical attention. Sulfadiazine, in a single oral dose of 1 Gm/day, is as effective as any of the other carefully tested oral regimens. The daily prophylactic dose of oral penicillin G or V is 200,000 to 250,000 u. once or twice/day.

The optimum duration of antistreptococcal prophylaxis is uncertain. Some authorities believe it should be maintained for life in every patient who has had rheumatic fever or chorea. Others recommend that prophylaxis be continued for the first few years after an acute attack, and in all patients under 18. Thereafter, prophylaxis can be discontinued in patients without cardiac damage, but maintained for life in patients with severe cardiac damage. In patients with mild cardiac damage (i.e., significant murmurs but no cardiomegaly or decompensation), prophylaxis can be maintained or else discontinued in favor of a find-then-treat approach to future streptococcal infections.

Dental coverage with additional antibiotics at the time of major dental work may prevent SBE in patients known to have had carditis and in those with rheumatic heart disease. The best regimen is penicillin 1.2 million u. plus streptomycin 1 Gm IM on the day of the dental work and on the day after.

Physical restrictions appear to confer no cardiac benefits in asymptomatic patients with or without residual rheumatic heart disease, and may create adverse psychosocial reactions. Accordingly, restrictions seem advisable only in patients with symptomatic cardiac decompensation—and the restrictions should be appropriate to reduce or remove the symptoms.

SYDENHAM'S CHOREA
(Chorea Minor; Rheumatic Chorea; St. Vitus' Dance)

A CNS disease, often of insidious onset but of finite duration, characterized by involuntary, purposeless, nonrepetitive movements, and subsiding without neurologic residua.

Etiology

Sydenham's chorea is generally regarded as an inflammatory complication of Group A streptococcal infections. After the infection, the time interval before onset of chorea (sometimes up to 6 mo) is longer than that of other rheumatic manifestations, and the chorea may begin as or after other clinical and laboratory features have returned to normal. If it is a sole clinical feature of post-streptococcal inflammation, Sydenham's chorea may thus appear to be an isolated, unrelated event.

The disease is more common in girls than boys; in childhood; and (for temperate climates) in the summer and early fall, after the spring and early summer peak incidence of rheumatic fever. Chorea occurs in about 10% of rheumatic attacks.

Symptoms and Signs

The patient develops rapid, purposeless, nonrepetitive movements that may involve all muscles except the eyes. Voluntary movements are abrupt, with impaired coordination. Facial grimacing is common. The patient may appear clumsy in mild cases, and may have slight difficulties in dressing and feeding. In extreme cases, the patient may need vigorous sedation and protection to avoid self-injury from flailing arms or legs. The neurologic examination shows no defect in muscle strength or sensory perception except for an occasionally pendulous knee jerk.

Course

The course of chorea is variable and difficult to measure because of its insidious onset and gradual cessation. A month or more may elapse before the movements become intense enough to make the patient or his parents seek medical attention. In many patients, the course is completed within 3 mo after a doctor is seen, but occasionally an episode may last 6 to 8 mo.

Laboratory Findings

Aside from occasional lingering evidence of previous streptococcal infection, chorea has no characteristic laboratory features. The CSF is usually unremarkable, and the EEG shows no more than nonspecific dysrhythmias.

Diagnosis

The athetoid movements of chorea are pathognomonic. They resemble those of cerebral palsy, from which they can be distinguished by the history of recent onset. Other conditions that must be differentiated are habit spasms, which are repetitive; and the movements of hyperkinetic children, which are purposeful. Huntington's chorea is usually associated with a family history and adulthood. The Parkinson-like side effects of tranquilizers, given to control the apparently "hyperactive" child, may confuse the diagnosis of chorea until the therapy is discontinued and the unaltered choreic movements can be noted.

Treatment

No known medication is consistently effective. Sedation with a barbiturate may be attempted when the movements are severe, in dosage adequate to make the patient barely drowsy. A tranquilizer—such as diazepam 5 mg 4 to 6 times/day—may be effective if barbiturates fail. A salicylate or a corticosteroid may be given in the dosage described for rheumatic fever if these two agents fail.

Chorea is best regarded and treated as a transitory, reversible form of cerebral palsy. It is most important to reassure patients and all those who deal with them—family, friends, nurses, teachers, classmates—that the ailment is self-limited, that it will ultimately subside without residual damage, and that the temporary impairment of motor functions will not affect intellectual capacity. Patients should miss school only if movements are uncontrollably severe; and should return to school as soon as they can manage the necessary locomotion, even if some residual dysfunction is still present. Many of the so-called psychologic effects ascribed to chorea in the past were due not to the disease itself, but to the associated scholastic deprivation and to the patients' anxiety and dismay at the bizarre movements and the reactions they invoke in people who do not understand.

Severe cardiac involvement is seldom present in patients with active chorea, but, if present, can be managed as described for rheumatic fever. After completion of an attack, antistreptococcal prophylaxis against recurrences of chorea (or rheumatic fever) should be maintained as described for rheumatic fever.

CAUSED BY GRAM-NEGATIVE ORGANISMS

SALMONELLA INFECTIONS

The 1400-odd salmonellas are classified according to their antigenic composition. Several are naturally pathogenic only for man (e.g., *Salmonella typhi*), but most are also pathogenic for (and therefore transmissible by) animals. *Salmonella* infection may occur as an asymptomatic carrier state, or as acute gastroenteritis, enteric fever, or a focal disease with or without associated septicemia. An endotoxin is produced, but its role in the varied symptomatology of salmonella infections is undefined. With the exception of typhoid fever, salmonella infections, especially gastroenteritis, are an increasing public health problem.

TYPHOID FEVER

A generalized infection caused by S. typhi (typhosa), *with involvement of the lymphatic tissues, and characterized by fever, bradycardia, rose-colored eruption, abdominal signs, and splenomegaly.* It is the prototype of the severe enteric salmonella infections.

Epidemiology and Pathology

The source of infection is the feces of asymptomatic carriers or the stool or urine of patients with active disease. Family contacts may be transient carriers. About 2 to 5% of patients become chronic carriers, women 3 times more often than men, and patients with preexisting cholecystitis and cholelithiasis in particular. In communities with poor sanitation, transmission is most frequently by water; next most often by food, especially milk. Transmission in modern urban areas is chiefly through food contaminated by food handlers who are healthy carriers. Flies may spread the organism from feces to food. Infection by direct contact probably does not occur.

The organism enters the body via the GI tract and invades the bloodstream via the lymphatic channels. Peyer's patches, especially in the ileum and cecum, are hyperplastic and often ulcerated. The ulcers heal without scarring. The kidneys and liver usually show cloudy swelling; the latter may show patchy necrosis. The spleen is enlarged and soft. Pulmonary infection is rare.

Symptoms and Signs

The incubation period (3 to 25 days) relates indirectly to the number of organisms ingested. Onset is usually gradual with chilly sensations (occasionally chills), malaise, headache, anorexia, epistaxis, backache, and constipation. Abdominal pain and tenderness to palpation dominate the clinical picture. Respiratory symptoms other than sore throat are uncommon; in untreated patients typhoid pneumonia or secondary pneumonitis may develop.

Without therapy, the temperature rises daily by steps for 7 to 10 days, maintains a peak for another 7 to 10 days, and then falls by lysis by the end of the 4th wk. Relative bradycardia and usually a dicrotic pulse are present. Discrete, rounded, rose-colored spots which blanch on pressure (the diagnostic **"rose spots"**) emerge in crops between the 7th and 10th days in about 10% of patients, most commonly on the abdomen and chest; they persist for 2 to 5 days, and then fade. Splenomegaly is usual by the end of the 1st wk. Florid diarrhea occurs late in the disease when intestinal lesions are most manifest. Delirium and stupor are common. Leukopenia and anemia are characteristic and are most marked by the end of the 3rd wk. Leukocytosis, except in children, usually indicates a complication. Albuminuria and casts are frequent.

Atypical clinical manifestations are common. Symptoms may be predominantly pharyngeal (sore throat), abdominal (nausea, vomiting, pain, rigidity), respiratory (bronchitis, pneumonia), renal (nephritis), or neural (meningismus, psychosis). In **ambulatory ("walking") typhoid,** patients are asymptomatic but have typhoid bacillemia.

Complications

Severe complications occur mainly in untreated patients or when treatment is delayed.

Intestinal hemorrhage may be occult, occasionally progressing to massive hemorrhage. Significant bleeding occurs during the 3rd wk and is indicated by a sudden fall in temperature or an abrupt rise in pulse rate, and by pallor, sweating, hypotension, and, rarely, abdominal pain. The mortality rate of symptomatic hemorrhaging patients is 25%, but this is an unusual complication and blood transfusions prevent death.

Intestinal perforation, the most frequently fatal complication, is most common during the 3rd wk and in adult males, especially those with pronounced abdominal signs. Sharp abdominal pain occurs suddenly, usually in the right lower quadrant, with nausea, vomiting, a fall in temperature, rapid pulse, and muscle spasms; leukocytosis is present. An upright abdominal x-ray showing free air may be helpful in diagnosis.

Relapses: Antibiotic therapy has *increased* the incidence of febrile relapses to 15% from a prior 8%. Fever occurs about 2 wk after cessation of treatment and may only last for several days. If antibiotic therapy is reinstituted, the fever abates rapidly, unlike the slow defervescence seen during the primary illness. Occasionally a second relapse occurs.

Diagnosis

This depends on demonstration of typhoid bacilli in the blood, urine, or feces, or development of a positive Widal reaction. Typhoid bacilli may be cultured from the blood during the first 2 wk; later cultures are less frequently positive.

The organism may be cultured from the urine or feces by the end of the 3rd wk. Cultures from bone marrow, rose spots, and liver biopsies have proved to be good sources of typhoid bacilli. The Widal agglutination test becomes positive during the 2nd wk; a progressive rise in agglutination titer is significant. Typhoid bacilli contain both H and O antigens which stimulate corresponding antibodies. Both H and O agglutination titers should be determined, though the O titer is of greater significance because the H agglutinins may remain elevated for years after typhoid immunization, whereas the O titer usually disappears within a year. The Widal test has several deficiencies. Many nontyphoidal strains have cross-reacting O and H antigens which will cause significant serum antibody levels, and cirrhosis of the liver induces circulating antibodies that react with Widal antigens.

Differential diagnosis should include other salmonella-induced enteric fevers, the major rickettsioses, leptospirosis, miliary tuberculosis, malaria, brucellosis, tularemia, infectious hepatitis, and abdominal Hodgkin's disease.

Prognosis

Mortality is less than 2% with prompt antibiotic therapy, but may be as high as 30% without specific treatment. Slight stresses during convalescence may cause 1- to 6-day recurrences of fever; these differ from the relapses that occur in about 15% of patients. Paradoxically, specific chemotherapy has increased the incidence of relapse.

Prophylaxis

Purification of drinking water, pasteurization of milk, preventing chronic carriers from handling food, and complete patient isolation technics are the most successful prophylactic measures. Compulsory surveillance and case-finding in an exposed population is essential for effective control of an epidemic.

Protection induced by typhoid vaccine is incomplete; therefore, recommendations vary. During an epidemic, only exposed persons need be vaccinated; widespread immunization is not indicated. Monovalent acetone-killed typhoid vaccine given s.c. in two 0.5-ml doses 1 mo apart is recommended; this vaccine has replaced the heat-killed, formalin-preserved typhoid-paratyphoid vaccine. Vaccination is not required for travel to endemic areas but it is advisable for travelers to epidemic areas. Care in selecting restaurants and avoidance of unsafe water, ice in beverages, and contaminated foods are more effective. Unless drinking water is known to be safe, it should be boiled or 2 to 4 drops of 4 to 6% chlorine bleach/L should be added ½ h before drinking. Raw leafy vegetables and foods that are kept or served at room temperature should be avoided. Recently prepared foods served hot or chilled, bottled carbonated beverages, and raw foods peeled by the consumer are generally safe.

Treatment

Specific: Chloramphenicol had been the drug of choice in all cases until a number of chloramphenicol-resistant strains were isolated during epidemics in Mexico and Southeast Asia. Patients acquiring typhoid fever in these areas should receive at least 6 Gm/day of ampicillin IV for 14 days; penicillin-allergic patients can be given trimethoprim 8 mg/kg/day with sulfamethoxazole 40 mg/kg/day in 3 divided doses/day for 10 days. Chloramphenicol is effective against strains acquired in other areas. It is given for 14 days—50 mg/kg/day in divided doses q 8 h until the temperature is normal; then 30 mg/kg/day for the remainder of the 2 wk.

Supportive: Despite antibiotics, skilled nursing care remains most important. Ideally, the patient should be isolated, but barrier screens suffice if explicit precautions are observed in the disposal of excreta and in hand cleansing. The patient's legs should be exercised regularly to prevent phlebothrombosis. Nutrition should be maintained with frequent, relatively high-caloric feedings. Blood replacement may be needed. Cathartics and laxatives should be **avoided;** persistent constipation or distention can be corrected by appropriate fluid and electrolyte therapy. Diarrhea is occasionally distressing, but may be controlled by a clear liquid diet and, if necessary, parenteral nutrition. Adequate fluid replacement is important with high fever. In severely ill patients, corticosteroids may reduce the severity of subjective complaints, delirium, and fever. Prednisone 20 to 40 mg/day orally (or equivalent), given for only the first 3 days of treatment, is sufficient. Management of perforation must be individualized.

Patients with febrile **relapses** should receive chloramphenicol 50 mg/kg/day in divided doses q 8 h for 5 days. If the strain is chloramphenicol-resistant, ampicillin or trimethoprim with sulfamethoxazole (in doses as for the primary disease) should be given for 5 days.

Convalescence

Prolonged bed rest is unnecessary in afebrile patients. Stool cultures should be repeated until they are permanently negative; typhoid bacilli may be isolated for as long as 3 mo after the acute illness.

Carriers

Persistent carriers (persons with positive stool cultures for 1 yr) must be reported to the local health department and prohibited from handling food. Antibiotic therapy rarely eliminates the carrier state and then only when the biliary tract is normal. If gallstones are present, cholecystectomy with pre- and postoperative antibiotic therapy are necessary; ampicillin 6 Gm/day IV for 6 wk is the optimal therapeutic agent.

OTHER SALMONELLA INFECTIONS

The epidemiology of other salmonelloses is similar to that of typhoid, though more complicated since disease may also occur in man by direct or indirect contact with numerous species of infected animals, their derived foodstuffs, and their excreta. The enormous reservoir of contaminated food products has caused a steady increase in the incidence of salmonellosis. Poultry products are a common source of infection. Pet turtles have become important in recent years. The most common salmonellas involved in the USA are *S. typhimurium, S. newport, S. montevideo, S. oranienburg, S. cholerae-suis, S. schottmuelleri (S. paratyphi B),* and *S. anatum.*

Certain types of *Salmonella* cause similar syndromes, including acute gastroenteric, typhoidal (enteric), or focal (with or without septicemia) syndromes, and a carrier state which may persist for weeks or months. The syndromes can occur in any patient singly, in combination, or in sequence. Patients with sickle cell disease or subtotal gastrectomies are prone to develop salmonella infections.

Acute gastroenteritis usually appears 12 to 48 h after ingestion of contaminated food. It may occur as only mild abdominal discomfort with minimal diarrhea lasting less than a day, or, rarely, may be protracted and cholera-like in severity. Fever may occur and persist for 24 h. The stools are usually loose and paste-like, but rarely contain blood or mucus. Diagnosis is confirmed by isolating a *Salmonella* strain from stool cultures. The true incidence of septicemia in patients with acute salmonella gastroenteritis is unknown. It does occur and is manifested by low-grade fever and mild abdominal pain; some patients develop localized infections in various body organs.

Focal manifestations of salmonellosis may occur as part of a septicemia or as isolated abscesses. The GI tract, including the appendix and the gallbladder, is frequently involved. Salmonellas tend to migrate to abnormal tissues (e.g., tumors), but can localize and cause necrosis in almost any part of the body (e.g., lungs, GU tract, soft tissues, CNS, upper respiratory tract, joints, bones, heart valves).

Paratyphoid: A few strains of salmonella other than *S. typhi* can cause enteric fever which mimics typhoid fever. Formerly called paratyphoid A and B, newer classifications identify these strains as *S. enteritidis* bioser. *paratyphi-A* or ser. *paratyphi-B*. The disease and its treatment are identical to that described above for typhoid fever.

Localized abscess caused by *S. cholerae-suis* is a form of salmonella infection that is rare in the USA. As the name implies, it is most often acquired from contaminated pork.

Prophylaxis

Case-reporting is imperative. Methods of controlling animal and human contamination of foodstuffs range from the careful preparation of bone-meal fertilizer to the proper cooking of poultry and poultry products, including eggs and foodstuffs containing dried eggs. Efforts to detect and control other infected animals (e.g., pet turtles) are also important in controlling the disease at its source. Human carriers do not seem to be major contributors to the large outbreaks of gastroenteritis.

Treatment

The routine use of antibiotics in uncomplicated acute salmonella gastroenteritis is unwarranted and will prolong the excretion of the organism in the stool. Symptomatic treatment with fluids, a bland diet, and antispasmodics or paregoric, if needed, usually suffices (see SHIGELLOSIS, below, and General Principles of Treatment in §7, Ch. 12). Patients with systemic or focal disease should be treated with antibiotics—either ampicillin or chloramphenicol in doses as for typhoid fever, or amoxicillin 50 to 100 mg/kg body wt/day orally in 3 divided doses; the therapeutic response in paratyphoid infection may be somewhat slower than in typhoid fever. Focal abscesses may require surgery.

Carriers should only be given prolonged ampicillin treatment (6 Gm/day IV for 6 wk) if they shed organisms for 1 yr. A diseased gallbladder will promote and perpetuate the carrier state; cholecystectomy plus ampicillin (6 Gm/day IV for 6 wk) is probably curative.

SHIGELLOSIS
(Bacillary Dysentery)

An acute infection of the bowel, caused by Shigella *organisms.*

Etiology and Epidemiology

The genus *Shigella* is divided into 4 major subgroups (A, B, C, and D), which are subdivided into serologically determined types. The genus is worldwide in distribution, but *Shigella flexneri* (B) and *S. sonnei* (D) are found more widely than *S. boydii* (C) and the particularly virulent *S. dysenteriae* (A).

The source of infection is the excreta of infected individuals or convalescent carriers. Direct spread is by the fecal-oral route; indirect spread, by contaminated food and inanimate objects. Waterborne disease is unusual. Flies serve as mechanical vectors.

Epidemics occur most frequently in overcrowded populations with inadequate sanitation. Bacillary dysentery is particularly common in younger children living in endemic areas; adults are relatively resistant to infection and usually have less severe disease.

Convalescents and subclinical carriers are significant infection hazards, but true long-term carriers are rare. Infection appears to impart little or no immunity, since reinfection with the same strain is possible.

Pathology and Pathophysiology

Shigella organisms penetrate the mucosa of the lower intestine and cause mucus secretion, hyperemia, leukocytic infiltration, edema, and often superficial mucosal ulcerations. The entire colon and often the lower ileum are involved in severe cases. The subacute form, seen almost exclusively in adults, is limited to the lower half of the colon.

Symptoms, Signs, and Course

The incubation period is 1 to 4 days. In younger **children,** onset is sudden, with fever, irritability or drowsiness, anorexia, nausea or vomiting, diarrhea, abdominal pain and distention, and tenesmus. Within 3 days, blood, pus, and mucus appear in the stools. The number of stools generally increases rapidly to 20 or more/day, and weight loss and dehydration become severe. The untreated child may die in the first 12 days; if not, acute symptoms subside by the 2nd wk.

Most **adults** are afebrile, with nonbloody and nonmucous diarrhea and little or no tenesmus. However, onset may be characterized by episodes of griping abdominal pain, urgency to defecate, and passage of formed feces, initially, which temporarily relieves the pain. These episodes recur with increasing severity and frequency. Diarrhea becomes marked, with soft or liquid stools containing mucus, pus, and often blood. Rectal prolapse and consequent fecal incontinence may result from severe tenesmus. The disease usually resolves spontaneously in adults: mild cases in 4 to 8 days, severe cases in 3 to 6 wk.

In the rare **choleriform type** of bacillary dysentery, onset is sudden, with ricewater or serous (occasionally bloody) stools. The patient may vomit and become rapidly dehydrated.

S. dysenteriae causes a rare form with delirium, convulsions, and coma, but little or no diarrhea; it may be fatal in 12 to 24 h.

Bacillary dysentery can induce significant dehydration and electrolyte loss with circulatory collapse and death, though this is largely limited to infants under age 2 yr and to debilitated adults.

Secondary bacterial infections may occur, especially in debilitated and dehydrated patients. Severe mucosal ulcerations may cause significant acute blood loss. Other complications are uncommon, but include toxic neuritis, arthritis, myocarditis, and, rarely, intestinal perforation. There is no convincing evidence that chronic bacillary dysentery is a clinical entity or that ulcerative colitis develops as a complication of shigella infection.

Laboratory Findings

The bacillus is found in the stools, but bacillemia and bacilluria are rare. Though the WBC count is often reduced at onset, it averages 13,000. Hemoconcentration is common. Plasma CO_2 is usually low, reflecting the diarrhea-induced metabolic acidosis.

Diagnosis

This is facilitated by a high index of suspicion during outbreaks and in endemic areas. Frequently, bacillary dysentery cannot be distinguished from salmonella gastroenteritis except by identification of the offending agent. Ulcerative colitis, diarrhea of nonspecific or viral origin, sprue, celiac disease, cholera, amebiasis, intestinal parasites, and infantile *Escherichia coli* diarrhea should be considered in the differential diagnosis.

Diagnosis is confirmed by isolation of *Shigella* from the stools. Proctoscopic examination is helpful since specific ulcers can be recognized and adequate culture material obtained. Smears of the stools should be examined for blood, pus, and parasites. Agglutinins develop too irregularly to be of diagnostic value.

Prophylaxis

To prevent spread by contaminated food, water, and flies requires good sanitation, with the following precautions: thorough handwashing before handling food; immersion of soiled garments and bedding of dysentery patients in covered buckets of soap and water until they can be boiled; use of screens on houses; use of mosquito netting. Patients and carriers should be managed by proper isolation technics (especially stool isolation). A live oral vaccine is being developed, and field trials in endemic areas seem successful.

Treatment

Fluid therapy: See §11, Ch. 6. Dysentery usually causes isotonic dehydration (equal salt and water loss), with metabolic acidosis and significant potassium loss. Thirst from dehydration can lead to a proportionately excessive water intake, causing hypotonicity.

In infants, especially in hot climates, the fluid lost through sweat and respiration, added to the severe diarrhea, may cause hypertonic serum (see DISORDERS OF WATER BALANCE IN CHILDREN in §11, Ch. 6). Premature administration of high-solute fluids (milk, tube feedings, "homemade" electrolyte mixtures) may cause damaging hypertonicity, including convulsions.

Infant feedings: See treatment of ACUTE INFECTIOUS GASTROENTERITIS in §10, Ch. 4.

Antibiotics: The decision to use antibiotics requires consideration of several factors, including the severity of the disease, age of the patient, adequacy of sanitation, the likelihood of further transmission, and the possibility of engendering antibiotic-resistant organisms. With proper fluid replacement, antibiotics are often unnecessary, and resistance to them is now widespread, varying with the species. *S. sonnei* isolates are likely to be resistant to ampicillin and tetracycline, but oxolinic acid 1500 mg/day (for adults) given for 5 days is effective. Trimethoprim with sulfamethoxazole (as for typhoid fever) will eradicate organisms quickly from the intestine. Ampicillin 3 Gm/day for 5 days will cure most *S. flexneri* infections.

Other treatment: A hot-water bottle helps relieve abdominal discomfort. Absorbent and demulcent methylcellulose preparations do little to alleviate diarrhea and tenesmus. Anticholinergics (e.g., propantheline, atropine) and paregoric should be avoided in patients with shigellosis. Opiates may induce intestinal stasis, prolong the febrile state, and permit continued organism excretion in the stool. However, codeine 30 mg q 4 h (for adults) may be necessary if pain, discomfort, and anxiety are pronounced.

The patient's progress should be followed until the stools are consistently free of *Shigella*.

CHOLERA
(Asiatic or Epidemic Cholera)

An acute infection involving the entire small bowel, characterized by profuse watery diarrhea, vomiting, muscular cramps, dehydration, oliguria, and collapse.

Etiology, Epidemiology, and Pathophysiology

The causative organism is *Vibrio cholerae*, a short, curved, motile, aerobic rod. Susceptibility varies among individuals. Since the vibrio is sensitive to gastric acid, hypo- and achlorhydria have been suggested as possible predisposing factors. Persons living in endemic areas gradually acquire a natural immunity.

Cholera is spread by the ingestion of water and foods contaminated by the excrement of persons with symptomatic or asymptomatic infection. Outbreaks of the disease may be explosive and brief or may be protracted. Cholera is endemic in Asia, the Middle East, and Africa. Cases have been imported into Europe, Japan, and Australia, resulting, in some instances, in localized outbreaks. Importation into the Western Hemisphere is a distinct possibility. In endemic areas, outbreaks usually occur during warm months and the incidence is highest in children; in newly infected areas, epidemics may occur during any season and all ages are equally susceptible. Both the El Tor and the classic biotypes of *V. cholerae* can cause severe disease; however, mild or asymptomatic infection is much more common with the El Tor biotype. A similar mild form of gastroenteritis caused by *V. parahaemolyticus* is discussed in §7, Ch. 12.

The manifestations of cholera result from the loss of isotonic, watery stools rich in bicarbonate and potassium. *V. cholerae* produces a protein enterotoxin, the enzymes mucinase and neuraminidase, and other less clearly defined substances. The enterotoxin induces hypersecretion of an isotonic electrolyte solution by an intact small bowel mucosa. The roles of mucinase and neuraminidase in pathogenesis are unclear. Mucinase may be important in reducing a protective effect of intestinal mucin, while neuraminidase may alter the structure of gangliosides in mucosal cell membranes, increasing the content of the specific ganglioside (GM_1) which binds the enterotoxin.

Clinical Course and Prognosis

The incubation period is 1 to 3 days. Cholera can be subclinical; a mild, uncomplicated episode of diarrhea; or a fulminant, rapidly lethal disease. Abrupt, painless, watery diarrhea with vomiting is usually the initial finding; stool loss may exceed 1 L/h but is usually much less. The resultant severe water and electrolyte depletion leads to intense thirst, oliguria, muscle cramps, weakness, and marked loss of tissue turgor with sunken eyes and wrinkled skin. Hypovolemia, hemoconcentration, anuria, and serious metabolic acidosis with potassium depletion (but with normal serum sodium concentration) occur, and if untreated, result in circulatory collapse, cyanosis, and stupor. Prolonged hypovolemia can cause renal tubular necrosis.

Uncomplicated cholera is self-limited; recovery is within 3 to 6 days. The fatality rate exceeds 50% in untreated severe cases but is reduced to less than 1% with prompt and adequate fluid and electrolyte therapy. Most patients are free of *V. cholerae* within 2 wk but a few patients become chronic biliary carriers.

Diagnosis

The diagnosis is confirmed by the isolation of *V. cholerae* in cultures from direct rectal specimens or fresh stools, and its subsequent identification through agglutination by specific antiserum. Cholera must be distinguished from clinically similar disease caused by enterotoxin-producing strains of *Escherichia coli,* and from watery diarrhea with dehydration that occasionally is produced by salmonella and shigella infections.

Prophylaxis

Proper disposal of human excrement and purification of water supplies are essential to the control of cholera. Cholera vaccine is beneficial in endemic areas, but booster injections are required every 6 mo. Precautions also include using boiled water and avoiding uncooked vegetables. Prompt prophylaxis with oral tetracycline is useful in preventing secondary cases among household contacts of cholera patients.

Treatment

Rapid correction of hypovolemia and metabolic acidosis, and prevention of hypokalemia are the objectives. IV infusion should be started promptly with either (a) a 2:1 mixture of normal saline and 0.17 M (⅙ M) sodium lactate; (b) Ringer's lactate solution; or (c) a solution of 8 Gm glucose, 4 Gm sodium chloride, 4 Gm sodium acetate, and 0.5 Gm potassium chloride per liter. Patients in shock require 100 ml/kg body wt; milder cases require only 50 to 80 ml/kg. The infusion should be given very rapidly until blood pressure is normal. The remainder is then given over a period of 2 h in adults; over 4 to 6 h in children. Water should also be given freely by mouth. Children also require potassium replacement. This is accomplished by adding potassium chloride 0.7 to 1 Gm/L to the IV solution or by giving potassium bicarbonate 1 ml/kg of a 100 Gm/L solution orally q.i.d.

Amounts for replacement of continuing stool loss are determined by measuring the stool volume and by frequent clinical evaluation of hydration (pulse rate and strength, skin turgor, and urine output).

Plasma, plasma volume expanders, and vasopressors do not correct the water and electrolyte loss and *should not be used.*

Initial IV rehydration followed by oral or nasogastric administration of a glucose-electrolyte solution is effective in replacing stool losses and is particularly useful in epidemic areas where supplies of parenteral fluids may be limited. Patients with mild disease and who are able to drink may be given the oral solution immediately, thus eliminating the need for IV infusion. A solution of 20 Gm glucose, 3.5 Gm sodium chloride, 2.5 Gm sodium bicarbonate, and 1.5 Gm potassium chloride per liter of boiled drinking water should be warmed to 25 to 37 C (77 to 99 F) and given ad libitum in amounts at least equal to stool and vomitus losses. Solid food should be withheld until vomiting stops and appetite returns.

Early treatment with tetracycline (500 mg orally q 6 h for 48 h) eradicates vibrios, reduces stool volume by 50%, and terminates diarrhea within 48 h.

WHOOPING COUGH
(Pertussis)

An acute, highly communicable bacterial disease, characterized by a paroxysmal or spasmodic cough which usually ends in a prolonged, high-pitched, crowing inspiration (the whoop).

Etiology and Epidemiology

The causative agent is *Bordetella pertussis,* a small, nonmotile, gram-negative coccobacillus. *B. parapertussis* closely resembles this organism; it causes **parapertussis,** which may be clinically indistinguishable from pertussis, but is usually milder and less often fatal.

Whooping cough is endemic throughout the world. In a given locality it becomes epidemic every 2 to 4 yr. It occurs at all ages, but about half of all cases occur before age 2, since infants usually have no protective antibodies. One attack does not confer natural immunity for life, but second attacks, if they occur, are usually mild and often unrecognized.

Transmission is by aspiration of *B. pertussis* sprayed into the air by a patient, particularly in the catarrhal and early paroxysmal stages. Transmission by contact with contaminated articles is rare. Patients are usually not infectious after the 8th wk.

Symptoms and Signs

The incubation period averages 7 to 14 days (maximum, 3 wk). *B. pertussis* invades the mucosa of the nasopharynx, trachea, bronchi, and bronchioles, causing an increased secretion of mucus, initially thin and later viscid and tenacious. The disease lasts about 6 wk and is divided into 3 stages: catarrhal, paroxysmal, and convalescent. Onset of the **catarrhal stage** is insidious, generally with sneezing, lacrimation, or other signs of coryza; anorexia; listlessness; and a troublesome, hacking nocturnal cough which gradually becomes diurnal. Fever is rarely present.

The cough becomes **paroxysmal** after 10 to 14 days. There are 5 to > 15 rapidly consecutive coughs followed by the whoop, a hurried, deep inspiration. After a few normal breaths another paroxysm may begin. Copious amounts of viscid mucus may be expelled (usually swallowed by infants and children) during or following the paroxysms. Vomiting subsequent to paroxysms, or due to gagging on the tenacious mucus, is characteristic. In infants, choking spells may be more common than whoops.

The **convalescent stage** usually begins within 4 wk; paroxysms are not so frequent or severe, vomiting decreases, and the patient looks and feels better. The paroxysmal coughing may be reinduced for months, usually by irritation from an upper respiratory infection.

The WBC count is usually between 15,000 and 20,000, but may be normal or as high as 60,000; there are usually 60 to 80% small lymphocytes.

Prognosis and Complications

Pertussis is serious in children under age 2; mortality is about 1 to 2% before age 1. The disease is troublesome but rarely serious in older children and adults, except in the aged.

The most frequent complications are respiratory, including asphyxia in infants. Bronchopneumonia and cerebral complications cause the majority of fatalities in infants and young children. Bronchopneumonia is also a frequent complication in the aged, and may be fatal at any age. Interstitial emphysema, subcutaneous emphysema, and pneumothorax are infrequent consequences of the increased intrathoracic pressure during paroxysms. Bronchiectasis, particularly in debilitated children, and residual emphysema can result. Atelectasis may result from occlusion of a bronchiole by a mucus plug. A primary tuberculous lesion may be extended by pertussis. Convulsions are not uncommon in infants, but are rare in older children. Hemorrhage into the brain, eyes, skin, and mucous membranes can result from severe paroxysms and consequent anoxia. Cerebral hemorrhage, cerebral edema, or encephalitis may result in spastic paralysis, mental retardation, or other neurologic disorders. An ulcer of the frenum of the tongue may develop from lower incisor trauma during paroxysms. Umbilical hernia and rectal prolapse occasionally occur. Otitis media is frequent.

Diagnosis

The catarrhal stage is often difficult to distinguish from bronchitis or influenza. Lymphocytosis of 70% or more in an afebrile or slightly febrile child over age 3 with a suspicious cough often suggests pertussis. Cultures of nasopharyngeal specimens are positive for *B. pertussis* in 80 to 90% of cases in the catarrhal and early paroxysmal stages. Best results are obtained with small sterile cotton swabs on 28-gauge, zinc-coated wire passed into the region of the middle turbinates or through the nostril to the nasopharynx. Standard Bordet-Gengou medium should be used, and the plates streaked with 1 loopful of aqueous solution of penicillin G (1000 u./ml) at the time of inoculation. Specific fluorescent antibody testing of nasopharyngeal smears is an accurate means of early diagnosis. Parapertussis is differentiated only by culture or by the fluorescent antibody technic.

Prophylaxis

Active immunization: See ROUTINE IMMUNIZATION PROCEDURES in §22.

Passive immunization is no longer recommended for exposed susceptible contacts since protection has not been shown to be reliable.

Recent studies suggest that oral erythromycin therapy commencing during the incubation period and continuing for 10 to 14 days might abort the infection.

Patients should be particularly quarantined from susceptible infants for at least 4 wk from onset of disease or until symptoms have subsided.

Treatment

Hospitalization is recommended for seriously ill infants because expert nursing care is important. Bed rest is unnecessary for older children with mild disease. Small, frequent meals are advisable. Parenteral fluid therapy may be required to replace salt and water losses if vomiting is severe. In infants, suction to remove excess mucus from the throat may be lifesaving, and tracheostomy is occasionally needed. O_2 therapy should be given if cyanosis persists after removal of mucus. Seriously ill infants should be housed in a darkened, quiet room and disturbed as little as possible, since any disturbance can precipitate serious paroxysmal spells with anoxia.

Drugs: Expectorant cough mixtures are of little value and may increase nausea and vomiting. Codeine 0.2 mg/kg orally t.i.d. is sometimes helpful but tends to constipate. A mild sedative (e.g., phenobarbital 1.5 to 2 mg/kg orally t.i.d. for infants and children) is useful for rest and sleep. Antibiotics should be used only for bacterial complications such as bronchopneumonia and otitis media. Hyperimmune globulin is of no therapeutic benefit.

BRUCELLOSIS
(Undulant, Malta, Mediterranean, or Gibraltar Fever)

An infectious disease characterized by an acute febrile stage with few or no localizing signs and a chronic stage with relapses of fever, weakness, sweats, and vague aches and pains.

Etiology and Epidemiology

The causative microorganisms of human brucellosis are *Brucella abortus* (cattle), *B. suis* (hogs), *B. melitensis* (sheep and goats), and *B. rangiferi* (*B. suis* biotype 4; Alaskan and Siberian caribou); *B. canis* (dogs) has caused sporadic infections. Brucellosis is acquired by direct contact with secretions and excretions of infected animals, and by ingesting cow, sheep, or goat milk or milk products (e.g., butter and cheese) containing viable *Brucella* organisms. It is rarely transmitted from person to person. Most prevalent in rural areas, brucellosis is an occupational disease of meat-packers, veterinarians, farmers, and livestock producers; children are less susceptible. Distribution is worldwide.

Clinical Course

The incubation period varies from 5 days to several months (average, 2 wk). Symptoms vary, especially in the early stages. Onset may be sudden and acute, with chills and fever, severe headache, pains, malaise, and occasionally diarrhea; or insidious, with mild prodromal malaise, muscular pain, headache, and pain in the back of the neck, followed by a rise in evening temperature. The total WBC count is usually normal or reduced, with a relative or absolute lymphocytosis. As the disease progresses, the temperature increases to 40 or 45 C (104 or 105 F), subsiding gradually to normal or near-normal in the morning, when profuse sweating occurs. Complications include SBE, meningitis, encephalitis, neuritis, orchitis, cholecystitis, hepatic suppuration, and bone lesions such as spondylitis.

The intermittent fever persists for 1 to 5 wk, followed by a 2- to 14-day remission with symptoms greatly reduced or absent; the febrile phase then recurs. This pattern may occur only once, but more often subacute or chronic brucellosis ensues, with repeated febrile waves (undulations) and remissions recurring over months or years. Constipation is usually pronounced; anorexia, weight loss, abdominal pain, joint pain, headache, backache, weakness, irritability, insomnia, mental depression, and emotional instability occur. Splenomegaly appears and lymph nodes may be slightly or moderately enlarged.

Patients with acute, uncomplicated brucellosis usually recover in 2 to 3 wk. The chronic disease may result in prolonged ill health, but it is rarely fatal.

Diagnosis

Recovery of the organism from the blood, CSF, urine, or tissues is diagnostic, but bacteriologic identification of the disease is not always possible. Agglutination titers of 1:100 or higher are significant; lower titers are highly significant if the agglutinins are IgG immunoglobulins. When the agglutination test is positive but a *Brucella* species cannot be isolated, diagnosis is based on a history of exposure to infected animals or animal products (e.g., ingestion of unpasteurized milk), epidemiologic data, and the characteristic clinical findings and course. Intradermal tests with *Brucella* antigens are of little value in diagnosing active brucellosis.

Prophylaxis

Pasteurization of milk and eating only aged cheese are the most important prophylactic measures. Persons handling animals or carcasses that are likely to be infected should wear rubber gloves and protect skin breaks from bacterial invasion. Every effort should be made to detect the infection in animals and control it at its source.

Treatment

Tetracycline 0.5 Gm is given orally q.i.d. for 21 days and should be repeated if relapses occur. Seriously ill patients are also given streptomycin 1 Gm IM q 12 h for 1 wk, then 0.5 Gm IM q 12 h for an additional 7 to 14 days. Prednisone 20 mg orally t.i.d. is given for 2 or 3 days if toxemia is present. Severe body pains, especially over the spine, may require codeine 15 to 60 mg orally or s.c. q 4 to 6 h.

Activity should be restricted in chronic cases, with bed rest enforced during febrile periods.

TULAREMIA
(Rabbit or Deer-fly Fever)

An acute infectious disease, often bizarre in its manifestations, but usually characterized by a primary local ulcerative lesion, profound systemic symptoms, a typhoid-like state, bacteremia, and not infrequently atypical pneumonia (see TULAREMIC PNEUMONIA in §5, Ch. 9).

Etiology and Epidemiology

The causative organism, *Francisella tularensis,* is a small, pleomorphic, nonmotile, nonsporulating, aerobic bacillus which enters the body by ingestion, inoculation, or contamination. It is able to penetrate unbroken skin. There are many animal hosts, but wild rabbits and rodents are the most important. Transmission among animals is by blood-sucking arthropods and by cannibalism.

Hunters, butchers, farmers, fur-handlers, and laboratory workers are most commonly infected. Most cases result from contact with infected wild rabbits; others follow handling of other infected animals or birds, contact with infected ticks or other arthropods, eating undercooked infected meat, and, occasionally, drinking contaminated water. Man-to-man transmission has not been reported.

Pathology

Characteristic focal necrotic lesions in various stages of evolution are scattered throughout the body. They are minute (1 mm) to large (8 cm), whitish-yellow, and commonly found in lymph nodes, spleen, liver, kidney, and lung. Externally, necrotic foci are seen as the primary lesions found on the finger, eye, or mouth; internally, they result in tularemic pneumonia and most gastrointestinal manifestations. Microscopically, the focal necrosis is surrounded by monocytes and young fibroblasts, in turn surrounded by large collections of lymphocytes. There is severe systemic toxicity, but no toxins have been demonstrated.

Symptoms and Signs

There are 4 clinical types of tularemia: **ulceroglandular,** 87% of cases, with primary lesions on the hands or fingers; **oculoglandular,** 3%; **glandular,** 2%, with regional lymphadenitis but no primary lesion; and **typhoidal,** 8%.

Onset occurs suddenly, 1 to 10 (usually 2 to 4) days after contact, with headache, chills, nausea, vomiting, fever of 39.5 or 40 C (103 or 104 F), and severe prostration. Extreme weakness, recurring chills, and drenching sweats develop. Within 24 to 48 h an inflamed papule appears at the infection site (finger, arm, eye, or roof of the mouth), except in glandular or typhoidal tularemia. The papule rapidly becomes pustular and ulcerates, producing a clean ulcer crater with a scanty, thin, colorless exudate. The ulcers are usually single on the extremities, but multiple in the mouth or eye. Usually, only one eye is affected. Regional lymph nodes enlarge, suppurate, and drain profusely. A typhoid-like state frequently develops by the 5th day, and the patient may show signs of an atypical pneumonia. A nonspecific roseola-like rash may appear at any stage of the disease. The spleen is often enlarged and perisplenitis may occur. Leukocytosis is common, but the WBC count may be normal with only an increased proportion of polymorphonuclears. Temperature remains elevated for 3 to 4 wk and falls by lysis in untreated cases. Mediastinitis, lung abscess, and meningitis are rare complications.

One attack confers immunity. Mortality is almost nil in treated cases, and about 6% in untreated cases. Death is usually from overwhelming infection, pneumonia, meningitis, or peritonitis. Relapses are uncommon, but occur in inadequately treated cases.

Diagnosis

A history of even slight contact with a wild rodent, the sudden onset of symptoms, and the characteristic primary lesion are usually diagnostic. Laboratory infections are frequently typhoidal or pneumonic, with no demonstrable primary lesion, and are difficult to diagnose. Recovery of the organism from the lesion, lymph nodes, or sputum is diagnostic. Skin sensitivity develops after the 3rd day in most cases. Agglutination tests become positive after the 10th day, never before the 8th day. The serum of brucellosis patients may also react positively to tularemic antigens, but usually to much lower titers.

Prophylaxis

Wild rabbits and other rodents should be handled with great caution, especially in endemic areas. The organisms may be present in the animal and in tick feces on the animal's fur. Protective clothing should be worn and all ticks removed at once. Wild birds and game must be thoroughly cooked before eating; any water that may be contaminated must be disinfected before use.

Treatment

The agent of choice is streptomycin, 0.5 Gm IM q 12 h until the temperature becomes normal; thereafter, 0.5 Gm/day for 5 days. Chloramphenicol or tetracycline 500 mg orally q 6 h may be given until the temperature is normal, and then 250 mg q.i.d. for 5 to 7 days; relapses occasionally occur with these 2 drugs, however, and they may not prevent node suppuration. Fluid balance and adequate nutrition must be maintained, especially in complicated, longstanding cases.

Continuous wet saline dressings are beneficial for primary skin lesions, and may diminish the severity of the lymphangitis and lymphadenitis. Large abscesses may be opened and drained, but this is rarely necessary unless therapy is delayed. In ocular tularemia, application of warm saline compresses and use of dark glasses give some relief; 1% homatropine 4 drops q 4 h may be instilled in severe cases. Intense headache usually responds to codeine 15 to 60 mg orally or s.c. q 3 to 4 h.

PLAGUE
(Bubonic Plague; Pestis; Black Death)

An acute, severe infection appearing in a bubonic or pneumonic form, caused by the bacillus Yersinia pestis.

Etiology, Epidemiology, and Transmission

The causative organism, *Y. pestis (Pasteurella pestis)*, is a short bacillus which often shows bipolar staining, especially with Giemsa stain, and may resemble "safety pins."

Plague occurs primarily in wild rodents (e.g., rats, mice, squirrels, prairie dogs), in whom it may be acute, subacute, or chronic, and murine or sylvatic depending on whether urban or rural rodents are infected. Massive human epidemics have occurred (e.g., the "Black Death" of the Middle Ages); more recently, infection has occurred sporadically or in limited outbreaks.

Plague is transmitted from rodent to man by the bite of an infected flea vector. Man-to-man transmission occurs from inhalation of droplet nuclei spread by coughing patients with bubonic or septicemic plague who have developed pulmonary lesions; primary pneumonic plague is the result. Asymptomatic pharyngeal carriers of *Y. pestis* have been recognized in bubonic plague but their epidemiologic significance is unknown.

Clinical Features

Bubonic plague is the most common form. The incubation period varies from a few hours to 12 days, but is usually 2 to 5 days. Onset is abrupt and often associated with chills; the temperature rises to 39.5 to 41 C (103 to 106 F). The pulse may be rapid and thready; hypotension may occur. Enlarged lymph nodes **(buboes)** appear with or shortly before the fever. The femoral or inguinal lymph nodes are most commonly involved (50%), followed by axillary (22%), cervical (10%), or multiple (14%) node involvement. The nodes are usually tender, firm, and fixed. The overlying skin is smooth and reddened but is not usually hot. Occasionally, a primary cutaneous lesion appears at the bite, varying from a small vesicle with slight local lymphangitis to an eschar. The patient may be restless, delirious, confused, and incoordinated. The liver and spleen may be palpable. The WBC count is usually 20,000 to 25,000 with neutrophilia. The nodes may suppurate in the 2nd wk. The mortality in untreated patients is about 60%, most deaths occurring from sepsis in 3 to 5 days.

Primary pneumonic plague has a 2- to 3-day incubation period, followed by abrupt onset of high fever, chills, tachycardia, and headache, often severe. Cough is not prominent initially but develops within 20 to 24 h, with sputum that is mucoid at first, rapidly shows blood specks, and then becomes uniformly pink or bright red (resembling raspberry syrup) and foamy. Tachypnea and dyspnea are present, but not pleurisy. Signs of consolidation are rare and rales may be absent. Chest x-rays show a rapidly progressing pneumonia. Most untreated patients die within 48 h after onset of symptoms.

Other forms of plague: Septicemic plague usually occurs with the bubonic form as an acute fulminant illness. It may be fatal before bubonic or pulmonary manifestations predominate. **Pharyngeal plague** and **plague meningitis** are less common forms. **Pestis minor,** a benign form of bubonic plague, usually occurs only in endemic areas, with lymphadenitis, fever, headache, and prostration that subside within a week.

Diagnosis

This is based on recovery of the organism, which may be cultured from blood, sputum, or lymph node aspirate. Needle aspiration of a bubo is preferable since surgical drainage may disseminate the organisms. *Y. pestis* can be grown on ordinary culture media or isolated by animal (especially guinea pig) inoculation. Serologic tests include CF, passive hemagglutination, and immunofluorescent staining of a node, secretions, or tissues. A vaccination history does not exclude plague in the differential diagnosis since clinical illness may occur in vaccinated individuals.

Prophylaxis and Treatment

Prevention is based on rodent control and the use of repellents to minimize flea attacks. Immunization with standard killed plague vaccine gives protection and is recommended for travelers to Southeast Asia.

Treatment should be immediate upon suspicion of plague; prompt treatment reduces mortality to below 5%. In septicemic or pneumonic plague, treatment must begin within 24 h. Streptomycin 0.5 Gm IM q 3 h for 48 h, followed by 1.5 to 2 Gm/day for 7 to 10 days, is preferred by many authorities. Others give tetracycline or chloramphenicol 500 mg IV q 3 h for 48 h, then 4 Gm/day orally for the next 48 h, and 3 Gm/day orally for an additional 4 to 5 days.

Routine aseptic precautions are adequate for patients with bubonic plague. Primary or secondary pneumonic plague requires strict isolation of the patient. All pneumonic plague contacts should be kept under medical surveillance; their temperatures should be taken q 4 h for 6 days. If this is not possible, chemoprophylaxis with tetracycline 1 Gm/day orally for 6 days is an alternative, but is not ideal, because of the potential danger of producing drug-resistant strains.

MELIOIDOSIS

A glanders-like infection of man and animals, endemic in Southeast Asia, caused by Pseudomonas pseudomallei. The causative bacillus can be isolated from soil and water. Man may contract melioidosis by contamination of skin abrasions or burns, by ingestion, or by inhalation, but not directly from infected animals or patients.

Clinical Manifestations

Illness may be asymptomatic or occur in various forms. Clinically inapparent infection may be latent for years. Mortality is less than 10%, except in the acute septicemic form.

Acute pulmonary infection, the most common form, varies from mild to an overwhelming necrotizing pneumonia. Onset may be abrupt or gradual, with headache, anorexia, pleuritic or dull aching chest pain, and generalized myalgia.

Fever is usually over 39 C (102 F). Cough, tachypnea, and rales are characteristic; sputum may be blood-tinged. Chest x-rays usually show upper lobe consolidation, frequently cavitating and resembling tuberculosis. Nodular lesions, thin-walled cysts, and pleural effusion may also be present. The WBC count ranges from normal to 20,000.

Acute septicemic infection: Onset may be abrupt, with disorientation, extreme dyspnea, severe headache, pharyngitis, upper abdominal colic, diarrhea, and pustular skin lesions. High fever, tachypnea, a bright erythematous flush, and cyanosis are present. Muscle tenderness may be striking. There may be signs of arthritis or meningitis. Pulmonary signs may be absent, or rales, rhonchi, and pleural rubs may be present. Chest x-rays usually show irregular nodular (4 to 10 mm) densities. The liver and spleen may be palpable. Liver function tests, SGOT, and bilirubin are often abnormal. The WBC count is normal or slightly increased.

Chronic suppurative infection: Secondary abscesses may develop in the skin, lymph nodes, or any organ. Patients may be afebrile. An **acute suppurative form** is uncommon.

Diagnosis

Culture of *P. pseudomallei* (which grows on most laboratory media in 48 to 72 h) and HA, agglutination, and CF tests on paired serums aid in diagnosis.

Treatment

Inapparent infection needs no treatment. Antibiotics—usually tetracyclines, chloramphenicol, kanamycin, and sulfonamides—are chosen by susceptibility studies. Mildly ill patients are given either tetracycline or chloramphenicol 40 mg/kg body wt/day orally, or sulfisoxazole 70 mg/kg/day orally, for a minimum of 30 days. Moderately ill patients are given two antimicrobials (e.g., tetracycline plus kanamycin or a sulfonamide) for 30 days, then tetracycline alone for 30 to 60 days. Patients with severe acute melioidosis are given a triple combination of tetracycline and chloramphenicol, 80 mg/kg/day of each orally or IV, and either sulfisoxazole 140 mg/kg/day orally or IV, kanamycin 30 mg/kg/day IM, or novobiocin 60 mg/kg/day orally.

CAUSED BY TOXIN-PRODUCING BACTERIA

DIPHTHERIA

An acute contagious disease caused by Corynebacterium diphtheriae, *characterized by the formation of a fibrinous pseudomembrane, usually on the respiratory mucosa, and by myocardial and neural tissue damage, secondary to an exotoxin.* Recently **cutaneous diphtheria** lesions have also been common.

Epidemiology

Three biotypes (*mitis, intermedius,* and *gravis*) of *C. diphtheriae* exist. Only toxigenic isolates produce exotoxin. Nontoxigenic organisms may produce symptomatic diphtheria, but the clinical course is usually milder than that caused by toxigenic isolates. Spread is chiefly by the secretions of infected persons, directly or via contaminated fomites. Sporadic cases usually result from exposure to carriers who may never have had apparent disease; cases occurring during an epidemic can usually be traced.

Cutaneous diphtheria can occur when any disruption of the integument is colonized by *C. diphtheriae.* Indigent adults living in an endemic area are particularly at risk, since poor personal and community hygiene contribute to the spread of cutaneous diphtheria.

Pathology

Ordinarily, the organisms lodge in the tonsil or nasopharynx and, as they multiply, produce exotoxins lethal to the adjacent host cells. Occasionally, the primary site is the skin or mucosa elsewhere. The exotoxin also damages cells in distant organs, to which it is carried by the blood. Pathologic lesions are found in the respiratory passages, oropharynx, myocardium, nervous system, and kidneys.

The diphtheria bacillus first destroys a layer of superficial epithelium, usually in patches, and the resulting exudate coagulates to form a grayish pseudomembrane containing bacteria, fibrin, leukocytes, and necrotic epithelial cells. The membrane is formed in the wake of the spreading infection, and the areas of bacterial multiplication and toxin absorption are wider and deeper than indicated by the size of the membrane.

The myocardium may show fatty degeneration or fibrosis. Degenerative changes in the cranial or peripheral nerves occur chiefly in the motor fibers. Anterior horn cells and anterior and posterior nerve roots may show damage in severe cases, in direct proportion to the duration of infection before antitoxin has been given. The kidneys may show a reversible interstitial nephritis with extensive cellular infiltration.

Symptoms and Signs

The incubation period (1 to 4 days) and prodromal period (12 to 24 h) are among the shortest in bacterial diseases. Initially, the patient with tonsillar or faucial diphtheria has only a mild sore throat, dysphagia, a low-grade temperature with an increased heart rate, and a rising polymorphonuclear leukocytosis. Nausea, emesis, chills, headache, and fever are more common in children.

The characteristic membrane is usually tonsillar, but may be found in other areas. Dirty grey, tough, and fibrinous, it may be firmly adherent so that removal causes bleeding. Depending on the duration of infection, the membrane may be punctate or extensive, and yellow-gray or creamy. In small children, who may not show any signs of illness until the disease is well established, a membrane is often present at the first examination. In older children and adults, complaints of sore throat and fatigue may antedate appearance of the membrane. Some patients never develop a membrane.

The disease may remain mild. When it progresses, dysphagia, signs of toxemia, and prostration become prominent. Edema of the pharynx and larynx obstructs breathing. If the membrane involves the larynx or the trachea and bronchi, it may partially obstruct the air passage, or, becoming detached, may suddenly cause complete obstruction. The cervical lymph glands are enlarged. In severe cases diffusion of exotoxin into the neck tissue may produce such edema that the patient appears "bull-necked." A serosanguineous nasal discharge, often unilateral, may appear if the nasopharynx is affected.

The lesions of **cutaneous diphtheria** are not morphologically specific. Any break in the skin can be secondarily infected with *C. diphtheriae;* lacerations, abrasions, ulcers, burns, and other wounds are potential reservoirs of the organism. The lesions occur most commonly on the extremities and if left untreated may become anesthetic due to local infiltration of the exotoxin. Cutaneous diphtheritic lesions usually also harbor β-hemolytic streptococci, *Staphylococcus aureus,* or both. A pseudomembrane is uncommon. Concomitant nasopharyngeal infection with the same biotype occurs in 20 to 40% of the cases.

Complications

Severe complications are especially likely when antitoxin is not given promptly. Myocarditis is usually manifest by the 10th to 14th day but can appear during the

1st to the 6th wk. Heart failure may follow; sudden death may occur. Insignificant ECG changes occur in 20 to 30% of patients. A-V dissociation, complete heart block, and ventricular arrhythmias are associated with a high mortality. Dysphagia and nasal regurgitation, from bulbar paralysis, may be seen in the 1st wk of illness; peripheral nerve palsies appear from the 3rd to the 6th wk. Kidney involvement may lead to albuminuria and oliguria.

Diagnosis

This is based on the clinical appearance, particularly of the membrane, pending confirmation by culture. Loeffler's or tellurite medium is preferred for primary isolation of the organism, but it grows well on other artificial media. The laboratory should be notified that isolation of this now rare organism may be expected. Cutaneous diphtheria should be suspected when a patient presents with skin lesions during a respiratory outbreak of diphtheria.

Immunization

Active immunization should be given routinely to all children, and to all susceptible contacts (see ROUTINE IMMUNIZATION PROCEDURES in §22). For previously immunized contacts, a booster dose is sufficient.

Schick test: Diagnostic diphtheria toxin (Diphtheria Toxin for Schick Test USP), 1/50 MLD (0.1 ml), is injected intradermally to determine susceptibility or immunity. The same amount of heat-inactivated test material (or toxoid) is injected simultaneously into the other arm to rule out sensitivity to bacterial proteins. Results are read 72 to 96 h later. An area, 1 cm or more in diameter, of inflammation and induration at the injection site **(positive test)** indicates susceptibility to the disease. If there is no local reaction **(negative test),** the subject may still contract diphtheria, but has an antibody level sufficient to neutralize the toxin and protect him against the toxigenic complications of diphtheria when exposed. A pseudoreaction or a combined reaction may occur. The Schick test yields a crude estimate of the level of circulating protective antitoxin. It is not recommended for general use, and it should not delay treatment of a symptomatic contact; it is discussed because some physicians still employ the test.

Treatment

Symptomatic patients are hospitalized in isolation rooms. Diphtheria antitoxin must be given early, since the antitoxin neutralizes only toxin not yet bound to cells. CAUTION: *Diphtheria antitoxin is derived from horses; hence, a skin test to rule out sensitivity should always precede administration* (see HORSE SERUM SENSITIVITY in §2, Ch. 5). If, after 30 min, no erythema or a flat erythema smaller than 0.5 cm in diameter appears about the site of injection, administration of antitoxin may proceed. The dose ranges from 20,000 to 100,000 u. The amount given is largely an empiric decision. Moderately symptomatic diphtheritic pharyngitis would require 20,000 to 40,000 u., while patients presenting with more severe symptoms or with complications would require larger doses.

Antitoxin may be given IM or IV. Doses above 20,000 u. may be added to 200 ml isotonic saline and given slowly IV over 30 to 45 min to facilitate delivery of the large volume.

An urticarial wheal in response to the skin test indicates sensitivity and mandates **extreme caution** in giving the antitoxin. The patient must first be desensitized with dilute antitoxin, given in graduated doses, as described in HORSE SERUM SENSITIVITY in §2, Ch. 5. Epinephrine 1:1000 should be available for immediate injection of 0.3 to 1 ml s.c., IM, or slowly IV if untoward symptoms appear. In the highly sensitive patient, IV administration of antitoxin is **contraindicated.**

Supportive treatment is important, particularly with the complications of diphtheria. Bed rest is necessary, as are careful nursing with emphasis on food and fluid intake, constant observation for signs that laryngeal intubation or a tracheostomy is needed, and frequent monitoring for cardiac and neurologic problems. Eradication of the organism with antibiotics is important. Adults may be given procaine penicillin G 600,000 u. IM q 12 h for 10 days or erythromycin 250 to 500 mg orally q 6 h for 7 days. Children weighing less than 25 kg should receive procaine penicillin G 300,000 u. IM q 12 h or erythromycin 40 mg/kg/day (maximum 1 Gm/day) orally or parenterally in 4 divided doses. Ampicillin is also effective, in a dosage of 75 mg/kg/day in 4 divided doses for children or 250 to 500 mg orally q.i.d. for adults. Clindamycin and rifampin have also been used.

Recovery from severe diphtheria is slow, and patients must be prevented from resuming activities too soon. Even normal physical exertion may be fatal to the patient recovering from myocarditis.

Management of an Outbreak

1. Isolate and treat all **symptomatic patients** as described above until 2 throat (or skin if appropriate) cultures are negative for *C. diphtheriae.* The cultures should be taken 24 and 48 h after cessation of antibiotics. If positive cultures persist after clinical recovery, re-treat for 10 days with erythromycin (2 Gm/day orally in 4 divided doses for adults). With current antibiotic regimens, tonsillectomy is no longer indicated for eradication of persistent foci.

2. Submit all isolates of *C. diphtheriae* to the local health department for biotyping and toxigenicity determination. Nontoxigenic and toxigenic biotypes may coexist in a community.

3. For all **close contacts** of known diphtheria patients, obtain appropriate cultures for *C. diphtheriae.* Examine their throats and integument; hospitalize *symptomatic* patients and treat as described above pending culture reports. Confine *asymptomatic* contacts with positive throat cultures for *C. diphtheriae* **(carriers)** at home, without visitors, for the duration of therapy, and give erythromycin orally, 250 to 500 mg q 6 h for adults; 40 mg/kg/day in 4 divided doses for children. Do *not* give antitoxin. The breadwinner may continue to work while taking antibiotics. *Recheck cultures after therapy.* Erythromycin treatment failures are usually due to failure to take the medicine rather than to drug resistance of the organism.

4. Update diphtheria immunization of **all contacts.** Schick tests are usually unnecessary in the management of a diphtheria outbreak.

5. Persons with negative cultures and full immunization may be presumed safe from both personal and public health standpoints.

CLOSTRIDIAL INFECTIONS

Clostridia are anaerobic, spore-forming, gram-positive bacilli that exist widely in nature, being found in dust, soil, vegetation, and the intestinal tracts of humans and animals. Though nearly 100 *Clostridium* species have been identified, relatively few cause disease in humans or animals (see TABLE 1-9). The pathogenic species, in the vegetative form, produce various tissue-destructive and neural exotoxins that have been biochemically and serologically delineated.

The most frequent clostridial infections in humans are benign, self-limited food poisoning (see *Clostridium perfringens* FOOD POISONING in §7, Ch. 12) and incidental wound contamination, which occurs in 10 to 30% of wounds. Lethal clostridial diseases, including gas gangrene (myonecrosis), tetanus, and botulism, are relatively rare but can follow trauma, injection of "street" drugs by addicts, and errors in food canning.

NEUROTOXIC CLOSTRIDIAL DISEASE

Botulism
(See in §7, Ch. 12)

Tetanus
(Lockjaw)

An acute infectious disease characterized by intermittent tonic spasm of voluntary muscles, and convulsions. Spasm of the masseters accounts for the name "lockjaw."

Etiology and Pathogenesis

Tetanus is caused by an exotoxin (tetanospasmin) elaborated by *Clostridium tetani,* a slender, motile, gram-positive, anaerobic, sporulating bacillus. The spores remain viable for years and can be found in soil and in animal feces.

Tetanus may follow trivial as well as overtly contaminated wounds, depending on a suitably reduced oxidation-reduction potential of the injured tissue. Drug addicts are particularly prone to develop tetanus, as are patients with burns or surgical wounds. Infection may also develop in the postpartum uterus and a newborn's umbilicus (**tetanus neonatorum**). Clinical disease does not confer immunity.

The toxin enters the CNS along the peripheral motor nerves, or it may be blood-borne to the nervous tissue. The tetanospasmin binds to the ganglioside membranes of nerve synapses and blocks the release of the inhibitory transmitter from the nerve terminals, thereby causing generalized tonic spasticity upon which intermittent tonic convulsions are usually superimposed. The toxin cannot be neutralized once fixed.

Symptoms and Signs

The incubation period ranges from 2 to 50 (usually 5 to 10) days. The most frequent presenting symptom is **stiffness of the jaw,** which must always be considered to be caused by tetanus until proved otherwise. Other presenting symptoms include difficulty in swallowing; restlessness; irritability; stiff neck, arms, or legs; headache; fever; sore throat; chilliness; or convulsions. Later, the patient has difficulty opening his jaws (**trismus**); spasm of the facial muscles produces a characteristic expression with a fixed smile and elevated eyebrows (**risus sardonicus**). Rigidity or spasm of abdominal, neck, and back muscles—even opisthotonos—

TABLE 1-9. CLOSTRIDIAL DISEASES

Disease	Agent	Major Types in Man	Exotoxin
Tetanus	C. tetani		Tetanospasmin
Botulism	C. botulinum	A, B, E	Neurotoxin (acetylcholine blocks)
Food poisoning	C. perfringens	A (variants?)	Enterotoxin
Necrotizing enteritis	C. perfringens	C (?)	
Histotoxic infections: local, uterine, wound infections (myositis, myonecrosis, anaerobic cellulitis)	C. perfringens, C. novyi, C. septicum	A–E A–D A	Lecithinase, protease, collagenase, fibrinolysin, hyaluronidase, deoxyribonuclease, leukocidin

may be present. Sphincteral spasm causes urinary retention or constipation. Dysphagia may interfere with nutrition. Painful convulsions with profuse sweating are characteristic and are precipitated by minor disturbances such as a draft or noise, or jarring the bed. The patient's sensorium is usually clear, but coma may follow repeated convulsions. During convulsions, chest wall rigidity or glottal spasm interferes with respiration, causing cyanosis or fatal asphyxia; since the patient is unable to speak or cry out, the immediate cause of death may not be apparent.

The patient's temperature is only moderately elevated except when a complicating infection, such as pneumonia, is present. The respiratory and pulse rates are increased. Reflexes are often exaggerated. Moderate leukocytosis is usual.

Localized tetanus can occur, with spasticity of a group of muscles near the wound but without trismus. The spasticity may persist for weeks.

Diagnosis

A history of a wound in a patient with muscle stiffness or spasm is suggestive. A slight wound may have been overlooked. Tetanus can be confused with meningoencephalitis of other bacterial or viral origin, but the combination of an intact sensorium and muscle spasms suggests tetanus. Trismus must be distinguished from local causes such as a peritonsillar or retropharyngeal abscess or another local infection. The phenothiazines can induce a tetanus-like rigidity but other signs of basal ganglia dysfunction are usually evident.

C. tetani can sometimes be cultured from the wound, but its absence does not negate the diagnosis.

Prognosis

The prognosis is poorer if the incubation period is short and symptoms progress rapidly, or if treatment is delayed. Mortality is highest in young and old patients and in drug addicts. The course tends to be milder when there is no demonstrable focus of infection.

Prophylaxis

Immunization: Primary immunization against tetanus with either the fluid or adsorbed toxoid is superior to giving antitoxin at the time of injury. For routine DTP immunization and booster recommendations, see ROUTINE IMMUNIZATION PROCEDURES in §22.

At the **time of injury,** 0.5 ml of toxoid elicits a protective antibody level in a *previously immunized patient;* this booster dose is not necessary if it is known beyond doubt that the patient has received a booster within the past 10 yr, or within the past 3 yr if the wound is severe and conducive to anaerobic infection. An *inadequately immunized patient* should be given tetanus immune globulin (human) 250 to 500 u. IM, depending on the wound potential and not on age or body wt. At the same time, the 1st of three 0.5-ml doses of adsorbed tetanus toxoid should be given s.c. or IM at another injection site. The 2nd and 3rd doses of toxoid are given at monthly intervals. Tetanus antitoxin 3000 to 5000 u. IM (CAUTION: *Made from horse or bovine serum; see* HORSE SERUM SENSITIVITY *in* §2, Ch. 5) should be used *only* if tetanus immune globulin (human) is not available.

Wound care: Prompt, careful wound debridement, especially of deep puncture wounds, is essential, since dirt and dead tissue promote multiplication of *C. tetani.* Penicillin and the tetracyclines are effective against *C. tetani* but are not substitutes for adequate debridement.

Treatment

Therapy involves maintenance of an adequate airway; early and adequate use of antitoxin; neutralization of nonfixed toxin; prevention of further toxin production; sedation; control of muscle spasm, hypertonicity, fluid balance, and inter-current infection; and continuous nursing care.

General principles: The patient should be kept in a quiet room. Tracheostomy should be performed early in moderate or severe cases. Mechanical ventilators may be necessary. O_2 should be humidified. An indwelling IV catheter is preferable to repeated IV administration of fluids and medication. Gastric intubation facilitates feeding; however, intravenous hyperalimentation avoids the hazard of aspiration secondary to feeding by gastric tube. Since constipation is usual, an initial cleansing enema is helpful; a rectal tube helps to control distention. Catheterization is required if urinary retention occurs. Changing the patient's position q 2 h and chest percussion q 12 h inhibit hypostatic pneumonia. Hypothermic measures help to reduce high fever. Codeine is useful for pain.

Antitoxin: The benefit of antiserum depends on how much tetanospasmin is already bound to the synaptic membranes. Tetanus immune globulin (human) 500 u. IM should be given initially, followed by daily doses of 500 to 1000 u., for a total dosage of 3000 to 6000 u. Antitoxin of animal origin is far less preferable since the patient's serum antitoxin level is not as well maintained and there is considerable risk of serum sickness. If horse serum must be used, however, the usual dose is 50,000 u. IM and 50,000 u. IV (CAUTION: *see* HORSE SERUM SENSITIVITY *in* §2, Ch. 5, *for necessary precautions*). Human immune globulin or animal antitoxin can be injected directly into the wound, but this is not as essential as proper wound excision and debridement.

Management of muscle spasms: Diazepam is excellent for controlling rigidity and spasms. Dosage and route vary markedly with the patient's age and the severity of the tetanus. The most severe cases may require 10 to 20 mg q 3 h by IV drip. Less severe cases can be controlled with 5 to 10 mg q 2 to 4 h orally. Alternatives include meprobamate (average adult dose, 400 mg IM q 4 h) or methocarbamol (1 Gm in 5% D/W given by slow IV drip). Chlorpromazine (average adult dose, 12.5 to 25 mg IM q 4 to 8 h) also helps to control convulsions and spasms, but requires close monitoring of the blood pressure since it can induce hypotension. Tetanospasms can be particularly frequent and severe in drug addicts and can be countered with morphine sulfate 5 to 35 mg IV or IM plus phenobarbital 50 to 200 mg IM or IV, both given q 3 to 4 h. Rarely, acute tetanospasm with respiratory arrest may require use of succinylcholine 80 mg IV for effective relaxation; assisted ventilation is essential.

Antibiotics: Penicillin G 2 million u. IV q 6 h or tetracycline 500 mg IV q 6 h should be given, although the role of antibiotic therapy is minor in contrast to wound debridement. It is not likely to prevent secondary infections (e.g., pneumonia). If pneumonia develops, cultures of the sputum or trachea should be taken, sensitivity tests performed, and an appropriate antibiotic given if necessary. If the patient has an indwelling urethral catheter, the urine should be cultured frequently and antimicrobial therapy given if indicated.

Immunization: Since immunity does not follow clinical tetanus, the patient should receive a full immunizing course of toxoid after he is discharged from the hospital.

HISTOTOXIC CLOSTRIDIAL DISEASE

Etiology and Pathogenesis

The ubiquitous and saprophytic clostridia become pathogenic when the tissues show a reduced oxidation-reduction potential, a high lactate concentration, and a low pH. Such an abnormal anaerobic environment may develop with primary arterial insufficiency or after severe penetrating or crush injuries. The deeper and more severe the wound, the more prone to anaerobic infection, especially if there has been even minimal foreign-particle contamination. Clostridial lesions tend to be self-perpetuating once the clostridia have assumed the vegetative form and are producing toxins.

Severe clostridial sepsis may complicate intestinal perforation and obstruction. *C. perfringens* infection may complicate simple appendicitis. Clostridia (usually *C perfringens* Type A) have been implicated in cholecystitis, peritonitis, ruptured appendix, meningitis, lung abscess, brain abscess, endocarditis, pyelonephritis and osteomyelitis. Clostridial infections may complicate initially aerobic local tissue or organ infections which have become anaerobic by extensive necrosis. Tumors, tissues devitalized by radiation, and even parenteral injection sites can also be susceptible to clostridial infection. Debilitated patients with neoplastic disease or leukemia and patients with diabetes mellitus (because of associated occlusive vascular disease) are at a high risk of developing clostridial infections. The anaerobic environment of intestinal lymphoma and carcinoma permits endogenous *C. perfringens* invasion and replication, resulting in severe local or, rarely, septicemic clostridial disease.

Clinical Types

Uterine Clostridial Infection

This may be a fatal complication of septic abortion; it can also follow relatively uncomplicated pelvic surgery or childbirth. The patient is toxic and febrile, the lochia is foul-smelling, and the uterus is tender. Gas is sometimes detected escaping through the cervix. Hemolytic anemia may develop as a result of clostridial septicemia and the effect of the toxin lecithinase on the RBC membrane. The patient becomes increasingly toxic and frequently develops acute renal failure within 1 or 2 days. When septicemia and overt hemolysis occur, the mortality rate is about 50%.

Early **diagnosis** requires a high index of suspicion. Early and repeated Gram stains and cultures of the lochia and blood are indicated, though it should be remembered that *C. perfringens* can occasionally be isolated from the healthy vagina and lochia. X-rays may show local gas production.

Treatment consists of debridement by curettage, and administration of penicillin G 10 million u./day for at least 1 wk. Hysterectomy may be necessary if debridement by curettage is insufficient. Early renal dialysis is needed if acute tubular necrosis develops.

Clostridial Wound Infections

These may occur as local cellulitis, local or spreading myositis, or, most seriously, progressive myonecrosis **(gas gangrene).** Infection develops hours or days after injury occurs, usually in an extremity after severe crushing or penetrating trauma that results in much devitalized tissue. Similar spreading myositis or myonecrosis may occur in operative wounds, particularly in patients with underlying occlusive vascular disease.

Clostridial cellulitis (anaerobic cellulitis) occurs as a localized infection in a superficial wound, usually 3 or more days after initial injury. Infection may spread extensively along fascial planes, but toxicity is much less severe than in patients with extensive myonecrosis. The exudate is foul-smelling, serous, and brown, with evident crepitation and abundant bubbling of gas. Discoloration and gross edema of the extremity are rare. In clostridial infections associated with primary vascular occlusion of an extremity, extension beyond the line of demarcation and progression to severe toxic myonecrosis are rare.

An initially localized deep **clostridial myositis** rapidly spreads by toxin production in an anaerobic environment, causing edema, gas production, and subsequent myonecrosis. In **myonecrosis,** the exudate is serous and brown, but not necessarily foul-smelling. Pain, tenderness, and edema are usually severe, with dramatic progression over a period of hours. Late in the course, gas crepitation can be felt in about 80% of cases. The wound site may appear pale initially, becomes red or bronze, and finally turns blackish-green. The affected muscle is a lusterless pink, then deep red, and finally gray-green or mottled purple. The patient becomes progressively toxic, though often alert until the terminal stage. In contrast to uterine clostridial infection, septicemia and overt hemolysis is rare with gas gangrene of the extremities, even in terminally ill patients.

Though localized cellulitis, myositis, and spreading myonecrosis may be sufficiently distinctive to permit clinical differentiation and appropriate treatment, precise **diagnosis** often requires thorough surgical wound exploration and visual evaluation of tissue involvement. X-rays may show local gas production. Appropriate anaerobic and aerobic cultures of wound exudate should be taken, primarily to identify the organism. Smears show gram-positive clostridial rods. Typically, there are few polymorphonuclear leukocytes in the exudate. Free fat globules may be demonstrated using Sudan stain. Many wounds, particularly if open, are contaminated with both pathogenic and nonpathogenic clostridia without evident invasive disease. The significance of this must be determined clinically.

Other anaerobic and aerobic bacteria, including members of the family Enterobacteriaceae and *Bacteroides, Streptococcus,* and *Staphylococcus* species, alone or mixed, frequently cause clostridia-like severe cellulitis, extensive fasciitis, or gas gangrene in traumatic and postoperative wounds. If polymorphonuclear leukocytes are abundant and the smear shows many chains of cocci, an anaerobic streptococcal or staphylococcal infection should be suspected. An abundance of gram-negative rods may indicate infection with one of the Enterobacteriaceae or a *Bacteroides* species.

It is to be emphasized that anaerobic wound infections, particularly those due to *Clostridium* species, can progress from initial injury through the stages of cellulitis to myositis to myonecrosis with shock, toxic delirium, and finally death within one to several days. Early suspicion and intervention are essential. Anaerobic cellulitis uniformly responds to treatment; however, established and progressive myositis with an associated systemic toxemia carries a mortality rate of 20% or more.

Appropriate **treatment** requires thorough wound debridement, including removal of foreign material and all devitalized tissue. Penicillin G 10 to 20 million u./day IV should be given as soon as clostridial disease is clinically suspected. Cephalothin 6 to 8 Gm/day IV or tetracycline 2 Gm/day IV may be substituted in penicillin-allergic patients.

The detection of specific antigenic toxins in the wound or blood is useful only in the rare instance of botulism acquired through a wound portal. For **wound botulism,** early administration of specific or polyvalent antitoxin (see BOTULISM in §7, Ch. 12) is valuable. Polyvalent heterologous antiserum is available for gas gangrene but its value is questionable compared to that of thorough wound debridement and use of penicillin. Hyperbaric O_2 is helpful in extensive myonecrosis as a supplement to antibiotics and surgery. However, few chambers large enough for surgical and nursing care are available.

Necrotizing Enteritis

In addition to *C. perfringens* food poisoning, clostridia occasionally cause acute inflammatory, sometimes necrotizing, disease in the small and large bowel. Preliminary observations suggest that such a process may occur in some patients being treated for leukemia. Such clostridial enterotoxemias can occur as isolated cases or as outbreaks and some appear due, at least in part, to contaminated meat. Pig-bel, for example, which occurs in New Guinea, presumably results from eating pork contaminated by *C. perfringens* Type C; it varies from mild diarrhea to fulminant toxemia with dehydration, causing shock and sometimes death.

CAUSED BY MYCOBACTERIA

TUBERCULOSIS

An acute or chronic infection caused by Mycobacterium tuberculosis *and, rarely in the USA, by* M. bovis. It is almost always initiated by inhalation. Pulmonary disease is most common, but disease can spread via the lymphatics and blood-stream to any other organ. TB is characterized clinically by a lifelong balance between the host and the infection in which pulmonary or extrapulmonary foci may reactivate at any time, often after long periods of latency; and pathologically by the formation of tubercles made up of giant cells and epithelioid cells, by a tendency for fibrosis to occur, and by caseation, a unique form of nonliquefying necrosis.

Etiology

M. tuberculosis is an acid-fast, nonmotile rod. *M. tuberculosis* organisms are characteristically sensitive to isoniazid **(INH)** and produce niacin and the enzyme catalase. INH-resistant mutants of *M. tuberculosis* generally lose their ability to produce catalase, but remain niacin-positive. *M. bovis* is also sensitive to INH, but does not produce niacin. All other mycobacteria are highly INH-resistant, cata-lase-positive, and niacin-negative. (See TABLE 1-10.)

Epidemiology

Infection occurs primarily by the aerosol route. Airborne droplets may remain infectious and suspended for long periods of time. They are small and reach the smallest airway without being trapped and removed by bronchial mucosal clearance mechanisms. In areas where bovine TB has not been eliminated, transmission may occur by ingestion of contaminated milk. Direct inoculation occasionally occurs in laboratory workers.

TABLE 1-10. CHARACTERISTICS OF MYCOBACTERIA

Organism	Produce Catalase	Produce Niacin	INH-Sensitive
M. tuberculosis	Yes	Yes	Yes
INH-resistant M. tuberculosis	No (generally)	Yes	No
M. bovis	Yes	No	Yes
Other mycobacteria (excluding M. leprae)	Yes	No	No

Progressive TB usually occurs in older individuals, particularly nonwhite males. In areas of the world with a very high prevalence of early infection, it is also common in very young children and particularly older adolescent and young adult females.

Pathogenesis

A nonsensitized host has no preexisting specific immunologic defense against TB. Therefore, when an infectious particle is inhaled into the terminal air passages, infection occurs and a colony of *M. tuberculosis* develops, usually in the lower or middle lung fields. With little host reaction and no symptoms, the bacilli spread readily to the draining lymph nodes and, via the bloodstream, throughout the body. With the development of tuberculin hypersensitivity 4 to 10 wk later, a small area of pneumonitis develops, further multiplication of intracellular bacilli is inhibited at the initial and metastatic foci, and the infection is usually arrested before symptoms develop. The process is bacteriostatic rather than bactericidal, however, and the bacilli may remain latent but viable for the life of the host. Foci of infection may be reactivated at any time by local factors, especially if cellular immunity wanes due to disease, corticosteroid or other immunosuppressant drug therapy, or old age.

Occasionally, the initial or metastatic infection evolves into clinical TB despite development of hypersensitivity. Local tissue destruction due to nonspecific lung abscess, carcinoma, or pulmonary resection; local joint tissue injury; gastric resection; and diabetes mellitus, particularly with ketoacidosis, favor progression of disease. Silicosis also favors progression by altering the host response. Leukemia, lymphoma, and Hodgkin's disease not only reduce immunity, but may often be confused with as well as complicated by TB. Pathogenesis is further discussed under the specific types of TB below.

Prophylaxis

Vaccination with BCG, an attenuated strain of *M. tuberculosis,* provides considerable protection against infection and tends to ameliorate the course of infection if it occurs. Successful BCG vaccination results in a positive tuberculin test, thus eliminating the diagnostic usefulness of this test, but this disadvantage is outweighed by the advantages of protection if the risk of infection is substantial. Vaccination of tuberculin-negative children is recommended in areas where the incidence of tuberculin-positive reactions in secondary school children is 20% or more.

Chemoprophylaxis usually consists of **INH** alone, 300 mg daily in adults, 6 to 10 mg/kg in children, for 12 to 18 mo, given as a single dose in the morning. Treatment of **tuberculin-negative** individuals prevents infection while the drug is being given, but is appropriate in only a few instances; e.g., when the brief exposure of an infant to a known infectious risk (e.g., the mother) cannot be avoided, or when exposed persons have a reduced immune response for any reason. Chemoprophylaxis is indicated in certain **tuberculin-positive** individuals in whom progressive disease is not apparent, including children under age 5; recent tuberculin converters, regardless of age; persons with exceptionally florid or necrotic reactions to low doses of tuberculin (> 20 mm of induration to 5 TU; see Diagnosis, in ADULT TYPE, below); individuals with pulmonary infiltrates of unknown etiology; some persons receiving corticosteroid therapy for more than a few weeks; post-gastrectomy patients with x-ray evidence of a quiescent or inactive focus of pulmonary TB; and all patients with silicosis.

Hospitalization or isolation of a patient under treatment for TB until the sputum is negative by laboratory tests is no longer considered necessary. TB is mainly spread before diagnosis, and a patient is unlikely to remain infectious after 10 days to 2 wk of effective drug therapy. However, an exception might reasonably be made when infants or young children might be exposed.

PULMONARY TUBERCULOSIS

Childhood Type

Clinical TB in young children, unlike that in adults, is characterized by hilar lymphadenopathy, pleural involvement, infrequent progression at the initial pulmonary focus, and hypersensitivity reactions.

Symptoms and Signs

Hilar lymphadenopathy is the hallmark of childhood pulmonary TB. Mediastinal nodes draining the initial area of pneumonitis become massively enlarged, usually unilaterally, causing bronchial compression resulting in a brassy, nonproductive cough or, particularly in very young children with flaccid small bronchi, atelectasis distal to bronchial compression. Complications or progressive disease may develop, including erosion of the bronchus by calcified nodes, often causing hemoptysis and occasionally resulting in spread of infectious material to distal parenchyma; traction diverticula of the mid-portion of the esophagus adherent to the nodes; and, rarely, erosion of the esophagus and bronchus adhering to the same node, with broncho-esophageal fistula formation. **Serofibrinous pleurisy** with effusion (see PLEURAL TUBERCULOSIS, below) occasionally occurs soon after infection. **Progressive primary TB,** though uncommon, occurs when the pneumonitis at the initial focus of infection progresses; caseation and, very rarely, cavity formation may result. **Hypersensitivity syndromes** include phlyctenular keratoconjunctivitis (a brisk ocular inflammatory reaction to locally deposited tubercle bacilli) and erythema nodosum. Both are rare, probably occur in association with the development of tuberculin hypersensitivity, are usually self-limited, and respond to corticosteroids.

Treatment

This is the same as for adults (see Treatment, in ADULT TYPE, below), except that the dose of INH (10 to 15 mg/kg body wt) is larger since children are much more resistant to INH induction of pyridoxine deficiency and resulting peripheral neuritis. Corticosteroids may be helpful when bronchial compression by enlarged nodes produces symptoms.

Adult Type

Pulmonary TB in adults is almost always initially manifested in the apical area of the lung after spreading hematogenously from a nonprogressive and often undetectable primary focus in the lower lung. Progression of the metastatic apical focus may occur after a long period of latency, but usually occurs within 2 yr of initial infection. The local environment of the apical-posterior area of the lung is favorable to bacillary multiplication; the infection progresses in this area while the initial focus of infection in the less favorable environment of the lower lung is healing. Caseous necrosis, liquefaction, and cavity formation are likely to occur in the apical areas, resulting in persistence of active infection, spread of infection via the bronchial tree to other areas of the same or opposite lung, and spread via the pulmonary secretions to uninfected individuals. Foci of infection that are spread via the bronchi are usually nonprogressive in the dependent areas of the lung, but tend to progress and form new cavities in the apical and subapical areas of the opposite lung.

Rarely, middle or lower lobe progressive TB occurs in adults. The former is usually due to erosion of the middle lobe bronchus by a hilar node with distal spread of infectious contents. The latter may represent progressive primary infection and usually occurs in individuals with lowered resistance due to such factors s severe diabetes mellitus, advanced age, or severe malnutrition.

Spontaneous healing most often involves closure of cavities, usually by obstruction of the broncho-cavitary junction, inspissation of cavity contents, and eventual fibrosis or calcification. Healing of open cavities rarely occurs except under the influence of chemotherapy.

Symptoms and Signs

Pulmonary TB is asymptomatic in the earliest stages. The symptoms and signs do not usually become apparent until after the lesions appear on x-ray. Onset is usually insidious; fever, malaise, and weight loss may occur when the mass of antigen reaches sufficient size.

Other symptoms are due to the local inflammatory reaction in the lung. **Cough** is due to irritative secretions draining into the bronchi from sloughing areas of lung tissue. It is therefore uncommon in early phases of the disease and is most frequently associated with cavitation. The cough at first occurs only in the morning as a result of material accumulated in the bronchi overnight, but becomes more severe as the disease progresses. **Sputum,** scanty at first, increases with progressive pulmonary excavation. In a caseous liquefying lesion, it is green and purulent. As the disease process becomes more chronic with less excavation, the sputum becomes yellowish and mucoid. **Hemoptysis** is occasionally the first symptom, and may be due to endobronchial involvement and granulation tissue formation, or to erosion of a pulmonary arterial branch by an enlarging cavity. It may vary from slight bloody streaking of the sputum to massive, though seldom fatal, hemorrhage. **Pleural** or **chest wall pain** aggravated by respiratory effort is due to pleural involvement. The pain may be referred to the shoulder or hypochondrium f the diaphragmatic pleura is irritated. **Dyspnea** is common during the acute febrile periods and in longstanding fibrogenic TB. Acute dyspnea may result from a spontaneous pneumothorax or a rapidly developing serous pleurisy. Rarely, endobronchial spread of infectious secretions causes oral ulcers, painful laryngeal involvement with hoarseness, or gastrointestinal TB which may first call attention to the pulmonary disease.

The pace of the illness varies widely. In some patients, particularly those from racial groups with low levels of genetic resistance to TB (e.g., Eskimos, American Indians, some blacks), the entire upper lobe may be involved and marked systemic symptoms may be present, suggesting lobar pneumonia. In others, symptoms may be minimal or absent despite extensive cavity formation and marked fibrosis. An undiagnosed and untreated patient may remain in relatively good health for prolonged periods while maintaining a high degree of infectiousness.

Complications

Extensive pulmonary TB always compromises pulmonary function. Patients in whom the infectious process is controlled by drugs may succumb to respiratory failure or to pulmonary hypertension and cor pulmonale, especially patients who have had thoracic surgery. Extrapulmonary TB is discussed below.

Diagnosis

Pulmonary TB is often accurately suspected on the basis of chest x-ray findings. An apical lesion is most common; characteristic x-ray findings of early reinfection consist of a small mottled density. Rarefaction may indicate beginning liquefaction and cavitation. Laminagrams are also helpful, particularly for visualization of cavities.

Microscopic identification of acid-fast rods on direct examination of sputum usually positive in the presence of cavitary disease with sputum production, i reliable but only presumptive evidence since it does not exclude other mycobac terial diseases. Histologic evidence of tubercle formation in pulmonary or extra pulmonary tissue is strong but also presumptive evidence for the same reason

Definitive diagnosis requires cultural identification of *M. tuberculosis,* var. *homi nis* or *bovis,* from pulmonary secretions, other body fluids, or tissue. Since the growth rate of *M. tuberculosis* is slow, culture is time-consuming and results may not be available for 3 to 6 wk. An early morning sputum collection is the mos productive. Alternatively, sputum expectorated and swallowed during the nigh may be obtained by aspirating gastric contents immediately after the patien awakens and prior to his leaving the bed. The specimen should also be plated or media containing various concentrations of INH, streptomycin, and, if possible other antituberculous drugs for initial drug sensitivity studies. A high degree of INH resistance, together with the ability to form catalase, is often the first evi dence that the infection is due to another mycobacterial species.

The **tuberculin test** is an important adjunct to diagnosis. Satisfactory materials for tuberculin testing are old tuberculin **(OT)** and a purified derivative **(PPD)** Since PPD rapidly deteriorates after mixing the powder with the diluent, a **stabi lized solution of tuberculin PPD** is usually used. If this is not available, the PPD is discarded after one use, or, alternatively, OT is used. First strength tuberculin (1 tuberculin unit or **TU**) is equivalent to 1:10,000 OT and is useful in individuals in whom a high degree of hypersensitivity might be anticipated, such as young children. Most epidemiologic data are based on 5 TU (1:2000 OT). Second strength PPD is 250 TU, approximately equivalent to 1:100 OT. Antigen can be applied by the scratch (Pirquet) test and by multiple-puncture Tine and Heaf tests, but the most satisfactory method is careful intradermal administration (Mantoux test). Palpable induration (not erythema) of over 10 mm 48 h after administration of 5 TU by the Mantoux technic is diagnostic of tuberculous infection, though not necessarily of *active* TB. A smaller reaction (5 to 9 mm of induration is labeled doubtful) to 5 TU is often due to infection with other myco bacteria. Many patients clinically ill with TB, and some not very ill, do not react to 5 TU; accordingly, no patient should be designated tuberculin-negative on the basis of tests with this strength only. Such patients must also be tested with 250 TU or its equivalent of OT. Some seriously ill patients are tuberculin-negative when initially tested, but usually revert to positive with clinical improvement. *Accordingly, a negative tuberculin test does not exclude a diagnosis of TB.*

Treatment

Principles of drug therapy: INH is the most effective, least toxic, and most easily administered antimicrobial used for TB. When drug resistance develops during drug therapy, the INH-resistant tubercle bacilli appear to be less invasive than INH-susceptible strains. Therefore, INH is recommended even when there is a high degree of in vitro resistance, since by maintaining a less virulent population, INH appears to have at least some suppressive effect in this situation. (1) Accord ingly, INH should be part of all treatment regimens except in the unusual circum stance of unacceptable drug toxicity, and probably when rifampin is being given for retreatment of INH-resistant TB. (2) At least 2 drugs are required for pulmo nary TB with cavitation, and perhaps in all cases of pulmonary TB. This is because the number of organisms initially resistant to 2 drugs is very small, even in a pulmonary cavity, and the likelihood that a drug-resistant infection will emerge is minimal. (3) Response to drug therapy and prognosis as to potential relapse can be predicted by the rapidity of sputum conversion from positive to negative. When this occurs within 3 mo, successful outcome without additional rugs or surgery is usual. When sputum conversion is delayed past 5 or 6 mo, the robability of an emerging drug-resistant population is more likely. If the sputum ulture produces only small numbers of colonies, one more effective drug should e added (streptomycin or rifampin); if the culture contains many colonies, two ew drugs (either streptomycin or rifampin and one other agent) should be dded; resection may be considered when anatomically possible in rare instances. 4) Therapy is continued at least 18 mo to 2 yr after sputum is negative for ubercle bacilli. Phases of therapy can be divided into an **active** and a **suppressive** hase. The disease is considered active for 3 mo after sputum is negative. Multile-drug regimens are required until active disease is controlled and the infection ecomes quiescent. Suppressive therapy, usually with INH alone, is recommend-d after the disease is quiescent or inactive. Indefinite suppressive therapy may be eeded when host factors are unfavorable. (5) Since most treatment failures are ased on lack of patient compliance, the least inconvenient and least disagreeable rug regimen is preferred.

Initial treatment regimens: (See TABLE 1-11, below.) In younger patients with ar advanced disease but normal renal function, INH plus daily streptomycin SM) is probably the most effective combination, but INH plus ethambutol **(EMB)** s usually used because of convenience. In patients with less advanced disease and n those over age 50 or with concomitant renal disease, EMB is the best and least oxic companion drug. Aminosalicylic acid **(PAS)** has been the traditional comanion drug, but it is much less well tolerated, much more toxic and allergenic, nd probably less effective than EMB. Triple therapy with INH, SM, and EMB is dvantageous in initially drug-resistant infections and should be used when initial drug resistance is unusually likely (e.g., in a patient living with another patient vho has active drug-resistant TB). Usually, SM 1 Gm/day (for adults) is added to NH and EMB for 2 mo or until sputum becomes negative. There is no advantage n using 3 drugs in patients with drug-sensitive infection, except in severe cavitary aseous disease where unusually large bacterial populations can be expected. ?MB is the preferred third drug in such cases.

Retreatment regimens: (See TABLE 1-11, below.) Principles of the therapy of reatment failures are complex. In general, if rifampin **(RMP)** has not been given reviously, it is the keystone of retreatment, in combination with at least one and referably two other drugs also not previously given.

Specific antimicrobial drugs: Isoniazid (INH) is the most potent, least toxic, least xpensive, and most easily administered antituberculous agent. It is almost alvays given at a dosage of 300 mg/day in adolescents and adults as a single dose n the morning (see TABLE 1-11 for children's dosages). INH given orally provides erum drug concentrations equal to those achieved after IV administration. Conentrations in the CSF are approximately 20% of those in the serum; with meninzeal inflammation, the concentration approaches that in the serum. Penetration nto other tissues is also excellent.

Toxic reactions are more common than previously thought. Hepatic injury is ommon though usually not progressive. Transient minor elevations of serum ransaminase occur in as many as 10% of patients; jaundice is seen in about 1%; atalities due to severe liver injury, histologically resembling chronic active hepaitis, occur in about 0.1% of some treatment groups. Older individuals are more at isk than younger patients. Minor transaminase elevations usually subside withut stopping the drug. Jaundice, usually associated with symptoms of hepatitis, equires stopping the drug and not giving it again. Most recorded fatalities have occurred when INH administration was continued despite hepatitis-like symp-oms.

INH-induced pyridoxine deficiency, which may cause peripheral neuritis, is dose-related, occurring in about 2% of patients taking 5 mg/kg/day, over 10% taking 10 mg/kg, and 40% taking 20 mg/kg. The toxicity and the fact that serum concentrations are almost always more than adequate have determined the conventional INH dosage. Routine administration of pyridoxine is usual with routine INH dosage and is mandatory for doses over 5 mg/kg.

INH hypersensitivity may be manifested by fever, skin rash, and, rarely, agranulocytosis. Hypersensitivity syndromes occur most frequently when INH has been administered with PAS, but may be seen with INH alone.

Streptomycin (SM) is the 2nd major antituberculous agent. It is given IM in a dosage of 1 Gm/day for adults; after the initial response to treatment has been established, the dosage may be reduced to 1 Gm 3 times/wk. (See TABLE 1-11 for children's dosages.) Since it is excreted virtually unchanged by the kidneys, compromised renal function is a relative contraindication to its use. When use of SM is mandatory despite the presence of azotemia, the dosage must be modified according to the principles of drug therapy in renal failure, and serum drug concentrations should be monitored. The minimal inhibitory serum concentration for sensitive strains of *M. tuberculosis* is 0.2 µg/ml, 20 to 50 times less than the peak serum concentration after a 1-Gm dose. CSF penetration is poor. Intrathecal SM is **not recommended.**

SM causes selective toxicity for the 8th cranial nerve, particularly the vestibular apparatus, and the vestibular injury tends to be permanent. Since patients over age 50 may become permanently ataxic, they should not be given SM if possible. Caloric testing of vestibular function and audiologic examination are recommended before and during treatment. SM may also cause allergic reactions including drug fever, agranulocytosis, and a serum-sickness–like illness. Flushing, itching, and fullness of the head immediately after injection are bothersome histamine-like reactions not necessarily associated with the more serious allergic and toxic manifestations.

Ethambutol (EMB) is the most desirable companion drug to INH. It is given orally and is well absorbed. The recommended adult dosage is 25 mg/kg/day for 2 mo (or until sputum becomes negative) with the patient under close supervision, reduced to 15 mg/kg/day for prolonged usage, particularly on an outpatient basis. Children's dosages are given in TABLE 1-11; however, some authorities do not give ethambutol to children. Optic neuritis with visual field constriction and loss of ability to distinguish the color green is a dose-related side effect, but is completely reversible when detected early.

Rifampin (RMP) is a relatively new antituberculous agent with a potency equal or perhaps superior to INH. It is most useful in retreatment of initial therapy failures; its use has changed the outlook for INH-resistant treatment failures from uncertain to usually excellent. The usual dosage for adults is 600 mg once/day, taken orally on an empty stomach (see TABLE 1-11 for children's dosages). It is always given with at least one other drug to which the infecting microbial population is sensitive. It has some hepatotoxicity which is augmented when it is given together with INH, and it may rarely induce hypersensitivity reactions including thrombocytopenic purpura and serum-sickness–like symptoms.

Aminosalicylic acid (PAS) is the most toxic and difficult to tolerate of the drugs. Even the usual adult dosage of 4 Gm t.i.d. orally of the acid form or 5 Gm t.i.d. orally of the sodium salt is poorly tolerated by most patients. GI intolerance is very common. Hypersensitivity reactions (hepatitis, serum-sickness–like syndromes, skin rashes, marrow toxicity, and an infectious-mononucleosis–like syndrome of fever, lymphadenopathy, and the appearance of atypical lymphocytes in the peripheral blood) may also occur. The prothrombin time in patients taking warfarin may be significantly prolonged. Goiter formation may rarely occur. Most disturbing is the fact that PAS may induce sensitivity to other drugs being given concurrently.

Capreomycin, pyrazinamide, ethionamide, cycloserine, viomycin, and **kanamycin** are effective and useful in special situations (see TABLE 1-11), but their use is limited by toxicity.

Other modes of therapy: Bed rest and **hospitalization** are indicated by the patient's general condition. Since patients receiving chemotherapy become noninfectious rapidly, most can quickly return to work and other normal activity. **Surgical resection** has limited usefulness. If sputum conversion is delayed, drug resistance emerges, or thick-walled cavities or dense confluent disease persists after 5 to 9 mo of effective chemotherapy, resection may be performed provided that lobectomy will suffice and that the remaining pulmonary tissue is such that

TABLE 1-11. SUGGESTED SCHEME OF TREATMENT FOR TUBERCULOSIS

	Recommended Regimen*
Initial Treatment, Pulmonary	
Chemoprophylaxis†	INH
Minimal disease	INH + EMB
Average moderately advanced or far advanced disease	INH + SM, or INH + EMB
Retreatment, Pulmonary	
Drug-sensitive	As above
INH-resistant‡	RMP + 2 other effective§ drugs
INH- + EMB- + SM- + RMP-resistant	3 effective§ drugs; preference, in order: capreomycin, pyrazinamide, ethionamide, PAS, cycloserine, viomycin, kanamycin
Extrapulmonary	
Miliary, meningeal, renal, spinal, pericardial	INH + SM**
Lymphatic; bone and joint (excluding spinal); pleural; peritoneal; GU (excluding renal); upper airways (laryngeal, oral, middle ear) in the absence of concomitant pulmonary disease (rare); GI in the absence of concomitant pulmonary disease (uncommon)	INH alone, or INH + EMB

* INH = isoniazid 300 mg/day (single dose) in adults, 10 to 30 mg/kg (single dose) in infants and small children.
EMB = ethambutol 25 mg/kg/day for 2 mo or while under close observation; otherwise 15 mg/kg/day (single dose in adults; divided dose in children).
SM = streptomycin 1 Gm/day (single dose) in adults; 20 mg/kg (single dose) in children.
RMP = rifampin 600 mg/day (single dose) in adults; 15 to 20 mg/kg (single dose) in children.
PAS = aminosalicylic acid (see text for dosage).
† Instances in which progressive infection has not been established (see chemoprophylaxis on p. 113).
‡ With exception of RMP-containing regimen, INH included in spite of in vitro resistance.
§ Effective here means that the infecting microbial population is sensitive to that drug.
** RMP may be substituted for SM in older individuals (see details on SM in text).

pulmonary function will not be seriously compromised. When resection is performed because of drug resistance, 2 drugs not previously given are administered together with the drugs previously given. When the infection has been under control for 2 or 3 mo, treatment is altered so that at least one major effective drug is given and 'continued for 1 to 2 yr.

Adjunctive corticosteroid therapy may be advantageous in some patients, including those with extensive disease and profound hypoxemia and toxicity (as in extensive miliary TB or extensive bronchogenic spread); those who remain toxic, anemic, catabolic, and febrile for many weeks despite effective chemotherapy; and those with tuberculous meningitis. For patients who remain toxic and catabolic, prednisone 30 to 40 mg/day is sufficient. In patients in whom the inflammatory response is life-threatening, as in extreme hypoxemia with extensive bronchogenic or miliary pulmonary TB or tuberculous meningitis, an initial larger dose (60 mg/day) of prednisone is advisable. Guided by whether or not the symptoms reappear, the dosage is progressively decreased after 2 or 3 wk, and discontinued. The use of corticosteroids in tuberculous pleurisy and pericarditis is controversial. Corticosteroids are also used for replacement rather than pharmacologic therapy in patients with coexistent Addison's disease.

EXTRAPULMONARY TUBERCULOSIS

Extrapulmonary TB may result from lymphohematogenous spread; dissemination of contaminated pulmonary secretions via the bronchi to the upper air passages, mouth, and GI tract (intracanalicular spread); or direct extension to contiguous tissue. Extrapulmonary infection due to lymphohematogenous spread is seeded prior to the onset of tuberculin hypersensitivity. It may remain undetectable for some time and then present as an isolated clinical syndrome, thus occurring in the absence of clinical pulmonary TB and leading to difficulty in diagnosis. Extrapulmonary lesions produced by intracanalicular spread respond promptly to drug therapy for the pulmonary disease and rarely achieve clinical prominence.

Treatment (see TABLE 1-11 and the preceding discussions of specific drugs for dosages and other details of drug regimens) differs from that of cavitary pulmonary TB. With the possible exception of cavitary renal TB, the bacillary populations are much smaller than in pulmonary cavities and there is less likely to be a large population of resistant organisms. The local environment of extrapulmonary foci is much less favorable to bacterial multiplication and the lesions are much more responsive to chemotherapy. The drug regimen is determined by urgency rather than by the possibility of emerging resistance. Prompt treatment with a multiple-drug regimen may be required when the anatomic location carries special risk, as in tuberculous meningitis, pericarditis, or spondylitis (Pott's disease). Initial treatment with INH alone is adequate when there is no immediate threat of loss of vital function, as in tuberculous lymphadenitis or peritonitis.

Miliary Tuberculosis
(Generalized Hematogenous or Lymphohematogenous Tuberculosis)

When metastatic foci are located near blood vessel lumens, the development of hypersensitivity and its attendant necrosis may result in secondary reseeding of the bloodstream, causing **early postprimary tuberculous septicemia (hyperacute miliary TB)**. High fever and general toxicity are usually present. Tuberculous meningitis is a common complication, particularly in young children. Early in the course, the chest x-ray may be negative due to the small size of the inflammatory foci; the tuberculin test may also be negative. Choroidal tubercles are usually present and are important in **diagnosis**. Cultures of sputum or gastric contents are often positive; urine cultures are occasionally positive even without demonstrable GU involvement. Examination and culture of the bone marrow may provide the only evidence of tuberculous infection. Maximally effective drug **therapy** is indicated, usually with INH and SM, or INH and RMP.

Late hematogenous dissemination or chronic hematogenous TB follows breakdown of a longstanding, previously quiescent and undetected, usually extrapulmonary focus of TB. Multiple, widely spaced episodes of bacteremic seeding may occur from these foci. When immunity wanes, cellular components of the inflammatory process may be lacking, as in **nonreactive TB** in which myriads of tubercle bacilli exist in the tissues with only a sparse nonspecific cellular response. The clinical manifestations may be extremely subtle, consisting simply of loss of appetite and weight, and failure to thrive. Fever may be present. Marrow involvement occasionally produces syndromes resembling such primary hematologic diseases as refractory anemia, thrombocytopenia, and leukemoid reaction. There is often no evidence of pulmonary disease and the tuberculin test is usually negative.

Diagnosis may be established by culture of any body fluid or tissue. Bone marrow examination is very important. The key to diagnosis is keeping the syndrome in mind, and, in the absence of contraindications, assessing results of a therapeutic trial of chemotherapy, usually with INH alone. Response is prompt; abrupt improvement in health, nutrition, and vigor generally supports the diagnosis. When the diagnosis is established on histologic or cultural grounds rather than by response to therapy with INH, double-drug **therapy** with INH and SM or INH and RMP is usually recommended.

Central Nervous System Tuberculosis

Tuberculous meningitis develops following rupture of a metastatic subependymal focus of TB into the subarachnoid space. When it complicates miliary disease, it usually develops several weeks after the initial manifestations of the miliary process, indicating that it is not due to direct bloodstream contamination of the CSF. Incidence is highest in children aged 1 to 5 yr, but the disease may occur at any age. Symptoms may be so acute as to resemble bacterial meningitis, or may be chronic with emphasis on headache and perhaps behavioral changes. Usually, however, there are significant alterations in consciousness ranging from drowsiness to stupor or coma; a variety of cranial nerve or long tract signs may be present. Permanent complications and sequelae may occur, including convulsive disorders, communicating hydrocephalus, subarachnoid block, mental retardation, and focal neurologic abnormalities.

Diagnosis is strongly suspected when there is a past history of TB or of exposure to someone with it, or when demonstrable tuberculous foci are present elsewhere in the body. The tuberculin test is usually positive. The key to the diagnosis, however, is CSF examination. Direct acid-fast staining of the solid pellicle which commonly forms over CSF fluid left standing in a tube for 3 h is helpful in 10 to 20% of cases. In most cases, the cell count is between 100 and 600/cu mm and is principally mononuclear. However, the pleocytosis may occasionally be predominantly polymorphonuclear, especially early in the course of the illness. Positive cultures have also been obtained from fluids with virtually no cellular content. CSF protein concentration is usually elevated. Simultaneous blood and CSF samples should be obtained for glucose determination. The CSF glucose content is typically less than half that of the simultaneously obtained blood. CSF culture is usually positive, but this is of little practical importance in determining initial therapy because of the long delay before results are available. A low CSF glucose content and mononuclear pleocytosis are most characteristic, but may also accompany fungal meningitis, meningeal involvement with carcinoma or lymphoma, and, rarely, partially treated bacterial meningitis.

Treatment consists of maximum chemotherapy, usually with INH and SM or INH and RMP. Adjunctive therapy with corticosteroids (e.g., prednisone 60 mg/day orally in 4 divided doses) is recommended for inflammatory complications. The symptoms of meningeal inflammation are an excellent guide to the duration of corticosteroid therapy and the rapidity of dosage tapering. Usually, corticosteroids are given at full dosage for about 2 wk and discontinued by 4 to 6 wk.

Tuberculomas produce symptoms of mass brain lesions, usually without evidence of infection, and are most often discovered at craniotomy. With **chemotherapy** (INH and RMP for 1 yr followed by 2 more yr of INH alone), the process can be expected to subside or cease to progress, and removal of function-compromising tissue without more radical tissue removal is adequate.

Pleural Tuberculosis

Pleural TB occurs in at least 2 forms differing in pathogenesis and clinical import. **Primary serofibrinous pleurisy with effusion** is an important clinical manifestation of TB, though pulmonary parenchymal disease may not be discernible. It most frequently occurs soon after initial infection. Due to the necrotizing effect of hypersensitivity, a previously quiet metastatic subpleural focus may suddenly become inflamed and rupture into the pleural space, producing an allergic effusion of mononuclear cells, protein, and pleural fluid enzyme (LDH) concentrations characteristic of exudates. Systemic symptoms may be marked or entirely lacking. A high degree of reactivity to tuberculin is commonly present. Direct inspection of the pleural cavity at thoracotomy or by thoracoscopy shows many small tubercles studding the surfaces. Tubercle bacilli are rarely seen on direct examination of the fluid; culture is positive in about $\frac{1}{3}$ of the cases. Pleural needle biopsy should be performed; histologic evidence of TB is present in most patients. Culture of the pleural biopsy specimen is also often positive. Pleural effusions with a mononuclear pleocytosis in a tuberculin-positive individual should be considered tuberculous unless proved otherwise. **Treatment,** usually with INH alone, is mandatory. Although the pleural involvement is usually self-limited and resolves with no visible residua, or, rarely, with some pleural fibrosis, most untreated patients develop progressive TB in the lung or elsewhere within 5 yr.

Tuberculous empyema is usually a chronic and generally progressive complication of an established focus of chronic pulmonary TB. The pleural fluid is frankly purulent and loculation is common. Bronchopleural fistula may occur as the initial cause or as a complication of the empyema. Resolution does not usually occur spontaneously or with chemotherapy, and surgical drainage is usually required. Though most often due to rupture of a noninfectious subpleural bleb, spontaneous pneumothorax followed by development of a tuberculous empyema or bronchopleural fistula suggests a tuberculous etiology and requires **treatment** as for established pulmonary TB in addition to surgical drainage.

Tuberculous Pericarditis

Tuberculous pericarditis is most commonly due to direct extension from involved mediastinal nodes, or, rarely, to generalized hematogenous dissemination. The initial presentation may be acute, with systemic symptoms and rapid development of compromised cardiac function, or may be extremely indolent, in some instances becoming clinically manifest only when scarring and retraction lead to constrictive pericarditis. There may be no clinical evidence of coexistent TB in the lungs or elsewhere. The tuberculin test is usually positive.

The **diagnosis** of tuberculous pericarditis is very difficult to establish. The presence of a pericardial effusion or constrictive pericarditis can be readily established, but it is extremely difficult to prove the etiology of the effusion. There is considerable risk of morbidity and some mortality associated with pericardiocentesis; the fluid obtained very rarely provides prompt evidence of TB and is culture-positive in less than half the cases. The clinical usefulness of a positive culture is compromised by the time necessary for the tubercle bacilli to grow. Pericardial biopsy considerably improves diagnostic accuracy by providing tissue for histologic study and culture, but false-negative reports may be obtained even then.

Infection usually responds to **therapy** with a maximal chemotherapeutic regimen, usually INH and SM. There is uncertainty concerning the proper use of corticosteroids and surgery in treatment. Combined administration of corticosteroids and antimycobacterials may prevent chronic scarring and constriction in some cases. The use of corticosteroids, however, requires a definitive diagnosis since other infectious processes unresponsive to antimycobacterial chemotherapy may occasionally produce a similar clinical picture. Pericardiocentesis may be necessary for relief or prevention of cardiac tamponade. Pericardectomy is advisable if the pericarditis becomes chronic or if hemodynamic evidence of constriction persists. If scarring, fibrosis, chronic constriction, and adhesion of the visceral pericardium to the myocardium have developed, pericardectomy may be technically difficult; performed earlier, it is simpler.

Genitourinary Tuberculosis

Tuberculous pyelonephritis begins as a small cortical focus seeded hematogenously. It does not progress until the infection reaches the medulla. Local symptoms may be subtle or absent (though fever and weight loss may be present) and the patient often appears to be in surprisingly good health. Renal cavities may be seen on IVP as calyceal deformities with areas of reflux of the dye from the pelvis to the interstitial area. When the process is longstanding, renal calcification and pyelographic evidence of pyelonephritis may constitute the only available clinical data. Symptoms of lower urinary tract involvement due to intracanalicular spread from the kidneys to the ureters, bladder, seminal vesicles, and even prostate are variable. Cystitis associated with pyuria without culturable bacterial urinary pathogens suggests tuberculous infection. Once the infection reaches the pelvis, inflammation of other genitourinary organs develops. Indolent draining perineal fistulas or an unexplained epididymal mass may be the first evidence of genitourinary TB.

Treatment consists of multiple-drug therapy, usually INH and SM or possibly, in older or uremic individuals, INH and EMB. Frequent pyelograms are indicated during the course of treatment to detect possible ureteral constriction. Nephrectomy is seldom indicated. Treatment with INH alone is satisfactory for TB localized to the epididymis, testes, or perineum.

Tuberculous salpingo-oophoritis is probably acquired hematogenously. It may remain clinically silent or may present as acute or chronic pelvic inflammatory disease. It has been a major cause of sterility. Laparotomy may be required for diagnosis. Culture of uterine scrapings or culture and biopsy of cervical lesions is occasionally diagnostic. Response to **chemotherapy** (INH alone) is usually prompt; surgery is unnecessary in most cases.

Tuberculosis of the Gastrointestinal Tract

Gastrointestinal TB may occur anywhere from the mouth to the anus as superficial mucosal ulcerations caused by continuous surface contamination, or as hyperplastic involvement of the wall of a viscus presenting as an obstructing lesion. The latter may occur without obvious active pulmonary TB, is almost always discovered during surgery for a suspected carcinoma, and heals promptly with chemotherapy (INH alone or INH plus EMB if there is coexistent pulmonary disease), even when the tissue has been interrupted at surgery. Where bovine TB is common, ingestion of contaminated milk may produce primary lesions in the GI tract, most frequently in the oropharynx. **TB of the stomach** is rare, usually presenting as a rigid hyperplastic wall involvement resembling linitis plastica due to carcinoma or lymphoma. Hyperplastic involvement of the **duodenum**, also rare, may resemble an obstructing lesion. Superficial mucosal involvement of the **small and large intestine** may result in profound malabsorption, but responds to drug therapy. TB of the **cecum**, probably the most frequent form of intestinal TB, may cause obstruction or bleeding with diarrhea.

Tuberculous Peritonitis

Tuberculous peritonitis may be due to spread from adjacent lymph nodes, a gastrointestinal focus, or tuberculous salpingo-oophoritis. Clinically, it ranges from an indolent illness with a doughy-feeling abdomen, local tenderness, and systemic signs of infection, to a process resembling acute bacterial peritonitis. The peritoneal exudate is usually mononuclear.

Diagnosis is reasonably established by prompt response to antituberculous **chemotherapy**, usually with INH alone. If invasive diagnostic technics are used, an open peritoneal biopsy is safer than a needle biopsy. The major differential diagnosis is peritoneal carcinomatosis.

Tuberculosis of the Adrenals

TB of the adrenals occurs occasionally as a result of hematogenous dissemination. The glands may be totally destroyed, causing adrenal cortical insufficiency (Addison's disease). **Treatment** with INH alone is adequate. Adrenal cortical hormone replacement therapy is also necessary.

Tuberculosis of Bones and Joints

TB of a peripheral joint is usually monarticular and involves the hip, knee, elbow, or wrist, producing a purulent arthritis from which organisms are easily recovered. Rarely, cystic areas of osteomyelitis due to TB are found in the long bones or digits. Response to **chemotherapy** (INH alone) is usually prompt. Immobilization and avoidance of weight bearing may be required to relieve pain.

Tuberculous spondylitis (Pott's disease) is a serious form of TB; neurologic damage frequently occurs. Symptoms are variable. Nagging local back pain may be present and may be referred to the anterior abdominal wall and mistaken for appendicitis or another abdominal disorder. A tender, prominent spinal process may develop due to anterior wedging of 2 vertebral bodies. A paraspinal abscess may extend and present as a mass in the groin or the supraclavicular space; symptoms may develop due to dissection of tissue by the abscess. Compression of the spinal cord by the paraspinal abscess or by intrusion of granulation tissue on the anterior aspects of the cord causes symptoms ranging from minor loss of bowel and urinary sphincter control to abrupt and irreversible paraplegia.

X-rays reveal anterior destruction of 2 or more adjacent vertebral bodies, loss of the intervertebral disc, anterior wedging of the vertebrae, and presence of a paraspinal abscess. Spondylitis due to staphylococci, gram-negative enterobacteria, and, less commonly, fungus infections such as blastomycosis may produce similar clinical and x-ray evidence. If active TB is or has been present elsewhere in the body, a strong presumptive **diagnosis** of tuberculous spondylitis can be made. However, surgical exploration of the lateral aspects of the vertebral column is often necessary to provide tissue for culture and histologic study.

Treatment with chemotherapy, usually INH and SM, and bed rest is usually satisfactory in neurologically uncomplicated disease. Posterior spinal fusion is safe and probably contributes to the firmness of healing (if instability of the spine is likely), but morbidity following prolonged immobilization is substantial. A major conflict surrounds the usual orthopedic recommendation that the spinal column be explored and debrided extensively along its anterior aspect. Serious worsening of the neurologic status of the patient has occurred and the procedure should be *avoided* if possible.

Tuberculous Lymphadenitis

Before the control of bovine TB, most tuberculous lymphadenitis occurred as **scrofula,** cervical lymphadenitis due to primary infection in the oropharyngeal lymphatic tissue. Scrofula, now rare in this context, is common in other mycobacterial infections. Currently, TB of the lymph nodes represents lymphohematogenous spread from a primary pulmonary focus. The process may be clinically disseminated, involving nodes in many parts of the body, or may be localized. Diagnosis is usually made by excisional biopsy. Response to INH alone is usually prompt and permanent.

Tuberculosis of the Mouth, Middle Ear, Larynx, and Bronchial Tree

TB of the mouth is almost always associated with a pulmonary cavity, but an oral ulcer or a tooth socket that does not heal after dental extraction may suggest an otherwise silent pulmonary cavitary lesion. **TB of the middle ear** represents extreme cephalad spread of the infection, presumably via the eustachian tube. Tuberculous otitis media is characterized by persistent drainage and multiple perforations of the tympanic membrane. Profound conductive hearing loss and intracranial complications may occur. **Tuberculous involvement of the larynx** is rare and usually due to cephalad extension of highly infectious bronchial secretions, or, occasionally, to hematogenous spread. Severe pain occurs on swallowing. Laryngeal carcinoma must be excluded. **Bronchial TB** is an invariable feature of cavitary pulmonary TB. The draining bronchi are superficially infected, granulation tissue forms, and, rarely, cicatrization and obstruction occur. Hemoptysis in pulmonary TB often originates from inflamed bronchial mucosa. Considerable bronchial distortion is almost always present following extensive pulmonary TB. Response of these types of TB to any INH-containing drug regimen is prompt and excellent.

OTHER MYCOBACTERIAL INFECTIONS RESEMBLING TUBERCULOSIS

Mycobacteria other than the tubercle and lepra bacillus cause disease in man pathologically and clinically similar to TB. They include *M. kansasii* and *M. marinum* (Group I), *M. scrofulaceum* (Group II), *M. intracellulare* and *M. avium* (Group III), and *M. fortuitum* (Group IV). *M. chelonei* subsp. *abscessus* is generally not included in this Runyon grouping. The organisms are INH-resistant, catalase-positive, and niacin-negative. They may cause chronic pulmonary disease and, rarely, (usually in immunologically compromised patients) disseminated disease in adults, cutaneous abscesses and granulomas, and, particularly in children, bone and joint involvement, lymphadenitis, and disseminated disease including meningitis. Person-to-person transmission has not been proved; the organisms presumably exist in the environment.

Pulmonary disease: *M. intracellulare* and *M. kansasii* are the usual etiologic agents. Most cases occur in white men over age 40. Systemic symptoms are frequently absent, but progressive pulmonary insufficiency occurs. Chemotherapy with 2 effective drugs or 3 or more partially effective drugs is based on demonstrating drug sensitivities of the organism. In the absence of drug sensitivity testing, RMP, EMB, and SM may be an effective combination, particularly in *M. kansasii* infection, though not in *M. intracellulare* infection. Resection of cavities may be helpful in *M. intracellulare* infections, but is seldom necessary in *M. kansasii* infections. Coexistent chronic lung disease and the anatomic extent of infection often make this impossible.

Cutaneous disease: "Swimming pool" granuloma is a protracted but self-limited superficial granulomatous ulcerating infection caused by *M. marinum* contracted from contaminated swimming pools and occasionally from home aquariums. The infection is pathologically similar to TB. Healing occurs spontaneously, though RMP may hasten healing. *M. abscessus* causes a deeper and more persistent cutaneous granulomatous abscess on the exposed parts of the body. Its epidemiology is unknown and the response to drug treatment is virtually nil.

Bone and joint involvement: Widespread lytic bone disease may rarely occur in children. Joint involvement, and, more rarely, cutaneous fistula formation may occur as complications. The infections are usually drug-resistant, but RMP, EMB, and SM may be tried.

Lymphadenitis: In the USA, these organisms probably cause infectious granulomatous lymphadenitis more frequently than does the tubercle bacillus. The portal of entry is probably the eye, pharynx, GI tract, or abraded skin. Many cases are due to local spread from the site of primary infection. Response to drug therapy varies; surgical excision is recommended when the process persists.

Disseminated disease is rare, occurring particularly in children and in immunologically compromised older individuals. It may resemble malignant reticuloendotheliosis, except that the causative organisms are readily recovered. Meningitis may also occur, and, rarely, extensive miliary-like pulmonary involvement. Treatment with maximum chemotherapy (INH, SM, RMP, or another combination based on sensitivity testing) is usually tried, almost always with disappointing results.

LEPROSY
(Hansen's Disease)

A chronic infectious disease caused by Mycobacterium leprae, *an organism with high infectivity but low pathogenicity and with a predilection for skin, mucous membranes, and peripheral nerves.*

Etiology and Distribution

M. leprae is an acid-fast bacillus that may appear as solids, fragmented rods, or granular bodies. Although prolonged, close (skin-to-skin) contact with infected persons has long been the proposed mode of transmission, it is now believed more likely that spread of the bacillus is respiratory, via bacilli-laden nasal discharges. Arthropods may play a role in transmission, but this has not yet been established.

Only a small percentage of exposed persons acquire the disease, although evidence suggests that many more have been infected but possess adequate immunity to prevent clinical disease. This can be detected by demonstrating the presence of *M. leprae* in an otherwise healthy individual or by measuring the individual's immunologic responsiveness against *M. leprae* as described below under Diagnosis.

Leprosy is found worldwide, but its major distribution is in a broad equatorial band that includes Africa, Southeast Asia, and South America. Of the estimated 12 to 20 million cases, about 2000 are in the continental USA. Endemic foci exist in Texas, Louisiana, and Hawaii. The disease is also seen in California, Florida, and New York City, primarily among immigrants.

Types and Clinical Course

Leprosy is classified as indeterminate, tuberculoid, dimorphous (borderline), and lepromatous. In all forms, skin and peripheral nerve lesions are the dominant clinical findings.

Indeterminate leprosy shows a nonspecific inflammatory cellular response and often goes unrecognized. The earliest skin lesion is usually a poorly defined, hypopigmented or erythematous macule 1 or 2 cm in diameter. The disease usually regresses, with spontaneous healing of the lesion, but may progress to one of the three distinct types.

Tuberculoid skin lesions tend to be large and well-defined, single or few in number, usually anesthetic, and asymmetric. Acid-fast bacilli are few and difficult to find. Breakdown products of *M. leprae* stimulate lymphocyte production with epithelioid and Langhans' giant cells histologically resembling a tubercle. The patient's resistance is high, and spontaneous recovery may occur.

Lepromatous lesions are numerous and small, with poorly defined margins. Macules are most common; papules, nodules, or plaques also occur. The entire body surface may be so diffusely involved that no distinct lesion is identifiable. Histologically, the lesions possess large numbers of bacilli occurring singly and in clumps. Collections of bacilli are present in macrophages with a honeycomb-like cytoplasm (termed "foamy histiocytes" or "leprae cells"). The patient's resistance to *M. leprae* is low, and untreated lepromatous leprosy is always progressive.

Dimorphous (borderline) lesions show clinical and histopathologic features of both the tuberculoid and lepromatous "polar" types; acid-fast bacilli may be numerous. Dimorphous leprosy is unstable; it may regress toward the tuberculoid form or progress toward the lepromatous form, depending upon whether treatment is received or not, with the shifts that occur reflecting the patient's immunologic status.

Nerve lesions: *M. leprae* invades peripheral nerves where the temperature is lower than core body temperature. Leprous neuritis may affect sensory or sensorimotor nerves or both, particularly the terminal cutaneous branches (producing anesthesia of a lesion) or the nerve trunk (producing anesthesia along the distribution of its cutaneous innervation). Both trunk and branches are involved in advanced cases, and complete "glove" or "stocking" anesthesia results.

Paralysis and deformity follow sensory loss. Facial paralysis is most often limited to lagophthalmos, which often ends in blindness if the cornea is insensitive. Claw hand follows paralysis of the intrinsic muscles of the hand. Wrist-drop is rare, but foot-drop and claw toe deformities are common and are often accompanied by wounds, especially plantar ulcers, and secondary infection. Destruction of the fingers, producing a mitten hand, and of the foot, resulting in a short foot with eventual collapse of the tarsus, are occasional late complications of trauma and infection imposed on a denervated extremity. At least 25% of patients have some disfigurement and disabling deformity.

Peripheral nerves in lepromatous disease may be enlarged, with numerous bacilli, yet show little clinical change and minimal pain. Paralysis and sensory loss develop insidiously over several years. Neural involvement in tuberculoid leprosy is more abrupt. Caseation necrosis destroys the nerve, producing sudden paralysis. Painful neuritides are usually associated with acute reaction episodes.

Reflexes are not affected. Deep-pain perception and proprioception are not lost until late in the disease.

Acute reactions: To simplify this complex subject, only the two most common categories, **reversal reactions** and **erythema nodosum leprosum (ENL)**, are described. Reversal reactions, seen in all but pure lepromatous leprosy, apparently are the result of a spontaneous shift in the patient's cell-mediated immunologic status toward *M. leprae* to a state of higher immunity. If, for example, the shift is from dimorphous toward tuberculoid, the lesions may become erythematous and edematous and may progress to ulceration. Multiple nerves may be damaged and fever is common. ENL, by contrast, does not seem to be associated with a cell-mediated immunologic shift, but instead is probably humoral and may be a manifestation of the Arthus phenomenon (see Type III Hypersensitivity Reactions in §2, Ch. 4). It is most common in lepromatous patients, but may also be seen in dimorphous cases. It usually presents as a fever, with multiple painful erythematous nodules that may appear wherever bacilli are present. A neuritis, iritis, lymphadenitis, leukocytosis, orchitis, and arthritis may accompany it.

Other manifestations are the result of progressive dimorphous and lepromatous disease. The face is commonly affected, and the nasal, oral, and pharyngeal mucosa may be involved. Nasal stuffiness and epistaxis are early occurrences; later, ulceration and necrosis destroy supporting cartilages, causing nasal deformity and collapse. Isolated lesions of the lip, tongue, and palate resemble malignancy. Loss of the eyebrows and enlarged earlobes are common.

The eyes are frequently involved, either by direct infection or in an acute reaction. Conjunctivitis, keratitis, corneal ulceration, iridocyclitis, anterior choroiditis, and glaucoma may occur and, if untreated, may lead to blindness.

Orchitis, often leading to testicular atrophy, and gynecomastia may occur in advanced lepromatous leprosy. Lymph nodes may enlarge and develop abscesses, particularly in the supraclavicular, axillary, and inguinal areas. Osteitis is only rarely identified radiographically, but bone marrow biopsy in lepromatous disease usually produces acid-fast bacilli. The spleen, liver, and kidney are involved in advanced lepromatous disease, and late in the course of the infection amyloidosis occasionally develops.

Diagnosis

Leprosy may mimic many other diseases involving the skin and peripheral nerves. Diagnosis is established by biopsy. Centrally anesthetic lesions should be biopsied at the margin where acid-fast bacilli are most likely to be found, although bacilli are sparse in indeterminate and tuberculoid leprosy. Skin smears are useful as a follow-up on treatment and as an indication of the extent of the disease.

The pathohistologic findings on skin biopsy best differentiate the type of leprosy. Another aid to differentiation is the **lepromin test** (intradermal injection of autoclaved bacilli from human lepromas), which is positive in tuberculoid and negative in lepromatous leprosy. A positive early lepromin reaction in tuberculin-negative children is considered evidence of infection with the leprosy bacillus. Definite in vitro evidence of immunologic responsiveness is provided by the lymphocyte transformation test and the leukocyte migration inhibition test. A positive lepromin test and these 2 in vitro tests apparently depend upon the same underlying mechanism: the cell-mediated immune response to the leprosy bacillus. Usually, this does not result in any clinical manifestations.

Prophylaxis

Control requires active case finding and early treatment. A patient is no longer thought to pose a public health problem once his disease is controlled by therapy. Prophylaxis with BCG vaccine or dapsone may be useful, but results to date are inconclusive. In the USA contacts without disease should be examined every 6 to 12 mo. Cure by immediate therapy can be expected should a lesion be found early.

Treatment

The sulfones are the drugs of choice. Though tuberculoid and indeterminate cases may heal spontaneously, every active case is treated. Response to therapy is variable, but the disease may be arrested in the great majority of cases. Generally, long-term therapy is required. Medication must be taken regularly since interrupted therapy may produce sulfone-resistant bacilli with exacerbation and progression of the disease.

Dapsone (4,4'-diaminodiphenyl sulfone, **DDS**), the parent sulfone, is generally prescribed. It is taken orally. Therapy is usually begun with 25 mg/wk for 2 wk, then increased by 25 mg every 2 wk until 100 mg/wk is reached. Dosage is then increased by 50 mg every 2 wk until the maintenance level is reached. Active indeterminate and tuberculoid leprosy are usually treated with 25 mg/day, continued for 2 yr after the disease becomes inactive. Dimorphous and lepromatous leprosy are treated with 50 mg/day, continued in dimorphous leprosy for 10 yr after the disease becomes inactive and for life in those with lepromatous disease. Side effects from dapsone 100 mg/day or less are infrequent. Mild hemolytic anemia is a common finding. Patients with G6PD deficiency, however, may experience more severe hemolysis. Agranulocytosis is a potentially serious but rare complication.

Sulfoxone is given if there is gastric intolerance to DDS; 330 mg are therapeutically equivalent to about 50 to 100 mg of DDS. Solapsone (solasulfone) and acedapsone (4,4'-diacetyldiaminodiphenyl sulfone, DADDS) are experimental drugs in the USA but are available elsewhere. Diphenylthiourea (thiocarbanilide) and streptomycin have been used in selected cases but lose their effectiveness within 2 yr.

Rifampin 600 mg/day for prolonged periods appears promising. It is bactericidal for *M. leprae* whereas all other drugs are bacteriostatic. At present it is used primarily in patients whose bacilli have become sulfone-resistant. Clofazimine 100 mg/day is also effective in these patients, but skin pigmentation limits its usefulness. Both drugs are considered experimental for use in leprosy. Rifampin is available commercially; clofazimine, from the USPHS Hospital at Carville, La.

Lepromatous leprosy may be difficult to control, and patients should be observed closely and frequently. If the disease is progressive despite therapy, drug resistance may have developed. This should be confirmed with mouse-footpad drug sensitivity studies before therapy is changed.

Mild **reactional states** are treated with bed rest and analgesics; more severe reactions may be managed with corticosteroids. Thalidomide, an experimental drug in the USA available through the USPHS Carville Hospital, is currently the treatment of choice for acute ENL reactions. Clofazimine 300 mg/day will also control ENL; though the pigmentation with these high doses is unacceptable to many patients, it may be the only alternative to prolonged high-dose corticosteroid therapy for severe reversal reactions.

The immediate recognition and treatment of **eye problems** is essential. Inadequate closure of the eyelids subjects the insensitive cornea to the drying effects of exposure and to trauma with infection and ulceration. Corneal dryness can be treated with commercial artificial teardrops, or ophthalmic mucin substitutes. Further management of lagophthalmos depends on many factors, but surgery may be beneficial. In general, the patient should be referred to an ophthalmologist for treatment of lagophthalmos associated with an insensitive cornea or intrinsic disease due to a leprous infiltrate or associated reaction.

Supportive care is important to protect insensitive or deformed eyes, hands, and feet from repeated injuries and infection that lead to mutilation. Deformities may be corrected surgically to improve function. Shoes are built to conform to residual deformity and to distribute weight-bearing evenly.

The patient must be educated to realize his problems and their potential dangers, to protect himself from trauma and infection, and to avert progressive destruction by daily inspection for early changes.

Physicians at the USPHS Hospital in Carville, La., are available to the medical profession at all times for consultation on leprosy-related matters.

CAUSED BY SPIROCHETES

SYPHILIS
(See §21, Ch. 1)

ENDEMIC TREPONEMATOSES
(Bejel, Yaws, and Pinta)

Chronic nonvenereal spirochetal infections, spread by body contact. Treponema pallidum II **(bejel)**, *T. pertenue* **(yaws)**, *and T. carateum* **(pinta)** *are morphologically and serologically indistinguishable from T. pallidum (syphilis).*

Epidemiology
Bejel is mainly found in Arab countries of the eastern Mediterranean and North Africa; yaws, in humid equatorial countries; and pinta, among the Indians of Mexico, Central America, and northern South America.

Clinical Course
Bejel (nonvenereal syphilis) begins as a mucous patch, usually on the buccal mucosa, followed by papulosquamous and erosive papular lesions of the trunk and extremities. Periostitis of the bones of the legs is common. Gummatous lesions of the nose and soft palate develop in later stages.

Yaws (frambesia) begins as a granulomatous lesion at the inoculation site, usually on the legs, after an incubation period of several weeks. The lesion heals but is followed by a generalized eruption of soft granulomas of the face, extremities, and buttocks, often at mucocutaneous junctions. These heal slowly and may relapse. Keratotic lesions may develop on the soles and cause painful ulcerations. Destructive lesions may develop years later, including periostitis (particularly of the tibia), proliferative exostoses of the nasal portion of the maxillary bone **(goundou)**, juxta-articular nodules, gummatous skin lesions, and, ultimately, mutilating facial ulcers, particularly around the nose **(gangosa)**.

Pinta begins at the inoculation site as small papules that progress to erythematous plaques in several months. Erythematous, squamous patches develop later, mainly on the extremities, face, and neck. After several years, slate-blue patches develop, usually symmetrically and generally on the face and extremities and over bony prominences; these later become depigmented, resembling vitiligo. Hyperkeratosis may occur on the soles and palms.

Diagnosis

Diagnosis is made from the typical appearance of lesions in persons from endemic areas. The VDRL and FTA-ABS tests are positive but do not distinguish these diseases from venereal syphilis. Early lesions are often darkfield-positive for spirochetes indistinguishable from *T. pallidum.*

Treatment

In each disease, a single IM injection of 2.4 million u. of procaine penicillin G in oil or benzathine penicillin G produces healing, with rapid disappearance of the spirochetes. Destructive lesions leave a scar.

RELAPSING FEVER
(Tick, Recurrent, Spirillum, or Famine Fever)

An acute infectious disease caused by several species of spirochetes, transmitted by lice and ticks, and characterized by recurrent febrile paroxysms lasting 3 to 10 days, with intervals of apparent recovery.

Etiology and Epidemiology

Relapsing fever is the term applied to a group of spirochetal fevers, clinically similar but etiologically distinct, caused by different *Borrelia* species. The insect vector may be the head and body louse or ticks of the genus *Ornithodoros,* depending on geographic location. The louse-borne relapsing fevers are endemic in Europe, Asia, and Africa; the tick-borne, in the Americas, Africa, Asia, and Europe. In the USA, the disease is generally confined to the western states.

The various species of spirochete are morphologically indistinguishable delicate threadlike organisms 8 to 30 μ long, with pointed ends and 4 to 10 large irregular coils. They appear in the blood during a paroxysm, and can be found in internal organs, especially the spleen and brain.

The louse is infected by feeding on a patient during the febrile stage. It usually infects man when spirochetes released from a crushed louse enter abraded skin or are transmitted to the conjunctiva by contaminated hands. Ticks acquire the spirochetes from animals acting as reservoirs, and infect man when spirochetes in the tick's saliva or coxal fluid (excreta) enter the skin as the tick bites.

Symptoms, Signs, and Prognosis

Following an incubation period of about 7 days, sudden chills usher in the disease, followed by high fever, tachycardia, severe headache, vomiting, muscle and joint pain, and often delirium. An erythematous rash may appear early over the trunk and extremities, followed by rose-colored spots; subcutaneous or submucous hemorrhages may be present. Urine contains albumin and casts during the febrile stage. Marked polymorphonuclear leukocytosis is present. Late in the course of the fever, jaundice, hepatomegaly, and splenomegaly may appear, especially in cases of louse-borne disease. Fever remains high for 3 to 10 days, then clears abruptly by crisis.

The patient is essentially asymptomatic for several days to a week or more; relapse then occurs with all the former symptoms and signs. Jaundice is more common during relapse. The illness clears as before, but from 2 to 10 similar paroxysms may follow at 1- to 2-wk intervals. The paroxysms usually become progressively less severe, and recovery eventually occurs as the patient develops immunity.

The mortality rate is generally low (2 to 8%) but may be considerably higher in very young, old, or debilitated persons, or during epidemics of louse-borne fever.

Diagnosis

Relapsing fevers may be confused with malaria, dengue, yellow fever, Weil's disease, typhus, influenza, smallpox, and the enteric fevers. Diagnosis is suggested by the recurrent fever and confirmed by the appearance of spirochetes in the blood during a paroxysm. Darkfield examination or thick and thin Wright- or Giemsa-stained blood smears will disclose the spirochetes. Intraperitoneal injection of the patient's blood into a mouse or rat usually produces large numbers of spirochetes in the animal's tail blood, examined in the same way on postinjection days 3 through 5.

Prophylaxis

Dusting the undergarments and inner surfaces of clothing with DDT, malathion, or lindane powders will protect against relapsing fever resulting from infestations of body or head lice. Tick-borne infections are more difficult to prevent because of the inadequacy of insect control measures (these are described under ROCKY MOUNTAIN SPOTTED FEVER in §1, Ch. 3).

Treatment

Therapy should be started early in the paroxysm or during the afebrile stage, but should be avoided near the end of a paroxysm because of the danger of a Herxheimer reaction. A tetracycline or chloramphenicol 0.5 Gm orally q 6 h is given for 5 to 10 days. The dose should be proportionately reduced in children. When vomiting or severe disease precludes oral administration, 500 mg in 100 or 500 ml of saline may be given IV once or twice/day.

In the rare instances when the spirochete is antibiotic-resistant, an arsenical (e.g., oxophenarsine 40 to 60 mg IV) may be given as fever is rising, or during the afebrile period.

Dehydration and electrolyte imbalance should be corrected with parenteral dextrose and saline. Codeine 30 to 60 mg orally q 4 to 6 h may be used to relieve severe headache. Nausea and vomiting should be treated with dimenhydrinate 50 to 100 mg orally or rectally (or 50 mg IM) q 4 h, or with prochlorperazine 5 to 10 mg orally or IM 1 to 4 times/day.

LEPTOSPIROSIS
(Weil's Disease or Syndrome; Infectious [Spirochetal] Jaundice)

An inclusive term applied to all infections due to an organism of the genus Leptospira, *regardless of serotype.* About 130 serotypes have been identified. A single serotype may cause a variety of clinical features, or a single syndrome (e.g., aseptic meningitis) may be caused by multiple serotypes.

Epidemiology

Leptospirosis, a zoonosis, occurs in several domestic and wild animal hosts, varying from an inapparent illness to a fatal disease. A carrier state exists in which animals shed leptospires in their urine for months. Human infections occur by direct contact with an infected animal's urine or tissue, or indirectly by contact with contaminated water or soil. Abraded skin and exposed mucous membranes (conjunctival, nasal, oral) are the usual portals of entry in man. Infection occurs at any age. At least 75% of those infected are males; in the USA ⅔ of infections occur from June through September. Leptospirosis can be an occupational disease (e.g., of farmers and sewer and abattoir workers), but most patients are exposed incidentally during recreational activities. Dogs, immersion (e.g., swimming) in contaminated water, and rats are the most common probable sources. From 40 to 140 cases are reported annually in the USA.

Clinical Features

The incubation period ranges from 2 to 20 (usually 7 to 13) days. The disease is characteristically biphasic. The **leptospiremic phase** is abrupt in onset, with headache, severe muscular aches, chills, and fever. Conjunctival suffusion is characteristic, usually appearing on the 3rd or 4th day. Spleno- and hepatomegaly are uncommon. This phase lasts 4 to 9 days with recurrent chills and fever that often spikes to > 39 C (102 F). Defervescence follows; then, on the 6th to 12th day of illness, the **second** or "**immune**" **phase** occurs, correlating with the appearance of antibodies in the serum. Fever and earlier symptoms recur and meningismus may develop. CSF examination after the 7th day discloses pleocytosis in at least 50% of the patients. Iridocyclitis, optic neuritis, and peripheral neuropathy occur infrequently. If acquired during pregnancy, leptospirosis may cause abortion even during the convalescent period.

Weil's syndrome is a form of severe leptospirosis with jaundice and usually azotemia, hemorrhages, anemia, disturbances in consciousness, and continued fever. Onset is similar to that of the less severe forms; the signs of hepatocellular and renal dysfunction appear from the 3rd to 6th day. Renal abnormalities include proteinuria, pyuria, hematuria, and azotemia. Hemorrhagic manifestations are due to capillary injury. Thrombocytopenia may occur.

Aseptic meningitis may occur with any serotype. The CSF cell count is between 10 and 1000/cu mm (usually < 500), with predominantly mononuclear cells. CSF sugar is normal; protein is < 100 mg/100 ml.

Mortality is nil in anicteric patients. With occurrence of jaundice, mortality is about 15%; in patients over 60, the rate is doubled.

Laboratory Findings

The WBC count is normal or slightly elevated in most cases but may reach 50,000. Leukocytosis above 15,000 suggests liver involvement. There are usually > 70% neutrophils, a finding which may help to differentiate leptospirosis from viral illnesses. In jaundiced patients, intravascular hemolysis may cause pronounced anemia. Serum bilirubin is usually < 20 mg/100 ml but may reach 40 mg/100 ml in severe infection; BUN is usually < 100 mg/100 ml.

Diagnosis

Meningitis or meningoencephalitis, influenza, hepatitis, acute cholecystitis, and renal failure must be included in the differential diagnosis.

Leptospires may be isolated from the blood, urine, or CSF during the first phase by inoculation onto Fletcher's medium. Serologic technics, including slide and microscopic agglutination tests, and an indirect fluorescent antibody method, may be used during the second phase.

Treatment

Antibiotics such as penicillin, streptomycin, the tetracyclines, chloramphenicol, and erythromycin are effective in experimental infections, but their value in man is uncertain. They are not beneficial if given later than 4 days after onset of the disease. In severe illness, penicillin G 6 to 12 million u./day IM or IV or tetracycline 2 Gm/day orally or IV is often recommended. Fluid and electrolyte therapy are necessary for azotemia or jaundice. Isolation is not required, but care is needed in disposing of urine.

RATBITE FEVER

Ratbite fever represents 2 clinically similar but etiologically distinct diseases that may follow a rodent bite. **Streptobacillary ratbite fever,** caused by the pleomorphic gram-negative bacillus *Streptobacillus moniliformis,* is more common in the USA than **spirillary ratbite fever,** caused by *Spirillum minor.* Ratbite fever may follow up to 10% of rat bites, and is therefore a disease of ghetto dwellers and of the socially deprived, although it has become a hazard to biomedical laboratory personnel. It may be mistaken for a viral infection.

Streptobacillary Ratbite Fever

S. moniliformis is found in the oropharynx of healthy rats. Epidemics have been associated with ingestion of unpasteurized, contaminated milk **(Haverhill fever),** but infection is usually from a wild rat or mouse bite.

The primary wound usually heals promptly, but after an incubation period of 1 to 22 (usually less than 10) days, the patient abruptly develops a viral-like syndrome with chills, fever, vomiting, headache, and back and joint pains. The WBC count ranges between 6000 and 30,000. A morbilliform, petechial rash appears on the hands and feet of most patients in about 3 days. Polyarthralgia or arthritis, usually asymmetrically affecting the large joints, develops in many patients within a week and may persist for several days or for months if untreated. SBE and abscesses in the brain or other tissues are rare but serious complications.

Streptobacillary ratbite fever can usually be differentiated on clinical grounds from spirillary ratbite fever, but can be confused with Rocky Mountain spotted fever, infection with Coxsackie B virus, and meningococcemia. **Diagnosis** is confirmed by culturing the organism from blood or joint fluid. Agglutinins develop during the 2nd or 3rd wk and are diagnostically important if the titer increases.

Treatment consists of procaine penicillin G 1.2 million u./day IM, or penicillin V 2 Gm/day orally for 7 to 10 days. Erythromycin 2 Gm/day orally or IM may be used as an alternative in cases of penicillin hypersensitivity.

Spirillary Ratbite Fever (Sodoku)

Spirillum minor infection is acquired through a rat or, occasionally, a mouse bite. The wound usually heals promptly, but inflammation recurs at the site after an incubation period of 4 to 28 (usually more than 10) days, accompanied by a relapsing fever and regional lymphadenitis. The WBC count ranges between 5000 and 30,000. VDRL tests are false-positive in half the patients. A roseolar-urticarial rash sometimes develops but is less prominent than the streptobacillary rash. Arthritis is rare. In untreated patients the disease usually runs its course in 4 to 8 wk but, rarely, febrile episodes may recur for more than a year. SBE is a rare complication.

Diagnosis is made by demonstration of the spirillum in blood smears or tissue from the lesions or lymph nodes, or by Giemsa stain or darkfield examination of blood from inoculated mice. In cases with a long incubation period, if the physician is unaware of a previous rat bite, he may easily confuse the disease with malaria, meningococcemia, or *Borrelia recurrentis* infection, all of which are characterized by relapsing fever.

Treatment consists of procaine penicillin G 1.2 million u./day IM, or tetracycline 2 Gm/day orally for patients allergic to penicillin, either drug given for 7 days.

ANTHRAX
(Malignant Pustule; Woolsorter's Disease)

A highly infectious disease of animals, especially ruminants, that is transmitted to man by contact with the animals or their products. Anthrax is an important animal disease. Overt disease in man is disappearing in most parts of the world, mainly occurring in countries without public health regulations that prevent industrial exposure to infected goats, cattle, sheep, and horses, or to their products. A vaccine, composed of a culture filtrate, is available for those at high risk (veterinarians, laboratory technicians, employees of textile mills where imported goat hair is processed).

Etiology and Epidemiology

The causative organism, *Bacillus anthracis,* is a large, gram-positive, facultatively anaerobic, encapsulated rod. The spores resist destruction and remain viable in soil and animal products for decades. Human infection is usually through the skin. Inhalation of spores under adverse conditions (e.g., the presence of an acute respiratory infection) may result in pulmonary anthrax **(woolsorter's disease),** which is often fatal. Systemic disease has followed ingestion of contaminated meat.

Diagnosis

The occupational history is most important. The organism may be demonstrated in cultures or in gram-stained smears from cutaneous lesions and, in the pulmonary form, from throat swabs and sputum. Mouse inoculation may permit isolation of the organism when primary cultures are unsuccessful.

Symptoms, Signs, and Treatment

The incubation period varies from 12 h to 5 days (generally, 3 to 5 days). The **cutaneous form** begins as a red-brown papule which enlarges with considerable peripheral erythema, vesiculation, and induration. Central ulceration follows, with serosanguineous exudation and formation of a black eschar. Local lymphadenopathy may be present, occasionally with malaise, myalgia, headache, fever, nausea, and vomiting. **Treatment** with procaine penicillin G 600,000 u. IM b.i.d. prevents systemic spread and induces gradual resolution of the pustule. Tetracycline 2 Gm/day orally is also effective.

Pulmonary anthrax follows rapid multiplication of spores in the mediastinal lymph nodes. Severe hemorrhagic necrotizing lymphadenitis develops and spreads to the adjacent mediastinal structures. Serosanguineous transudation, pulmonary edema, and pleural effusion occur. Initial symptoms are insidious and influenza-like. Fever increases; within a few days, severe respiratory distress develops, followed by cyanosis, shock, and coma. Hemorrhagic meningoencephalitis may develop. Lung x-ray may show diffuse patchy infiltration; the mediastinum is widened due to enlarged hemorrhagic lymph nodes. Death is common. Antibiotic therapy is of little value when given at the toxic stage, but early and continuous IV **therapy** with penicillin G 10 million u./day may be lifesaving. Corticosteroids may be of value, but have not been adequately evaluated.

ERYSIPELOID

An acute, but slowly evolving, skin infection caused by Erysipelothrix rhusiopathiae.

Etiology

Erysipelothrix rhusiopathiae (insidiosa), a gram-positive, noncapsulated, nonsporulating, nonmotile, microaerophilic bacillus with worldwide distribution, is primarily an animal pathogen, especially for swine. Infection in man is chiefly occupational and typically follows a penetrating hand wound in persons who handle fish or animal tissues (e.g., butchers).

Symptoms, Signs, and Diagnosis

Within a week of injury a characteristic raised, purplish-red, nonvesiculated, indurated maculopapule appears, accompanied by itching and burning. Local swelling, though sharply demarcated, may inhibit use of the hand. The border of the lesion may slowly extend outward. Regional lymphatic involvement is absent. The disease is usually self-limiting; discomfort and disability may persist for 2 to 3 wk. Bacteremia is rare but may result in infection of joints or previously damaged heart valves.

The characteristic lesion and its course are diagnostic. Culture of a needle aspirate or biopsy specimen taken from the advancing edge of a lesion may yield *Erysipelothrix*.

Treatment

Benzathine penicillin G 1.2 million u. IM (600,000 u. in each buttock), or erythromycin 0.5 Gm q.i.d. orally for 7 days, is curative.

LISTERIOSIS

Infection caused by Listeria monocytogenes *with manifestations that vary according to pathogenesis, site, and age of the patient.*

Etiology, Incidence, and Epidemiology

L. monocytogenes is a gram-positive, noncapsulated, nonsporulating, motile, microaerophilic bacillus of worldwide distribution that afflicts mammals, birds, arachnids, and crustaceans. Of the 7 major serotypes, Types 1b (about 25%), 4b (about 20%), and 1a (about 15%) account for most human listerioses in the USA. Incidence is highest in neonates and in persons over 40, and peaks in July and August. The only proven transmission is antepartum and intrapartum, from mother to child, but a human carrier state exists and may be epidemiologically important. That 25% of listeriosis patients have a preexisting disease (e.g., cirrhosis, cancer) may also be significant.

Clinical Forms

Antepartum infection occurs transplacentally. Abortion, premature birth, or stillbirth usually results. Focal abscesses or granulomas are present in the fetal liver and may be found in any other organ. Listerias may be present in the meconium of live infants—the one specific finding in neonates with cardiorespiratory distress, nausea and vomiting, hypothermia, hepatosplenomegaly, and granulomas of the oropharynx and skin. **Intrapartum infection** usually results in meningitis following a 1- to 4-wk incubation period.

In the adult, **meningitis** is the most common form of listeriosis. **Endocarditis** is a rare form, as is **typhoidal listeriosis** with bacteremia and high fever and without localizing symptoms and signs. **Oculoglandular** infection, with ophthalmitis and regional lymph node involvement, follows conjunctival inoculation; if untreated, it may progress to bacteremia and meningitis.

Diagnosis

Listerial infections cannot be identified clinically, and isolation of *L. monocytogenes* is necessary for diagnosis. The laboratory must be informed of the possibility of listeriosis when specimens are sent for culture. In neonatal listeriosis specimens should be taken from cord blood, the infant's CSF and meconium, the mother's lochia and cervical and vaginal exudates, and grossly diseased parts of the placenta. In all forms, IgG agglutinin titers peak 2 to 4 wk after onset.

Treatment

For neonatal listeriosis, penicillin G should be given IV for 2 to 3 wk: 80,000 u./kg body wt q 12 h for infants under 1 wk old, and 110,000 u./kg q 8 h for those 1 to 4 wk old.

For meningitis in the adult, tetracycline has been used most often: 25 to 40 mg/kg body wt/day is divided into 4 equal doses given orally q 6 h until 1 to 2 wk after defervescence. However, erythromycin and penicillin G are more active and may be preferable. For meningitis, penicillin G 240,000 u./kg/day is given IV and continued for 1 wk after defervescence. For endocarditis and typhoidal listeriosis, both penicillin G 160,000 u./kg/day IV and erythromycin 25 to 30 mg/kg/day orally in divided doses q 6 h are given until 4 wk after defervescence. Oculoglandular listeriosis should respond to oral erythromycin or tetracycline in the above dosages, continued until 1 wk following defervescence.

---

6.   SYSTEMIC FUNGUS DISEASES
(Systemic Mycoses)

The important systemic mycoses are discussed in this chapter. Dermatophytoses and other skin infections can be found in §16, Ch. 5; pulmonary disorders caused by hypersensitivity to fungi are discussed in §5, Ch. 12.

General Diagnostic Principles

Several considerations are important in the diagnosis of the deep mycoses.

1. Many of the causative fungi are "opportunists," not usually pathogenic unless they enter a compromised host. Opportunistic fungus infections are apt to occur and should be anticipated in patients with azotemia, diabetes mellitus, bronchiectasis, emphysema, tuberculosis, Hodgkin's disease or other lymphoma, leukemia, or burns; after ionizing (x-) irradiation; and during therapy with corticosteroids, immunosuppressives, or antimetabolites. Candidiasis, aspergillosis, phycomycosis, nocardiosis, and cryptococcosis are typical opportunistic infections.

2. Fungus diseases occurring as primary infections may have a typical geographic distribution. For example, in the USA, coccidioidomycosis is virtually confined to the southwest, while histoplasmosis occurs in the east and midwest, especially in the Ohio and Mississippi River valleys. Blastomycosis is restricted to North America and Africa; paracoccidioidomycosis, often called South American blastomycosis, is confined to that continent. However, travelers can develop a symptomatic infection some time after returning from such endemic areas.

3. The major clinical characteristic of virtually every deep mycosis is its chronic course. Septicemia or an acute pneumonia is rare. Lung lesions develop slowly. Months or years may elapse before medical attention is sought or a diagnosis is made.

4. Symptoms are rarely intense; fever, chills, night sweats, anorexia, weight loss, malaise, and depression may all be present.

5. When a fungus disseminates from a primary focus in the lung, the manifestations may be characteristic. Thus, cryptococcosis usually appears as meningitis, progressive disseminated histoplasmosis as hepatic disease, and blastomycosis as a skin lesion.

6. Delayed cutaneous hypersensitivity tests and serologic tests are available for only 3 or 4 of the infections discussed in this chapter. Even in these, the tests

become positive either so late (e.g., coccidioidomycosis) or so infrequently (e.g., blastomycosis) that they are of no diagnostic value for the acutely ill patient.

7. The diagnosis is usually confirmed by isolation of the causative fungus from sputum, bone marrow, urine, blood, or CSF, or from lymph node, liver, or lung biopsy. When the fungus is a commensal of man or is prevalent in his environment (e.g., *Candida, Aspergillus)*, it is difficult to interpret its isolation from such specimens as sputum, and confirmatory evidence of tissue invasion is helpful.

8. Fungal infections, in contrast to viral and bacterial diseases, can be diagnosed histopathologically with a high degree of reliability. It is the distinctive fungal morphology, not the tissue reaction to the fungus, that permits specific etiologic identification.

9. Even when the microorganism has been demonstrated histopathologically in tissues, the activity of the disease must be established before treatment is begun. Culture of the causative microorganism or such clinical and laboratory findings as fever, leukocytosis, elevated ESR, abnormal liver function, worsening of chest film findings, or elevated serum globulins are helpful as indications for therapy.

General Therapeutic Principles

General medical care, surgery, and chemotherapy constitute modes of treatment for systemic fungus infections. Because it is used in many of the systemic mycoses, amphotericin B is covered in detail here. Indications and directions for other therapeutic measures are given in the discussions of the specific mycoses below.

Amphotericin B, a fungicidal antibiotic, has reversed the prognosis of many fungus infections. An initial IV dose of 0.25 mg/kg body wt/day is increased by 0.25 mg/kg every few days until 1.0 mg/kg (but not exceeding 50 mg/dose) is given daily or every other day. The antibiotic is dissolved in 5% D/W (optimal concentration, 0.1 mg/ml). (CAUTION: *Saline solution precipitates the drug and should not be used. Follow the manufacturer's instructions in preparing and storing solutions.*)

The drug should be given over a 2- to 6-h period. Reactions are usually mild, but some patients may experience chills, fever, headache, anorexia, nausea, and occasionally vomiting, particularly with the initial injections. The severity of reactions may be reduced by giving aspirin or an antihistamine (e.g., diphenhydramine 50 mg) before, after 3 h, and at the end of treatment. If these are ineffective, hydrocortisone 25 to 50 mg IV may be given at the beginning of the amphotericin B infusion.

Chemical thrombophlebitis may occur; adding heparin to the infusion (or into the tubing just prior to starting the injection) may lessen the incidence.

The BUN or serum creatinine should be determined before and periodically during treatment. A slight increase can be ignored. A moderate rise may be reversed by giving the drug on alternate days, but if not, treatment should be discontinued until the levels approach normal. If this requires only a few days, treatment can be resumed with the previous dose, but if a longer period is necessary, therapy should be restarted with a smaller dose. Serum potassium should also be determined regularly since hypokalemia is common and occasionally is dramatic and dangerous. Oral liquid supplements are usually sufficient; rarely, potassium IV (**not** added to the amphotericin B infusion) may be necessary (see DISTURBANCES IN POTASSIUM METABOLISM, in §11, Ch. 6).

Intrathecal injection may be indicated in meningitis, but great care must be taken to ensure proper dose and volume: 50 mg of amphotericin B should be painstakingly dissolved in 10 ml of sterile water. The total volume should then be diluted in a 250-ml bottle of 5% D/W from which 10 ml has been removed. From

0.5 ml (0.1 mg) to 5.0 ml (1.0 mg) should then be drawn into a 10-ml syringe, further diluted to 10 ml with CSF, and injected *slowly* (over at least 2 min). A lumbar, cisternal, or (directly or by an Ommaya reservoir) ventricular site may be used.

HISTOPLASMOSIS

An infectious disease caused by Histoplasma capsulatum, *characterized by a primary pulmonary lesion, and occasional hematogenous dissemination, with ulcerations of the oropharynx and GI tract, hepatomegaly, splenomegaly, lymphadenopathy, and adrenal necrosis.*

Etiology and Incidence

H. capsulatum in tissue is an oval budding cell 1 to 5μ in diameter. Infection follows inhalation of dust which contains the spores. Severe disease is more frequent in males.

Chest x-ray surveys in certain geographic areas have demonstrated many residents with symptomless, nontuberculous, occasionally calcified pulmonary lesions; delayed cutaneous hypersensitivity reactions to histoplasmin suggest widespread but subclinical infection. The highest incidence of such hypersensitivity is in the Ohio and Mississippi River valleys.

Symptoms and Signs

There are 3 recognized forms of the disease. The **primary acute form** causes symptoms (fever, cough, malaise) indistinguishable in endemic areas (except by culture) from otherwise undifferentiated URI or grippe-like disease. The **progressive disseminated form** follows hematogenous spread from the lungs and is characterized by hepatomegaly, lymphadenopathy, splenomegaly, and, less frequently, oral or GI ulceration. Addison's disease is an uncommon but serious manifestation. Addison's disease of other etiology, lymphoma, Hodgkin's disease, leukemia, and sarcoidosis must be differentiated. The **chronic cavitary form** produces pulmonary lesions indistinguishable, except by culture, from cavitary TB. The principal manifestations are cough, increasing dyspnea, and eventually disabling respiratory embarrassment. That histoplasmosis is a cause of uveitis has been postulated but not proved.

Diagnosis

Demonstration of *H. capsulatum* by culture is diagnostic. Specimens for culture may be obtained from sputum, lymph nodes, bone marrow, liver biopsy, blood, urine, or oral ulcerations. Tissues may also be examined microscopically after staining (Gomori's methenamine silver, periodic acid–Schiff, or Gridley). Delayed cutaneous hypersensitivity and CF tests are of no diagnostic value since they are usually negative early in the disease.

Prognosis and Treatment

The acute primary form is usually benign; it is fatal only in those rare cases with massive infection. The progressive disseminated form has a high mortality. In the chronic cavitary form, death results from severe respiratory insufficiency.

Primary acute disease rarely requires chemotherapy. The disseminated form responds to amphotericin B (see General Therapeutic Principles, above); in the chronic cavitary form, the fungi disappear with therapy, but fibrotic lesions show little change.

COCCIDIOIDOMYCOSIS
(San Joaquin or Valley Fever)

An infectious disease, caused by the fungus Coccidioides immitis, *occurring in a* **primary form** *as an acute, benign, self-limiting respiratory disease, or in a* **progressive form** *as a chronic, often fatal, infection of the skin, lymph glands, spleen, liver, bones, kidneys, meninges, and brain.*

Etiology, Incidence, and Pathology

The disease is endemic in the southwestern USA and occurs most frequently in men aged 25 to 55. Infection is acquired by inhalation of spore-laden dust. Individuals contracting the disease while traveling through endemic areas may not develop manifestations until later, after leaving the area.

The basic pathologic change is an acute, subacute, or chronic granulomatous process with varying degrees of fibrosis. Lesions may show central necrosis; the organisms are surrounded by lymphocytes and by plasma, epithelioid, and giant cells. Cavitation or granuloma ("coin lesion") formation may occur in chronic lung infection.

Symptoms and Signs

Primary pulmonary coccidioidomycosis, the more common form, may occur asymptomatically, as a mild URI, as acute bronchitis, occasionally with pleural effusion, or as pneumonia. Symptoms, in descending order of frequency, include fever, cough, chest pain, chills, sputum production, sore throat, and hemoptysis. Physical signs may be absent, or occasional scattered rales and areas of dullness to percussion may be present. Leukocytosis is present and the eosinophil count may be high. Some patients develop **"desert rheumatism,"** a more recognizable form with conjunctivitis, arthritis, and erythema nodosum.

Progressive coccidioidomycosis develops from the primary form; evidence of dissemination may appear a few weeks, months, or occasionally years after primary infection or long residence in an endemic area. Symptoms include continuous low-grade fever, severe anorexia, and loss of weight and strength. Progressive cyanosis, dyspnea, and mucopurulent or occasionally bloody sputum are present in the pulmonary type. The bones, joints, skin, viscera, brain, and meninges may be involved as the disease spreads.

Diagnosis

Coccidioidomycosis should be suspected in a patient with an obscure illness who has been or is in an endemic area. Diagnosis is established by finding the characteristic spherules of *C. immitis* in sputum, gastric washings, pleural fluid, CSF, pus from abscesses, biopsy specimens, or exudates from skin lesions by direct examination or culture. In the tissues, the fungus appears as thick-walled nonbudding spherules 20 to 80μ in diameter.

A delayed cutaneous hypersensitivity reaction to coccidioidin usually appears 10 to 21 days after infection, but is characteristically absent in progressive disease. Precipitating and CF antibodies are present regularly and persistently in the progressive form but only transiently in acute primary cases.

Prognosis and Treatment

Treatment is not needed and the outlook is excellent for primary pulmonary coccidioidomycosis, but the progressive type is fatal in 55 to 60% of cases. Amphotericin B (see General Therapeutic Principles, above) is the only effective drug and is indicated in all patients with the progressive form. Results are less satisfactory than in blastomycosis or histoplasmosis. Meningitis requires prolonged intrathecal administration, usually for years. Untreated meningitis is fatal.

CRYPTOCOCCOSIS
(Torulosis)

An infectious disease due to the fungus Cryptococcus neoformans *(formerly Tor-ula histolytica), with a primary focus in the lung and characteristic spread to the meninges and occasionally to the kidneys, bone, and skin.*

Incidence and Pathology

Distribution is worldwide. In the USA, more cases occur in the southeast, in adults aged 40 to 60, and in men more often than in women.

CNS lesions include diffuse meningitis, meningeal granulomas, endarteritis, in-farcts, areas of softening, increase in neuroglia, or extensive tissue destruction. Cutaneous lesions appear as acneiform pustules or granulating ulcers. Subcutane-ous and visceral lesions are deep nodules or tumorlike masses filled with gelat-inous material. Acute inflammation is minimal or absent, but infiltration with lymphocytes and fibroblasts, and with plasma, "foam," and giant cells, is seen occasionally.

Symptoms and Signs

Meningitis with headache is the most common form. The patient seeks medical care because of blurred vision or is brought to the physician because of such mental disturbances as confusion, depression, agitation, or inappropriate speech or dress. CSF examination shows elevated protein and cell count (mostly lympho-cytes) in about 90% of patients, and decreased glucose in 50%; *C. neoformans* can be seen on India ink examination in 60%.

Though the infection is acquired via the respiratory route with a primary focus in the lung, it has only recently been recognized that a benign, rarely progressive, pulmonary form occurs, often as a complication of other lung disease. Cough or other symptoms of the underlying pathologic changes in the lung are usually present.

The kidney is the next most common organ involved. *C. neoformans* can be cultured from the urine in about 30% of patients with cryptococcal meningitis. Although renal infection is usually asymptomatic, pyelonephritis with renal papil-lary necrosis has been reported.

Skin lesions (pustules or ulcers) and bone lesions (osteomyelitis) are seen less frequently.

Diagnosis

This is strongly suggested by finding, with an India ink preparation, the bud-ding yeast surrounded by a clear capsular area in sputum, pus, other exudates, or CSF. Similar encapsulated yeast forms, seen on proper staining of fixed tissues, are also diagnostic. Isolation in culture and identification of the causative fungus confirm the diagnosis.

Prognosis and Treatment

Treatment with amphotericin B (see General Therapeutic Principles, above) has reduced the fatality rate of the meningeal form to about 15%. Though daily and total dosages are not firmly established, a 2- to 3-Gm total dose seems reason-able. Patients with nonprogressive pulmonary disease may need no treatment. Skin, bone, and renal infections require therapy, though these forms are interme-diate in severity.

Alternatively, once sensitivity has been demonstrated, flucytosine 150 mg/kg body wt/day orally in 4 equal doses may be given, continued for at least 6 wk. Since the drug is excreted by the kidney, impaired renal function calls for dosage modification. Leukopenia and, occasionally, elevated SGOT have been encountered, which can be due to the drug, to underlying disease, to the infection, or to a combination of all three.

Early data suggest that combined amphotericin B and flucytosine therapy is optimal in meningitis.

BLASTOMYCOSIS
(North American Blastomycosis, Gilchrist's Disease)

An infectious disease caused by the fungus Blastomyces dermatitidis, *primarily involving the lungs and occasionally spreading hematogenously, characteristically to the skin.*

Etiology and Incidence

B. dermatitidis is a fungus of unknown natural source. Most reported cases are from the USA, chiefly the southeastern states and the Mississippi River valley, and occur in men aged 20 to 40. A sufficient number of cases from widely scattered sites in Africa now precludes geographic limitation of the disease name.

Symptoms and Signs

Pulmonary form: Primary pulmonary blastomycosis frequently forms patches of bronchopneumonia which appear, on chest x-ray, to fan out from the hilum like a neoplastic growth. Onset is usually insidious. A dry hacking or productive cough, chest pain, fever, chills, drenching sweats, and dyspnea are initial symptoms.

Systemic form: Sites of hematogenous spread include skin, prostate, epididymis, testis, bone, subcutaneous tissue, and, rarely, oral or nasal mucosa. The vertebrae, tibia, and femur are more commonly involved than other bones; swelling, heat, and tenderness are present over the lesion. Genital tract lesions are characterized by painful swelling.

Skin lesions begin as papules or papulopustules on exposed surfaces and spread slowly. Painless miliary abscesses, varying from pinpoint to 1 mm in diameter, develop on the advancing borders. Irregular, wartlike papillae form on the surfaces. As the lesions enlarge, the center heals with a typical atrophic scar. A fully developed individual lesion appears as an elevated verrucous patch measuring 2 cm or larger with an abruptly sloping, purplish-red, abscess-studded border. Ulceration may occur if bacteria are present.

Diagnosis

Isolation in culture and identification of *B. dermatitidis* is diagnostic. Diagnosis is almost as certain if thick-walled budding yeasts, about 15μ in diameter and without a capsule, are seen on direct examination of pus, sputum, or exudate, or after appropriate tissue fixation and staining. Skin and serologic tests are of no value.

Pulmonary disease must be distinguished from tuberculosis, other fungus infections, and bronchogenic carcinoma. Skin lesions resemble sporotrichosis, tuberculosis, iodism, or, especially, basal cell carcinoma. Genital involvement mimics tuberculosis.

Prognosis and Treatment

In most untreated patients, the disease is slowly and fatally progressive. Amphotericin B (see General Therapeutic Principles, above) is highly effective. Improvement begins within a week, with a rapid disappearance of organisms.

Hydroxystilbamidine is occasionally useful for this infection (e.g., in patients with a renal disorder or with nonprogressive blastomycosis limited to the skin). However, storage and administration are problematic, and the manufacturer's instructions for use of the drug must be carefully followed. Dosage is begun with

25 mg/day and increased in increments of 25 mg/day until 225 mg/day is reached; this dose is continued until a total of 8 Gm has been given. Alleviation of symptoms usually begins after 14 days, but little improvement in the lesions is noted before 30 days. Improvement usually continues for 3 to 6 mo after the last dose. Occasionally, the course of treatment must be repeated. Rarely, facial numbness in the sensory distribution of the 5th cranial nerve occurs. Fever occurring near the end of the first week of therapy suggests a Herxheimer-like reaction.

PARACOCCIDIOIDOMYCOSIS
(South American Blastomycosis)

An infectious disease of the skin, mucous membranes, lymph nodes, and internal organs, caused by the fungus Paracoccidioides brasiliensis *(formerly* Blastomyces brasiliensis*).* The disease occurs only in South and Central America, most frequently in men aged 20 to 50, and especially in the coffee-growers of Brazil.

Symptoms and Signs

There are 4 clinical forms. (1) The **cutaneous form** occurs most often on the face, frequently at the nasal and oral mucocutaneous borders. The typical lesion is a slowly expanding ulcer with a granular base and numerous pinpoint yellowish-white areas in which the fungus is abundant. Regional lymph nodes enlarge, become necrotic, and discharge through the skin. (2) In the **lymphatic form,** there is massive painless enlargement of the cervical, supraclavicular, or axillary lymph nodes. (3) In the **visceral form,** the liver, spleen, and abdominal lymph nodes enlarge. Abdominal pain may be the first symptom. (4) In the **mixed type,** cutaneous, lymphatic, and visceral lesions are present simultaneously.

Diagnosis and Treatment

Identification of *P. brasiliensis* in pus, biopsy, or culture is diagnostic. Treatment with amphotericin B (see General Therapeutic Principles, above) is effective; sulfonamides are suppressive but not curative.

SYSTEMIC CANDIDIASIS
(Candidosis; Moniliasis)

Invasive disease caused by Candida *spp., especially* C. albicans, *and manifested by septicemia, endocarditis, meningitis, or rarely osteomyelitis.* Topical *Candida* infections are discussed in other appropriate sections of THE MANUAL.

Etiology and Incidence

The infections are usually caused by *C. albicans.* Superficial candidiasis is universal, but patients with leukemia, or with organ transplants, or receiving immunosuppressive or antibacterial therapy are especially prone to *Candida* septicemia. *Candida* endocarditis is related to intravascular trauma such as cardiac catheterization, surgery, or indwelling venous catheters.

Symptoms and Signs

Candida **endocarditis** resembles bacterial disease, with fever, heart murmur, splenomegaly, and anemia; large vegetations and emboli to major vessels are frequently present and are differential features. Renal involvement is usually found on laboratory and autopsy examination. *Candida* **septicemia** resembles gram-negative bacterial sepsis in frequency of fever, shock, azotemia, oliguria, renal shutdown, and fulminant course. *Candida* **meningitis** is chronic, like cryptococcal meningitis, but lacks the latter's usually fatal outcome when untreated. *Candida* **pyelonephritis** and pulmonary disease are less well characterized. **Osteomyelitis** is rarely encountered; it resembles that due to other microorganisms.

Diagnosis

Because *Candida* species are commensals of man, their culture from sputum, mouth, vagina, urine, stool, or skin must be interpreted cautiously. To confirm the diagnosis, the culture must be complemented by a characteristic clinical lesion, exclusion of other etiology, and histologic evidence of tissue invasion. Isolation from blood or CSF, however, establishes the presence of *Candida* infection and supports the appropriate clinical impression: septicemia, endocarditis, or meningitis.

Treatment

Such predisposing conditions as diabetic acidosis or prolonged antibacterial therapy must first be controlled. In systemic candidiasis, amphotericin B must be given IV (see General Therapeutic Principles, above). As an alternative, flucytosine may be given as for cryptococcosis (see above) if the isolate is sensitive to it.

ASPERGILLOSIS

An infectious disease of the lung, with occasional hematogenous spread, caused by various species of Aspergillus, *especially* A. fumigatus. A noninvasive pulmonary disorder may also occur as an allergic reaction to *A. fumigatus* (see ALLERGIC BRONCHOPULMONARY ASPERGILLOSIS in §5, Ch. 12).

Etiology, Symptoms, and Signs

The fungus, an "opportunist," appears after antibacterial or antifungal therapy (to which it is usually resistant) in bronchi damaged by bronchitis, bronchiectasis, or tuberculosis. The "fungus ball" (aspergilloma), a characteristic form of the disease, appears on the chest x-ray as a dense round ball capped by a slim meniscus of air in a cavity, and is composed of a tangled mass of hyphae, fibrin, exudate, and a few inflammatory cells. Aspergillomas usually occur in old cavitary disease (e.g., tuberculosis) or, rarely, in patients with rheumatoid spondylitis. Symptoms (cough, productive sputum, dyspnea) and findings on physical examination or chest film are usually those of the underlying disease. However, hemoptysis has been a disturbing and even occasionally fatal complication. In the presence of leukemia, organ transplantation, or corticosteroid or immunosuppressive therapy, dissemination to the brain and kidneys is characteristic. The clinical picture in this form is a typical septicemia: fever, chills, hypotension, prostration, and delirium.

Diagnosis and Treatment

Because it is a commensal of man, culture of a species of *Aspergillus* from sputum, mouth, or bowel must not be considered diagnostic unless a clinically compatible illness is present, other causes have been eliminated, and tissue invasion has been demonstrated. In disseminated and pulmonary disease, amphotericin B should be given IV (see General Therapeutic Principles, above), although tolerated doses are usually ineffective since most strains are resistant.

PHYCOMYCOSIS
(Mucormycosis)

A term that includes numerous clinical conditions associated with the presence of broad, nonseptate hyphae. In most cases, the fungus has been visualized in tissues only microscopically. When cultured, it has been either a *Rhizopus* or *Basidiobolus* species. One form of the disease, subcutaneous phycomycosis, occurs in southeast Asia and Africa as a self-limited, multiple, grotesque, subcutaneous swelling of the neck and chest. **Rhinocerebral phycomycosis**, more familiar in the USA, is a fulminant and usually fatal primary infection of the nose, sinus, or orbit seen in patients with diabetic acidosis. Severe pain, fever, orbital cellulitis, proptosis, purulent nasal drainage, and gangrenous and necrotic destruction of septum, palate, or orbital or sinus bones are usually present. Early invasion of vessels and spread to the brain causes convulsions, aphasia, and hemiplegia. The clinical appearance is diagnostic, but bacterial abscesses, histoplasmosis or tuberculosis of the oral cavity, or lethal midline granuloma occasionally mimic rhinocerebral phycomycosis. It has been difficult to culture the fungi clearly present in tissues at biopsy or autopsy. **Treatment** includes control of the underlying acidosis and amphotericin B therapy, given empirically since the causative fungus has not usually been available for sensitivity studies.

ACTINOMYCOSIS
(Lumpy Jaw)

A chronic infectious disease characterized by multiple draining sinuses and caused by the anaerobic gram-positive microorganism Actinomyces israelii, *often present as a commensal on the gums, tonsils, and teeth.*

Etiology, Incidence, and Pathology

The disease is seen most often in adult males. In the cervicofacial form, the most common portal of entry is decayed teeth; pulmonary disease results from aspiration of oral secretions; abdominal disease, from a break in the mucosa of a diverticulum or the appendix.

The characteristic lesion is an indurated area of multiple, small, communicating abscesses surrounded by granulation tissue. Disease spreads to contiguous tissue and, rarely, hematogenously. Bacteria are usually also present.

Symptoms and Signs

There are 4 clinical forms of actinomycosis. (1) The **cervicofacial form,** accounting for about half the cases, usually begins as a small, flat, hard swelling, with or without pain, under the oral mucosa or the skin on the neck, or as a subperiosteal swelling of the jaw. Subsequently, areas of softening appear and develop into sinuses and fistulas with a discharge that contains the characteristic "sulfur granules" (rounded or spherical, usually yellowish, granules up to 1 mm in diameter). The cheek, tongue, pharynx, salivary glands, cranial bones, meninges, or brain may be affected, usually by extension. (2) In the **thoracic form,** involvement of the lungs resembles tuberculosis. Extensive invasion may occur before chest pain, fever, and productive cough appear. Perforation of the chest wall, with chronic draining sinuses, may result. (3) The **abdominal form** affects the intestines (usually the cecum and appendix) and the peritoneum. Pain, fever, vomiting, diarrhea or constipation, and emaciation are characteristically present. An abdominal mass with signs of partial intestinal obstruction appears, and draining sinuses and fistulas may develop in the abdominal wall. (4) In the **generalized form,** hematogenous spread occurs to the skin, vertebral bodies, brain, liver, kidney, and ureter, and, in women, to the pelvic organs.

Diagnosis

This is based on clinical symptoms, x-ray findings, and demonstration of *A. israelii* in sputum, pus, or biopsy specimen. In pus or tissue, the microorganism appears as tangled masses of branched and unbranched wavy filaments, or as the distinctive "sulfur granules." These consist of a central mass of tangled filaments, pus cells, and debris, with a midzone of interlacing filaments surrounded by an outer zone of radiating, club-shaped, hyaline and refractive filaments that take the eosin stain in tissue.

Lung lesions must be distinguished from tuberculous lesions and neoplasms. Lesions in the abdomen occur most frequently in the ileocecal region and are difficult to diagnose except at laparotomy, or when draining sinuses appear in the abdominal wall. A tender, palpable mass suggests appendiceal abscess or regional enteritis. Nodules in any location may simulate malignant growths.

Prognosis and Treatment

The disease is slowly progressive. Prognosis relates directly to early diagnosis, is most favorable in the cervicofacial form, and is progressively worse in the pulmonary, abdominal, and generalized forms.

Most cases will respond to medical treatment but, owing to the extensive induration and relatively avascular fibrosis, response is slow and treatment must be continued for at least 8 wk and occasionally for more than a year. Extensive and repeated surgical procedures may be required. Aspiration is indicated for small abscesses and drainage for large ones. Penicillin G, at least 12 million u./day IV, should be given initially; penicillin V 1 Gm orally q.i.d. may be substituted after about 2 wk. Tetracycline 500 mg orally q 6 h may be given instead of penicillin. Treatment must be continued for several weeks after apparent clinical cure.

NOCARDIOSIS

An infectious, often disseminated, granulomatous-suppurative disease caused by the aerobic microorganism Nocardia asteroides. Though closely related to *Actinomyces israelii*, *N. asteroides* is not clubbed and becomes arranged in loose clusters of interlacing, slender, branching filaments rather than in the true "sulfur granule" form. Pulmonary nocardiosis may resemble actinomycosis, but *N. asteroides* usually disseminates hematogenously with abscess formation in the brain or, less frequently, in the kidney or in multiple organs. Diagnosis is by identification of the microorganism in tissue or culture. Sulfonamide **treatment** (e.g., with sulfadiazine 4 to 6 Gm/day orally) must be continued for several months since most cases respond slowly.

MADUROMYCOSIS
(Madura Foot; Mycetoma)

A fungus infection of the feet (and occasionally the upper extremity), characterized by chronicity, tumefaction, and multiple sinus formation, and progressing until ended by excision, amputation, or death.

About half the cases are caused by *Nocardia* species, the remainder by some 20 different fungi. The disease is most prevalent in the tropics and southern USA and is usually contracted between ages 21 and 40.

Symptoms, Signs, and Diagnosis

The first lesion may be a small papule, a deep-seated fixed nodule, a vesicle with an indurated base, or an abscess that ruptures and produces a fistula. Early lesions are granulomatous but are later surrounded by a dense fibrous capsule and intersected by fibrous trabeculae. Lesions are usually nontender unless secondary infection is present. The disease progresses slowly; 6 to 8 papules or abscesses may form in succession and then disappear. Months or years may pass before muscles, tendons, fascia, and bone are destroyed.

In advanced cases, the foot characteristically appears as a grotesque, swollen, club-shaped mass of cystlike areas with multiple draining and intercommunicating sinuses and fistulas that discharge an "oily" or serosanguineous fluid. Characteristic fungus granules in the discharge measure 0.5 to 2 mm, are irregularly shaped, and vary in color. The patient is able to walk until deformity or muscle wasting intervenes. Systemic symptoms are rare. The course may be prolonged for 10 yr or longer, the patient eventually dying from sepsis or intercurrent disease unless the infecting organism is sensitive to an antimicrobial agent. Diagnosis is made from the clinical course, appearance, and demonstration of the characteristic colored granules in the exudate.

Treatment

Cases caused by *Actinomyces* should be treated with penicillin or a tetracycline (see ACTINOMYCOSIS, above); those caused by *Nocardia* with a soluble sulfonamide (see NOCARDIOSIS, above). No specific treatment is known for other types. Amputation of the limb may be required to prevent fatal spread of secondary bacterial infection.

SPOROTRICHOSIS

An infectious disease caused by the plant saprophyte Sporotrichum schenckii, *and characterized by the formation of nodules, ulcers, and abscesses, usually confined to the skin and superficial lymph channels.* Farm laborers and horticulturists, especially those handling barberry bushes, are most often infected.

Symptoms and Signs

The most common form, cutaneous-lymphatic, occurs characteristically on the arm and hand. The primary lesion, usually on the finger, begins as a small, movable, nontender, subcutaneous nodule that slowly enlarges, adheres to the skin, becomes pink and later necrotic, and finally ulcerates. In a few days or weeks, similar discolored subcutaneous nodules appear along the course of the lymphatics draining the area. Local pain, heat, and general symptoms (fever, chills, malaise, or anorexia) are notably absent.

Inhalation of the microorganism apparently can cause pneumonia, localized infiltrates, or cavities (sometimes bilateral). Symptoms are relatively mild, and the course is chronic.

Though *S. schenckii* has only rarely been cultured from the blood, it seems reasonable to explain other extracutaneous disease as hematogenous dissemination either from a subclinical cutaneous lesion or, perhaps more likely, from a pulmonary focus. Bone, periosteum, or synovium is involved in 80% of such cases; muscle and eye, in others. Involvement of the spleen, liver, kidney, genitalia, or CNS is rare.

Diagnosis

Isolation and identification of *S. schenckii* in culture is diagnostic. Unlike other pathogenic fungi, *S. schenckii* can rarely be seen in fixed tissue, even with special stains.

Prognosis and Treatment

The cutaneous-lymphatic form is chronic, indolent, and rarely fatal. It responds readily to potassium iodide saturated solution: initially 1 ml orally t.i.d., increased by 1 ml/day to an optimal dose of 3 to 4 ml t.i.d. The solution may be diluted in water or other beverage and should be taken after meals. Therapy must be continued and may be well tolerated for prolonged periods. However, iodism may appear at any time as irritative phenomena of the skin and mucous membranes (e.g., rashes, coryza, conjunctivitis, stomatitis, laryngitis, bronchitis). When symptoms develop, the dose should be decreased or the drug temporarily stopped. After a 1- to 2-wk interruption, the drug may be cautiously resumed at a lower dosage. It may be considered essential to continue iodide medication despite iodism; in such cases, iodide sensitivity may lessen or disappear despite continued therapy.

In disseminated disease, IV amphotericin B (see General Therapeutic Principles, above) is necessary, since about 30% of iodide-treated patients die, some despite extensive treatment.

CHROMOMYCOSIS
(Chromoblastomycosis; Verrucous Dermatitis)

An infectious disease caused by Hormodendrum pedrosoi, H. compactum, *or* Phialophora verrucosa, *and characterized by warty cutaneous nodules which slowly develop into large papillomatous vegetations that tend to ulcerate.* Incidence is worldwide, but highest in the tropics. The disease is prevalent from age 30 to 50, primarily in men.

Symptoms, Signs, and Diagnosis
The infection, usually unilateral, begins on the foot and leg, or sometimes on other exposed parts, especially where the skin is broken. The early lesion is a small, itching, enlarging papule resembling ringworm. The patch is dull red or violaceous in color, is sharply demarcated, and has an indurated base. New crops projecting 1 or 2 mm above the skin may appear several weeks or months later along the paths of lymphatic drainage. Hard, dull red or grayish cauliflower-like nodules may develop in the center of the patch and gradually cover the infected extremities. Lymphatics may be blocked, itching may be present, and secondary infection may lead to ulceration. From 4 to 15 yr may elapse before the entire extremity is involved.

In late cases, the diagnosis is made from the clinical appearance. Early lesions may be mistaken for dermatophytoses and must be differentiated by finding the characteristic dark brown septate bodies in pus or biopsy specimens.

Prognosis and Treatment
The disease is rarely fatal but cure is possible only in the earliest forms, where complete surgical excision is the treatment of choice. A few reports suggest that amphotericin B, instilled into the lesion, may be effective even in advanced cases.

RHINOSPORIDIOSIS

An infectious disease caused by Rhinosporidium seeberi, *and characterized by large, friable, sessile or pedunculated polyps on the mucous membranes of the nose, eyes, larynx, and vagina, and occasionally on the skin of the ears or penis.* The disease, apparently contracted by swimming in stagnant water, occurs most often in boys and young men in India and Ceylon. The diagnosis is established by identifying the ovoid spores (measuring 7 to 9μ) in smears, or by demonstrating the characteristic spore-filled sporangia (200 to 300μ) in biopsy material.

Prognosis and Treatment
The disease is rarely fatal but the patient may die of secondary infection. Complete excision of the early lesions is curative.

GEOTRICHOSIS

A variety of conditions, none yet characterized or studied, existing in a patient from whom Geotrichum candidum *has been cultured.* Since the microorganism is a commensal of man, its isolation from the mouth and bowel is etiologically meaningless. No clinical condition has been consistently associated with *Geotrichum*, although there have been rare reported cases of fungemia.

PENICILLIOSIS

A term used to include the rarely encountered, disparate instances when a species of apparently multiplying Penicillium *has been recovered from deep tissues* (e.g., the brain, orbit, or kidney). Like *Candida* and *Geotrichum, Penicillium* is a commensal in the bowel and is found in stool.

---

7. OPPORTUNISTIC INFECTIONS

Infections ranging from minor to fatal, caused by normally nonpathogenic organisms in patients whose host defense mechanisms have been compromised.

Etiology

Host defense mechanisms—physiologic, anatomic, or immunologic—may be altered or breached by disease or trauma, or by procedures or agents used for diagnosis or therapy. Thus, opportunistic infection may occur if antimicrobial therapy alters the normal relationship between host and microbe, or if the host defense mechanisms have been altered by burns, anemia, neoplasms, metabolic disorders, irradiation, foreign bodies, immunosuppressive or cytotoxic drugs, corticosteroids, or diagnostic or therapeutic instrumentation. The underlying alteration predisposes the patient to infections from his endogenous microflora or from organisms acquired by contact with other patients, hospital personnel, or equipment.

1. Antibiotic resistance and impaired anatomic host defense mechanisms: Antimicrobial treatment alters the normal microflora of the skin, mucous membranes, and GI tract. It may result in **superinfection** (invasion by endogenous or environmental organisms that are resistant to the antibiotic being given) which is demonstrable by microbiologic and clinical evidence. Factors predisposing to superinfection include extremes of age, chronic infection or other debilitating disease, excessive doses of a single antimicrobial, and the use of one or a combination of broad-spectrum antibiotics. The wider the antimicrobial spectrum, the greater the danger of opportunistic infection. Superinfections usually appear on the 4th or 5th day of chemotherapy and may convert a benign, self-limited disease into a serious, prolonged, or even fatal one. They are most often caused by endogenous gram-negative enteric bacilli, fungi, and resistant staphylococci. The diagnosis of superinfection by a normally commensal organism is certain only when the organism is recovered from blood, CSF, or body cavity fluid.

Nosocomial (hospital-acquired) infections are usually acquired from the hospital environment or personnel, the patient's own microflora, or inadequately sterilized equipment, and are commonly due to *Enterobacter, Klebsiella, Serratia, Pseudomonas, Proteus, Paracolobactrum,* or *Candida*. They may replace strains of *Escherichia coli* and many gram-positive organisms, especially when a susceptible patient is given a broad-spectrum antibiotic or massive doses of any antibiotic. Patients with extensive **burns** or those undergoing diagnostic or therapeutic **procedures** which breach normal anatomic barriers to infection (e.g., tracheostomy, inhalation therapy, urinary tract instrumentation, indwelling urethral or IV catheters, surgery, and surgical prostheses) are vulnerable to infection by endogenous or environmental antibiotic-resistant organisms. Gram-negative bacteria, particularly *Pseudomonas* and *Serratia,* alone or in combination with staphylococci, cause bacteremia in severely burned patients. Significant bacteriuria develops in patients with indwelling urethral catheters, thus increasing the risk of cystitis, pyelonephritis, and gram-negative rod bacteremia. Polyethylene IV catheters may cause sepsis, especially when thrombophlebitis from irritating IV solutions is present. Sepsis ranging from local suppuration to systemic infection and death may arise in current or prior IV infusion sites, due to gram-negative organisms alone or in combination with staphylococci and *Candida*. Patients with endotracheal tubes or tracheostomies and others who require repeated tracheal suctioning or inhalation therapy with equipment containing a reservoir of nebulization fluid may develop bronchopulmonary infection with nosocomial gram-negative organisms or staphylococci.

2. Impaired cellular or humoral host defense mechanisms: Such **neoplastic and immunodeficiency diseases** as leukemia, Hodgkin's disease, myeloma, and macroglobulinemia are characterized by selective defects in host resistance. Patients with hypogammaglobulinemia, myeloma, macroglobulinemia, or chronic lymphatic leukemia tend to have deficient humoral immune mechanisms and to develop pneumococcal and staphylococcal pneumonia and gram-negative genitourinary infections. Patients with Hodgkin's disease or acute leukemia, and those receiving intensive **immunosuppressive** or **irradiation therapy** frequently develop gram-negative septicemia secondary to pneumonia. Since these patients also tend to have depressed cellular immune mechanisms, serious infection with *Aspergillus, Candida, Cryptococcus, Histoplasma, Mucor, Nocardia,* or *Staphylococcus* is frequent; herpes zoster, cytomegalovirus, *Pneumocystis,* and *Toxoplasma* infections also occur.

Cytotoxic drugs enhance the susceptibility of tissues to infection by direct cytotoxic action, resulting in severe leukopenia and thrombocytopenia; depression of the primary immune response, including antibody production and delayed hypersensitivity; and an altered inflammatory response.

Corticosteroids probably affect host defenses at the vascular bed by inhibiting the movement of leukocytes into the inflammatory exudate. Corticosteroids may reactivate healed pulmonary TB, histoplasmosis, coccidioidomycosis, and blastomycosis. Patients receiving corticosteroid treatment for RA, ulcerative colitis, asthma, sarcoidosis, SLE, and pemphigus, and patients with **Cushing's syndrome** have an increased susceptibility to infection from usual and unusual bacteria; from *Aspergillus, Candida, Cryptococcus, Mucor,* and *Nocardia;* and from spread of varicella-zoster virus.

Prophylaxis

Understanding and minimizing the underlying host defect is essential, as is pretreatment evaluation of the benefits and risks of therapy in compromised hosts. Awareness and control of opportunistic infection may be increased by continuous epidemiologic hospital surveillance.

Use of broad-spectrum antibiotics, massive doses of any antibiotic, or prophylactic use of systemic antibiotics may ultimately result in infection with resistant bacteria and should be avoided. Most primary infections can be treated with conservative doses of one antibiotic. Patients receiving antimicrobial therapy should be watched for signs of superinfection. Constant microbiologic monitoring of the patient for any changes in his microflora that may signal superinfection is important and should be instituted if possible. The appearance or increase in numbers of a specific organism without clinical evidence of superinfection usually responds to withdrawal of the antimicrobial in use.

Hypogammaglobulinemia may require maintenance with immune serum globulin. Tuberculin sensitivity should be determined before a patient is treated with immunosuppressive or corticosteroid agents, and isoniazid (INH) treatment should be considered in tuberculin-positive patients.

Strict **asepsis** should be maintained in diagnostic and therapeutic manipulative procedures. **Urethral catheters** must be connected to closed sterile drainage bags and the system kept closed. The initial use of triple-lumen indwelling urethral catheters continuously irrigated with an antibacterial solution of neomycin-polymyxin B (neomycin 40 mg, polymyxin B 20 mg in 1 L of isotonic saline/24 h by constant drip) will markedly decrease the incidence of bacteriuria.

Attendants should wear sterile gloves during **endotracheal** or **tracheostomy suctioning,** and suction catheters should be sterile, disposable, and used only once. Reservoir nebulizer jars on **inhalation machines** should be filled daily with 0.25% acetic acid solution until the tube leading to the nebulizer jet is covered. The solution is aerosolized through the machine for 10 min, the remaining solution from the nebulizer jar is discarded, and the jar is rinsed with water and refilled with the desired medication. Alternatively, the inhalation tubing, valve assembly, and reservoir nebulizer can be replaced daily with sterile units which have been washed, rinsed, and immersed in 2% glutaraldehyde solution for 15 min, then rinsed again. Some have found the use of copper pads in the reservoir to be helpful; the elution of copper is inhibitory and bactericidal for microorganisms.

When possible, **IV therapy** should be given through conventional metal needles. IV catheters should be inserted securely, covered with a sterile protective dressing, and removed after 48 h or at the first sign of phlebitis. An antibiotic ointment of neomycin, polymyxin B, and bacitracin should be applied daily to the cannulation site and the emerging catheter. Thrombophlebitis usually responds to catheter withdrawal and local application of hot compresses.

Treatment

The organisms of opportunistic infection tend to be resistant to most commonly used antibiotics and are difficult to treat once established. Cultures, and possibly tissue biopsy (e.g., for *Pneumocystis* infections—see in §5, Ch. 9), should be obtained before starting or altering antibacterial treatment, but at times one may have to begin therapy on the basis of clinical-bacteriologic diagnosis and presumptive sensitivity while awaiting laboratory results. When possible, corticosteroid dosage should be reduced while treating an opportunistic infection except in patients with *Pneumocystis* pneumonia. Severely leukopenic patients should be given granulocyte transfusions, if available.

Therapy may be merely suppressive unless the underlying condition can be corrected (e.g., removal of urethral or IV catheters, or tracheostomy closure).

---

8. PARASITIC INFECTIONS

(NOTE: Several of the drugs mentioned in this chapter are not available commercially in the USA but may be obtainable as investigational drugs from the Parasitic Diseases Branch of the Center for Disease Control in Atlanta, Georgia.)

PROTOZOAL DISEASES

AMEBIASIS
(Entamebiasis)

An infection of the colon caused by Entamoeba histolytica. It is most commonly asymptomatic, but symptoms ranging from mild diarrhea to dysentery may occur.

TABLE 1-12. COMMONLY ENCOUNTERED

Condition	Causative Organism (Synonyms or Varieties)	Geographic Distribution	Source of Infection	Portal of Entry (& Stage)
Roundworms Ascariasis	Ascaris lumbricoides (Giant intestinal roundworm)	Cosmopolitan, more common in warm moist climates	Fecal contamination of soil (eggs) Contaminated vegetables	Mouth (embryonated eggs)
Hookworm infection	a) Ancylostoma duodenale (Old World type) b) Necator americanus (Tropical type)	a) Temperate & warm moist climates b) Warm moist climates	Fecal contamination of soil (larvae)	Skin, usually feet, possibly mouth (filariform larvae)
Strongyloidiasis	Strongyloides stercoralis (Threadworm)	Southern USA, moist tropics	Fecal contamination of soil (larvae)	Skin, usually feet (filariform larvae)
Trichuriasis	Trichuris trichiura (Whipworm)	Warm moist climates Uncommon in USA	Fecal contamination of soil (eggs)	Mouth (embryonated eggs)
Enterobiasis	Enterobius vermicularis (Oxyuris vermicularis; Pinworm, seatworm)	Cosmopolitan, esp. in children	Eggs from contaminated fomites	Mouth (embryonated eggs)
Tapeworms Dwarf Tapeworm infection	Hymenolepis nana	Southern USA, in children Cosmopolitan	Eggs contaminating environment	Mouth (eggs)
Beef Tapeworm infection	Taenia saginata	Cosmopolitan	Poorly cooked or raw infected beef	Mouth (cysticercus larvae in infected beef)
Pork Tapeworm infection	Taenia solium	Rare in USA; common in Latin America, Asia, USSR, E. Europe	Poorly cooked infected pork	Mouth (cysticercus larvae in infected pork)
Fish Tapeworm infection	Diphyllobothrium latum	Northern Minn. & Mich.; Canada Cosmopolitan	Infected freshwater fish	Mouth (larvae in infected freshwater fish flesh)

INTESTINAL PARASITIC INFECTIONS

Most Common Symptoms	Diagnostic Findings	Therapeutic Agents	Remarks
Bronchial symptoms, eosinophilia* (larval stage) Colicky pains, "acute abdomen"	Immature eggs in stool Worms evacuated in stool, occasionally vomited	Piperazine citrate Pyrantel pamoate Thiabendazole	May block intestine, biliary or pancreatic duct
Abdominal pain, melena, anemia, cardiac insufficiency, retarded growth	Immature eggs in stool	Pyrantel pamoate Tetrachloroethylene Bephenium hydroxynaphthoate Thiabendazole	Prophylaxis: Use sanitary latrines, wear shoes, treat infected persons
Radiating pain in pit of stomach, diarrhea	Larvae in stool	Thiabendazole	Prophylaxis: As for hookworm
Diarrhea, abdominal pain, anemia, weight loss	Immature eggs in stool	Mebendazole Hexylresorcinol enema Thiabendazole	May produce dysenteric syndrome or acute appendicitis; rectal prolapse in children
Perianal & perineal pruritus	Eggs in perianal swabs; adult worms per anum	Pyrvinium pamoate Pyrantel pamoate Thiabendazole Piperazine citrate	Often involves entire family
Diarrhea, abdominal discomfort, dizziness, inanition in children	Eggs in stool	Quinacrine Niclosamide†	May be symptomless
Systemic toxemia, abdominal distress, "acute appendix"	Proglottids of adult worms in stool; eggs near anus	Niclosamide† Quinacrine Bithionol†	May be symptomless Prophylaxis: Thoroughly cook all suspected beef
Similar to T. saginata	Eggs and proglottids of adult worms in stool; eggs near anus	Quinacrine Niclosamide†	May be symptomless Ingested eggs may produce human cysticercosis Prophylaxis: Thoroughly cook all pork in infected areas
Mild GI symptoms; may cause pernicious anemia	Immature eggs in stool	Niclosamide†	May be symptomless Prophylaxis: Thoroughly cook or freeze fresh-water fish

* Note: Eosinophilia often accompanies intestinal helminthiasis.
† Available in USA from Center for Disease Control.
‡ Not available in USA.

TABLE 1-12. COMMONLY ENCOUNTERED

Condition	Causative Organism (Synonyms or Varieties)	Geographic Distribution	Source of Infection	Portal of Entry (& Stage)
Tapeworms Sparganosis	Diphyllobothrium mansoni	Several areas, incl. southern USA Cosmopolitan	Drinking water containing infected Cyclops (primary host)	Usually mouth (larval stages)
Protozoa Amebiasis	Entamoeba histolytica (E. dysenteriae, Endamoeba histolytica)	Cosmopolitan; common in warm moist climates	Feces-contaminated water, food, fomites	Mouth (cyst)
Giardiasis	Giardia lamblia (G. intestinalis, Lamblia intestinalis)	Cosmopolitan	Human feces	Mouth (cyst)
Flukes Intestinal	a) Fasciolopsis buski b) Heterophyes, Metagonimus c) Echinostoma ilocanum et al	In USA only as rare infections imported from Orient or tropics	a) Vegetation b) Fresh-water fish c) Snails	Mouth (encysted metacercarial larva)
Hepatic	a) Fasciola hepatica (sheep liver fluke) b) Clonorchis sinensis	a) Cosmopolitan in sheep-raising countries b) Orient	a) Watercress containing metacercarial cysts b) Fresh-water fish	a) Mouth (encysted metacercarial larva) b) Mouth (encysted larva)
Pulmonary	Paragonimus westermani (Oriental lung fluke)	a) Nigeria b) Orient, extensive foci	Crabs or crayfishes containing metacercarial cysts	Mouth (encysted metacercarial larva)
Blood (Schistosomiasis)	a) Schistosoma japonicum b) S. mansoni c) S. haematobium	a) Orient b) Africa, Latin America c) Africa, Near East	Infested water containing fork-tailed larvae from snail hosts	Skin (active fork-tailed cercariae)

INTESTINAL PARASITIC INFECTIONS *(Cont'd)*

Most Common Symptoms	Diagnostic Findings	Therapeutic Agents	Remarks
Inflamed subcut. tissue containing sparganum larva	Sparganum larva in subcut. tissues	Surgical excision	Adult worm in intestine of various nonhuman mammals

a) Intestinal
  1. Mild
  2. Dysentery
 	
b) Amebic hepatitis and abscess
	Trophozoite stage or cyst in stool	a) 1. Diiodohy-droxyquin & Tetracycline
		  2. Metronidazole *or* Emetine, Tetracycline, & Diiodohydroxyquin
		b) Metronidazole *or* Emetine and Chloroquine phosphate
			Amebiasis may be asyndromic in individuals or populations

Mucous diarrhea, abdominal pain, weight loss	Vegetative stage or cyst in stool	Metronidazole Quinacrine	Prevalent in children and patients with immunoglobulin deficiencies. A cause of "travelers' diarrhea"
Intestinal toxemia, at times intestinal obstruction	Eggs in stool	a) Tetrachloroethylene Niclosamide† b) Tetrachloroethylene Hexylresorcinol c) Tetrachloroethylene Aspidium oleoresin	Primary intermediate hosts are fresh-water snails
Hepatic colic, cholecystiasis	a) Immature eggs in stool or biliary drainage b) Eggs in stool & duodenal contents	a) Bithionol† b) None	a) Sheep infected in USA, but only 1 confirmed human infection b) Infections in USA from imported dried or pickled fish
Peribronchiolar distress, with hemoptysis	Immature eggs in stool or sputum	Bithionol†	Related species in wild mammals and hogs in USA
Dysentery, fibrosis of intestinal or bladder walls, hepatic fibrosis (a,b), hematuria (c)	Embryonated eggs in stool (a,b), or urine (c)	a) Antimony potassium tartrate b, c) Stibophen, Stibocaptate†, Niridazole†, Hycanthone‡	Related flukes cause "swimmer's itch" in bathers in USA and elsewhere

† Available in USA from Center for Disease Control.
‡ Not available in USA.

Etiology, Epidemiology, and Incidence

There are 2 forms of *E. histolytica:* the motile trophozoite and the cyst. The trophozoite is the parasitic form and dwells in the bowel lumen where it feeds on bacteria or tissue. With diarrhea, the fragile trophozoites pass unchanged in the liquid stool and rapidly die. If diarrhea is not present, the organisms usually encyst before leaving the gut. The cysts resist environmental changes and are the infective form of the organism.

Infection is acquired by ingesting the cysts in food or water contaminated by feces. Asymptomatic carriers (particularly food handlers if the area is highly sanitated) are the principal source of infection. Transmission may involve direct contact with unwashed hands or contaminated food. Extensive waterborne epidemics have resulted from faulty hotel and factory plumbing. Flies and cockroaches may spread the cysts if sanitary latrines are not used. Eating raw vegetables and fruits that have been fertilized with human feces or washed in polluted water may result in amebiasis. Patients with amebic dysentery rarely transmit the disease. The infection rate in the USA is about 1 to 5%. The carrier rate may exceed 50% in poorly sanitated areas of the world.

Pathogenesis

Excystation of ingested cysts occurs in the small intestine. The released trophozoites are carried to the colon where they grow and multiply in the bowel lumen as commensals. Change in the organism's virulence or the host's resistance may lead to tissue invasion and disease.

The trophozoites penetrate the mucous membrane mainly in regions of fecal stasis—the cecum, appendix, ascending colon, sigmoid colon, and rectum. The earliest lesion is a small abscess, usually in the submucosa; later, ulcers form which tend to be ragged and undermined. The lesions are focal and discrete in mild cases, but may spread and become confluent, with hemorrhage, edema, and sloughing of large areas of mucosa. Although the muscular coat limits penetration by the ameba, it is occasionally destroyed and perforation results; amebas enter the radicles of the portal vein, and are carried to the liver. Most of the amebas are probably destroyed, but one or more large hepatic abscesses develop if the survivors are numerous and multiply. Further spread of the disease is usually by direct extension from the liver into the pleura, right lung, and pericardium.

Symptoms and Signs

Because of the infrequency of tissue invasion, most patients, particularly those living in temperate climates, are asymptomatic. Symptoms occur with tissue invasion. These may be so vague as to be recalled only after successful therapy, but more often intermittent diarrhea and constipation, flatulence, and cramping abdominal pain occur. There may be tenderness over the liver and ascending colon, and the stools may contain mucus and blood.

Amebic dysentery, common in the tropics but uncommon in temperate climates, is characterized by episodes of frequent semifluid or fluid stools, often containing blood, flecks of mucus, and hordes of active trophozoites. Slight fever may be present. Between relapses, symptoms diminish to recurrent cramps and loose or very soft stools due to colitis, yet emaciation and anemia increase.

Complications and Sequelae

Hepatic amebiasis: Tender hepatomegaly frequently accompanies amebic colitis. This syndrome was formerly termed "diffuse amebic hepatitis," but probably reflects a nonspecific periportal inflammation and not amebic liver infection. **Liver abscess** may develop during or 1 to 3 mo after an attack of dysentery, or may be unassociated with dysentery. Abscesses occur most frequently in adult males. The abscesses are usually single and develop insidiously, though the onset of symptoms may be abrupt. Symptoms include pain or discomfort over the liver, aggravated by movement and occasionally referred to the right shoulder; intermittent fever; sweats; chills; nausea; vomiting; weakness; and weight loss. Jaundice is unusual, except in mild degree. The abscess may perforate into the subphrenic space, right pleural cavity, right lung, and other adjacent organs.

Symptoms of **subacute appendicitis** may occur during clinical or subclinical amebic infection as a result of diffuse amebic invasion of the appendix and cecum. Surgery in such cases often results in peritonitis and death. If there is reasonable suspicion that the symptoms are of amebic origin, it is advisable to delay surgery for 48 to 72 h in order to observe the effects of emetine or metronidazole (see Treatment, below).

The lungs, brain, and other organs are occasionally infected by **hematogenous spread** from the intestines. Skin lesions, especially around the perineum and buttocks, and particularly traumatic and operative wounds, are occasionally infected with amebas.

Healing of intestinal lesions sometimes causes excessive scar formation and partial obstruction.

Diagnosis

Intestinal amebiasis is suggested by the clinical picture and epidemiologic setting, and confirmed by the demonstration of *E. histolytica* in the stool or tissues. Wet mounts of liquid and semiformed stools should be examined immediately for trophozoites. Bloodstained flecks of mucus in the stool are likely specimens. Formed stool should be examined for the presence of cysts by direct and concentration methods. If examination is delayed, a portion of the stool should be placed in a preservative for cysts (10% formalin) and trophozoites (polyvinyl alcohol). Diagnosis may require examination of 3 to 6 stool specimens. Since antibiotics, antacids, antidiarrheal agents, enemas, and intestinal radiocontrast agents may interfere with recovery of the parasite, their administration should be postponed until after the stool is examined.

Proctoscopy often demonstrates mucosal lesions in symptomatic patients. The lesions should be aspirated and the material examined for trophozoites. Biopsy specimens from the lesions may also show trophozoites.

Extraintestinal amebiasis is more difficult to diagnose. Stool examination is usually negative and recovery of the trophozoite from pus is uncommon. In patients suspected of having an amebic liver abscess, a therapeutic trial of amebicides may be the single most helpful diagnostic tool.

Serologic tests are positive in almost all patients with amebic liver abscess and in more than 80% of those with acute amebic dysentery. However, since antibody titers may persist for months or years, serologic tests are less helpful in endemic areas. The tests are positive in only about 10% of asymptomatic carriers, suggesting that tissue invasion is a prerequisite of antibody formation. The indirect HA test appears to be the most sensitive test available.

Differential Diagnosis

Amebic dysentery may be confused with bacillary or balantidial dysentery, schistosomiasis, ulcerative colitis, regional enteritis, tuberculous enterocolitis, and carcinoma of the large bowel. In contrast to bacillary dysentery, the stools in amebic dysentery are more fecal and less frequent, watery, or purulent. They characteristically contain tenacious mucus and flecks of both fresh and altered blood. Balantidiasis, caused by *Balantidium coli* and occasionally contracted from pigs, can be identified by finding the protozoon by stool culture.

Hepatic amebiasis and amebic abscess must be differentiated from other hepatic infections, including abscesses due to bacterial infection and infected echinococcus cysts. Fever, local pain and tenderness, and hepatomegaly are significant findings. Serologic tests are usually positive in hepatic amebiasis; amebas are found in the stools in about ⅓ of cases.

When an abscess is present, the liver is usually enlarged and tender, but it may not be palpable. X-rays may show elevation and fixation, or impaired excursion of the right leaf of the diaphragm. Radioisotopic liver scanning may show the extent of the abscess. The ESR, BSP, and alkaline phosphatase may be elevated. The abscesses contain thick, semifluid material ranging in color from yellow to chocolate, and composed of cytolyzed remains of tissue. A needle biopsy may show pus, but motile amebas are difficult to find in the abscess material and cysts are not present.

Prophylaxis

Controlling the spread of *E. histolytica* requires preventing access of human feces to the mouth. The high incidence of asymptomatic carriers complicates the problem.

Treatment

General: This is directed at relief of symptoms, replacement of blood, and correction of fluid and electrolyte losses.

Chemotherapy:

Course A (for acute amebic dysentery): Metronidazole is effective against both intestinal and hepatic amebiasis, and is the drug of choice. For adults, 750 mg orally t.i.d. for 10 days is recommended; for children aged 1 to 13, 50 mg/kg body wt/day orally for 10 days. Paromomycin 25 to 35 mg/kg/day orally for 5 to 10 days may also be used for intestinal, but not for extraintestinal, amebiasis.

Amebic liver abscesses have been reported in patients previously treated with metronidazole for amebic dysentery. For this reason, some authorities still prefer the following regimen: Emetine 1 mg/kg/day (maximum, 65 mg) by deep s.c. or IM (*never* IV) injection for 3 to 5 days, followed by tetracycline 250 to 500 mg orally q.i.d. for 10 days, and then diiodohydroxyquin 650 mg orally t.i.d. for 20 days. (CAUTION: *Emetine is toxic; patients receiving it should be confined to bed. Therapy should be stopped promptly if such signs of toxicity as tachycardia, hypotension, muscular weakness, marked gastrointestinal effects, or dermatoses appear.*) Emetine may cause an increase in diarrhea, often with nausea. Pregnancy and cardiac disease are **contraindications;** in these patients, chloroquine phosphate 1 Gm (600 mg base)/day orally for 2 days, and then 500 mg (300 mg base)/day for 2 wk should be given concurrently with the above course of tetracycline and diiodohydroxyquin.

Course B (for carriers, patients with mild symptoms, and those without acute dysentery or symptoms of hepatitis): Diiodohydroxyquin 650 mg orally t.i.d. for 20 days plus tetracycline 250 mg orally q.i.d. for 10 days is recommended.

Course C (for chronic, intractable cases resistant to ordinary therapy): Amebic infections resistant to other therapy may respond to glycobiarsol 500 mg orally t.i.d. for 7 days, or to the following drugs, though these are not approved for use in the USA: diloxanide furoate 500 mg orally q.i.d. for 10 days, clefamide (chlorphenoxamide) 500 mg orally t.i.d. for 8 days, or emetine bismuth iodide 65 mg orally t.i.d. for 10 days.

Amebic liver abscess: A favorable response to chloroquine or emetine is so characteristic that it constitutes an important diagnostic aid. A therapeutic trial of metronidazole, however, may lead to an erroneous diagnosis since it is also effective against many anaerobic bacteria which commonly cause pyogenic liver abscess.

If the diagnosis of amebic liver abscess is established by serologic tests, liver aspiration, or a dramatic response to chloroquine or emetine, then metronidazole 750 mg orally t.i.d. should be given for 10 days. Alternatively, emetine 1 mg/kg/day (maximum, 65 mg/day) by deep s.c. or IM injection is given for 10 days, concurrently with chloroquine phosphate 1 Gm (600 mg base)/day orally for 2 days, and then 500 mg (300 mg base)/day for 2 wk.

Criteria of cure: Ideally, the patient should not be discharged until 3 stool examinations, performed daily for 3 days after completion of treatment, are negative. One of the specimens should be obtained after catharsis. Since amebiasis tends to relapse, stools should be reexamined with reasonable frequency; if feasible, at 1, 3, and 6 mo after treatment. Recurrence of GI symptoms does not require amebicidal drug therapy unless parasitic relapse has been proved by demonstration of *E. histolytica*.

MALARIA

A protozoan infection characterized by paroxysms of chills, fever, and sweating, and by anemia, splenomegaly, and a chronic relapsing course.

Etiology and Epidemiology

Malarial parasites of 4 types, each with a different biologic pattern, may affect man: *Plasmodium vivax, P. falciparum, P. malariae,* and *P. ovale.* Infection occurs through the bite of an infected anopheles mosquito, transfusion of blood from an infected donor, or use of a common syringe by drug addicts.

Most hyperendemic malarious areas are in the tropics. Chemotherapeutic agents and insecticides have made autochthonous malaria rare in the USA and many other parts of the world, but visitors from malarious areas may introduce the infection; returning armed forces personnel have caused small sporadic epidemics.

Pathogenesis

The life cycle of the malarial parasite begins when a female anopheles mosquito, feeding on a patient with malaria, ingests blood containing gametocytes. These undergo sexual development (sporogony) within the mosquito, to end as sporozoites located in the insect's salivary glands. The mosquito injects the sporozoites into man, and the parasite multiplies asexually in the liver parenchymal cells. Little is known of the pathologic changes accompanying this asymptomatic fixed-tissue **(exoerythrocytic)** phase. After a period of maturation ranging from days to months (average, 2 to 4 wk), merozoites are released and invade the RBCs, initiating the clinical or **erythrocytic** phase of the disease. *P. vivax, P. malariae,* and, presumably, *P. ovale* exoerythrocytic parasites persist in the liver cells, periodically "seeding" the bloodstream with new merozoites to cause a relapse. Since *P. falciparum* does not persist in the liver cells, it does not cause relapse and responds readily to prophylaxis and therapy.

All 4 parasites multiply asexually within the RBCs (schizogony) to produce a new generation of merozoites. The RBCs rupture and these merozoites are released into the circulating plasma to enter intact RBCs and repeat the erythrocytic cycle. Gametocytes rather than merozoites are formed in some RBCs. These cannot self-replicate, and die unless ingested by the anopheles mosquito for completion of the sexual cycle.

Pathology

After prolonged untreated malarial infection or repeated relapses, a persistent hepatosplenomegaly develops. The spleen is usually soft and full of malarial pigment. The sinusoids are filled with numerous parasitized RBCs and the macrophages contain ingested malarial pigment. The Kupffer cells may be distended with parasites and pigment. There are no characteristic changes in other organs except the presence of scattered malarial pigment in macrophages. In fatal falciparum malaria, however, the brain is slate gray and punctate hemorrhages are often scattered throughout the brain substance. The capillaries are choked with parasite-infected RBCs.

Symptoms and Signs

The incubation period is usually 10 to 35 days, often followed by a short (2 to 3 days) prodrome of irregular low-grade fever, malaise, headache, myalgia, and chilly sensations that is frequently misidentified and treated as influenza.

In **vivax** and **ovale malaria**, the primary attack begins abruptly with a shaking chill, followed by fever and sweats with irregularly remittent fever. Within a week the typical paroxysmal pattern of the disease is established. The initial chill may be preceded by a short period of malaise or headache. The fever lasts from 1 to 8 h; after it subsides, the patient feels well until the next rigor. A rigor occurs every 48 h in uncomplicated vivax malaria.

In **falciparum malaria**, there may be a chilly sensation rather than a shaking chill; the temperature rises gradually and falls by lysis. The paroxysm may last 20 to 36 h, there is more prostration than in vivax malaria, and headache is prominent. During intervals between paroxysms, which are exceedingly variable (36 to 72 h), the patient usually feels miserable and has a low-grade fever.

In **malariae malaria**, the disease more frequently begins abruptly with a paroxysm which then recurs at 72-h intervals.

In falciparum malaria, fever of 40 C (104 F) or the presence of severe headache, drowsiness, delirium, or confusion may indicate impending **cerebral malaria**, usually a fatal complication. Delirium may accompany high fever in vivax malaria, but cerebral manifestations are uncommon.

In both falciparum and vivax malaria, the periodicity of the chills and fever is influenced by numerous factors, including dual infection (by more than one plasmodium species), strain differences, and immunity. The WBC count is usually normal, with an increase in the percentage of lymphocytes and monocytes. Mild jaundice usually develops if the disease persists untreated, and the spleen and liver become enlarged.

Chronic malaria with low-grade parasitemia occurs in partially immune subjects in hyperendemic areas, and may be accompanied by malaise, listlessness, periodic headache, anorexia, fatigue, and mild fever. These symptoms may culminate in acute attacks of chills and fever, considerably milder and of shorter duration than in the primary attack.

Blackwater fever, a rare complication, is characterized by intravascular hemolysis and hemoglobinuria. It occurs, perhaps exclusively, in chronic falciparum malaria, especially in patients treated with quinine. Primaquine may cause hemolysis in individuals with G6PD deficiency (see Curative Therapy, below).

Diagnosis

Periodic attacks of chills and fever without apparent cause always suggest malaria, particularly if the individual has been in a malarious area within the year and if the spleen is enlarged. Diagnosis depends on demonstration of the parasite in the stained blood smear; more than one smear may be required since the intensity of parasitemia often varies. It is important to identify the type of plasmodium as this will influence therapy and prognosis.

If fever persists after adequate antimalarial therapy in patients with suspected malaria, the original diagnosis was in error.

Prognosis

Untreated vivax malaria subsides spontaneously in 10 to 30 days, but may recur at variable intervals. The prognosis becomes less favorable if intercurrent infection supervenes, or if the individual was in poor condition when the attack began. Antimalarial therapy produces excellent results in vivax and falciparum malaria. Untreated falciparum malaria has a high mortality rate.

Prophylaxis and Suppression Therapy

Attempts to induce immunity with vaccines of killed parasites have failed. Patients with malaria, however, develop a gradual immunity which considerably modifies the clinical course. This immunity has a degree of strain specificity.

Preventive measures include control of mosquito breeding places; use of residual insecticide sprays in homes and outbuildings, and screens on doors and windows, or mosquito netting where screens are not feasible; and use of mosquito repellents and sufficient clothing, particularly after sundown, to protect as much of the skin surface as possible against mosquito bites. Contact between malaria patients and mosquitos must be prevented to avoid further spread of infection.

Chloroquine phosphate 500 mg (300 mg base) orally once or twice/wk protects travelers to malarious areas by suppressing the erythrocytic infection and thus the clinical manifestations of malaria. The drug should be started 1 wk before arrival in the area, and it should be continued for 6 to 8 wk after leaving since this continued use results in eradication of sensitive strains of *P. falciparum.* In other types of malaria, primaquine must be given in addition to chloroquine (see Curative Therapy, below).

Treatment

1. Treatment of the acute attack: The drug of choice in all types of malaria except drug-resistant falciparum malaria is chloroquine. The dose is 1 Gm of chloroquine phosphate (600 mg base) orally, followed by 500 mg (300 mg base) in 6 h, and then 500 mg (300 mg base)/day for 2 days. The total dose is 2.5 Gm (1.5 Gm base). Patients who are comatose or vomiting may be given chloroquine hydrochloride 250 to 375 mg (200 to 300 mg base) IM q 6 h. Oral therapy with chloroquine phosphate should be resumed as soon as possible.

Chloroquine-resistant strains of *P. falciparum* (any case contracted in Central or South America or the Far East may be resistant) should be treated with quinine, pyrimethamine, and a sulfonamide, all given concurrently. Quinine sulfate 600 mg t.i.d. is given orally for 10 days. If oral therapy is precluded, 600 mg of quinine dihydrochloride may be diluted in 300 ml saline or glucose and given IV over 30 min. The dose may be repeated q 8 h, but oral therapy should be restarted as soon as possible. In cases with renal failure, the dose is limited to 600 mg once/day. Quinine may cause tinnitus and, occasionally, drug fever or allergic purpura. Pyrimethamine 25 mg b.i.d. is given orally for 2 days. It is a folate antagonist and may cause or accentuate anemia. Sulfadiazine 500 mg orally q.i.d. is given for 5 days.

2. Curative therapy: Because *P. falciparum* parasites do not have a persistent hepatic (exoerythrocytic) phase, the disease is cured once the acute attack is adequately treated as outlined above.

In other types of malaria, the exoerythrocytic and erythrocytic parasites must be eradicated to prevent relapse. Primaquine phosphate 26.3 mg (15 mg base)/day orally for 14 days accomplishes this in 80 to 90% of primary infections. It may be given at the same time as chloroquine or afterwards. A second course of primaquine may be given if relapse occurs. Primaquine may cause intravascular hemolysis in patients with G6PD deficiency, but this is infrequent and generally benign if the recommended therapeutic doses are given. Abdominal cramps and methemoglobinuria may also occur with primaquine.

3. Gametocidal therapy: Gametocytes usually appear 2 to 3 days after onset of the erythrocytic phase and may persist for long periods, particularly in falciparum malaria. They do not produce symptoms, but indicate preexisting infection and serve as a source of infection for the anopheles mosquito.

P. vivax and *P. malariae* gametocyte development can be prevented by suppression with chloroquine (see Prophylaxis and Suppression Therapy, above), or by adequate and prompt treatment of the acute attack. *P. falciparum* gametocytes, once developed, are resistant to suppressive drugs, but are susceptible to primaquine; 15 mg (base)/day for 3 days or a single 45-mg dose will sterilize the gametocytes.

LEISHMANIASIS

A group of conditions caused by a species of Leishmania *and transmitted by several species of sandfly* (Phlebotomus). Depending on the causative species, the disease may manifest itself as **kala-azar** *(L. donovani),* **oriental sore** *(L. tropica),* or **American leishmaniasis** *(L. braziliensis, L. mexicana).* The strain of infecting organism and the host's immunologic status apparently can greatly modify the clinical manifestations. The incubation period is weeks to months.

Diffuse cutaneous leishmaniasis is a form of the disease characterized by widespread skin lesions resembling those of lepromatous leprosy. It presumably results from a specific defect of cell-mediated immunity to the leishmanial organism. In South America, it is caused by *L. mexicana* var. *pifanoi;* in Ethiopia, by *L. tropica.* The diagnosis is made by demonstrating the organisms in the skin lesions. The disease is resistant to treatment.

KALA-AZAR
(Visceral Leishmaniasis; Dumdum Fever)

Epidemiology, Pathogenesis, and Findings

Kala-azar occurs in India, China, Russia, Africa, the Mediterranean basin, and several South and Central American countries. Children are particularly susceptible. The protozoa invade the bloodstream and localize in the reticuloendothelial system, causing fever, pronounced splenomegaly, emaciation, and pancytopenia. The fever is seldom sustained and recurs irregularly. The liver and lymph nodes may become enlarged. Hypergammaglobulinemia is present. The parasite may be demonstrated in needle biopsy of the liver, spleen, bone marrow, or lymph nodes, or in cultures from these tissues or from blood. Sensitive serologic tests have been developed but are not generally available. The leishmanin skin test is negative during active disease. The fatality rate is 90% in untreated cases but generally below 10% in treated cases.

Treatment

General: Bed rest, oral hygiene, and good nutrition are important. Transfusions are useful for anemia; antibacterial chemotherapy is indicated for bacterial complications.

Specific: Pentavalent antimony compounds and aromatic diamidines are the drugs of choice. Sodium antimony gluconate (sodium stibogluconate) is given once daily, slowly IV or IM in distilled water. The generally accepted dosage is 0.1 ml (10 mg antimony)/kg body wt/injection (maximum, 600 mg antimony/day; minimum, 200 mg/day) for 6 to 10 days. If toxic effects (nausea, vomiting) appear, the drug should be given on alternate days, its dosage reduced, or its administration stopped. Three 10-day courses as above, separated by 10-day intervals, may be given in resistant cases.

The usual dosage of ethylstibamine is 200 mg IV the first day, then 300 mg IV daily or every other day for 16 doses (total, 5 Gm). Relapses, if they occur, usually appear in 2 to 6 mo and require further intensive treatment with ethylstibamine 500 mg/day IV for 20 days (total, 10 Gm).

Kala-azar encountered in the Sudan is resistant to antimony; pentamidine 4 mg/kg/day IM for up to 15 days must be used instead.

ORIENTAL SORE
(Cutaneous Leishmaniasis; Tropical Sore; Delhi or Aleppo Boil)
Epidemiology and Findings

Oriental sore occurs in China, India, the Near East, the Mediterranean basin, and Africa as far south as Nigeria and Angola. It is characterized by single or multiple sharply demarcated, ulcerating, granulomatous, autoinoculable skin lesions. Secondary infection is usual. There are no systemic symptoms except those due to secondary infection. *Leishmania tropica* may be demonstrated in smears or cultures of curettings from the sides or base of the ulcer. The leishmanin skin test is positive. Healing occurs spontaneously in 2 to 18 mo, leaving a depressed scar.

Treatment

Excellent results are obtained by infiltrating the indurated edge and base of the ulcer with 6 ml of sodium antimony gluconate 3 or 4 times every other day. CO_2 snow, infrared therapy, and radiotherapy may also be effective. When lesions are numerous, sodium antimony gluconate should be given parenterally as for kala-azar, above. Antibiotics or sulfonamides are indicated for secondary infections.

AMERICAN LEISHMANIASIS
(Espundia; Forest Yaws; Uta; Chiclero Ulcer)

This disfiguring disease, which causes ulcerative lesions of the nose and pharynx, occurs in southern Mexico and Central and South America. Untreated, the disease may persist for years, with death resulting from secondary infection. **Diagnosis** is by demonstrating the parasites in biopsy material or by culture of material from the ulcer edge.

Treatment of the early cutaneous lesions is as recommended above for oriental sore. The extensive lesions of later stages require sodium antimony gluconate or ethylstibamine as for kala-azar (see above).

TRYPANOSOMIASIS
(African Sleeping Sickness; Chagas' Disease)

A chronic disease caused by protozoa of the genus Trypanosoma. *T. brucei* var. *gambiense* and *rhodesiense* produce African sleeping sickness (Gambian and Rhodesian trypanosomiasis); *T. cruzi* causes Chagas' disease (South American trypanosomiasis), seen in South and Central America. The African forms of trypanosomiasis are spread by the bite of the tsetse fly (genus *Glossina*). Chagas' disease is transmitted by contamination of the bite wound of the "assassin" or "kissing" reduviid bugs (*Triatoma* and related Reduviidae) with the infected feces of the insect.

Symptoms, Signs, and Course

African trypanosomiasis is characterized by irregular fever, generalized lymphadenopathy (particularly of the posterior cervical chain), cutaneous eruptions, and areas of painful localized edema. CNS symptoms, such as tremors, headache, apathy, and convulsions, later predominate and progress to coma and death. Rhodesian trypanosomiasis is more severe and more often fatal than Gambian trypanosomiasis.

Acute **Chagas' disease** occurs predominantly in young children and is characterized in the early stages by fever, lymphadenopathy, hepatosplenomegaly, and facial edema. Rarely, meningoencephalitis or convulsive seizures may occur, sometimes causing permanent mental or physical defects or death. Acute myocarditis is common and may be fatal. Chronic Chagas' disease may be mild or even asymptomatic, or may be accompanied by myocardiopathy, megaesophagus, and megacolon, with fatal outcome. These late manifestations probably result from neuropathies caused by the destruction of nerve ganglions during the acute stage of the disease. In Brazil and Argentina the disease is often severe; in Chile, usually mild.

Diagnosis

Recognition of African trypanosomiasis depends on demonstration of the trypanosomes. Early in the disease, they may be found in smears of peripheral blood or in fluid aspirated from an enlarged lymph node. In advanced stages, they may be found only in the CSF.

Chagas' disease is identified by demonstration of trypanosomes in the peripheral blood or leishmanial forms in a lymph node biopsy, or by animal inoculation or culture, xenodiagnosis, or CF tests.

Prophylaxis

Prophylaxis against African trypanosomiasis includes protection against the vector flies, avoidance of endemic areas, or chemoprophylaxis. Pentamidine 4 mg/kg body wt IM every 2 to 6 mo confers a high degree of protection against the Gambian form of disease. Its use in the Rhodesian variety is controversial.

Reduviid bugs, the vectors of Chagas' disease, inhabit poorly constructed houses and outbuildings. Residual spraying with 5% γ-benzene hexachloride is most effective in controlling the vector.

Treatment

There is no known treatment for Chagas' disease.

Early stages of Gambian African trypanosomiasis (before CNS involvement) should be treated with pentamidine 4 mg/kg/day in 3 ml of sterile distilled water IM for 10 days. Suramin is the drug of choice for early Rhodesian trypanosomiasis. It is given IV as a 10% solution in distilled water; an initial test dose of 100 mg (to exclude hypersensitivity) is followed by 1 Gm on the next day and on days 3, 7, 14, and 21, for a total of 5 Gm. (CAUTION: *Renal irritation.*)

Melarsoprol, a trivalent arsenical, is more toxic than the above drugs, but is effective in all stages of Gambian and Rhodesian trypanosomiasis. It should be used when the CNS is involved. Patients with minimal to moderate neurologic involvement are given two 3-day courses of 3.6 mg/kg/day IV, each course 2 wk apart. Melarsoprol causes the usual arsenical toxicity: gastrointestinal, neurologic, and renal.

Patients with severe neurologic involvement may develop a reactive encephalopathy when given melarsoprol. Prior treatment with suramin may help to avert this complication, which is apparently due to release of trypanosomal antigen. Suramin is given in 2 to 4 alternate-day doses of 250 to 500 mg IV. Melarsoprol is then given in 3 daily or alternate-day doses of 1.5, 2.0, and 2.2 mg/kg IV. After a 7-day interval, 3 doses of melarsoprol, 2.5, 3.0, and 3.6 mg/kg/day, are given; after another 7-day interval, a third course of 3.6 mg/kg/day is given for 3 days.

TOXOPLASMOSIS

A severe generalized or CNS granulomatous disease caused by Toxoplasma gondii. Asymptomatic infections are common; serologic surveys show that 7 to 94% of various populations are infected. The disease occurs worldwide.

Etiology and Pathogenesis

T. gondii is a small intracellular protozoan parasite that can infect any warm-blooded animal. It invades and multiplies asexually within the cytoplasm of nucleated host cells. With the development of host immunity, multiplication slows and tissue cysts are formed. Sexual multiplication occurs in the intestinal cells of cats (and apparently only cats); oocysts form and are shed in the stool. Transmission may occur transplacentally, by ingestion of raw or undercooked meat containing tissue cysts, or, perhaps most importantly, by exposure to oocysts in cat feces.

Symptoms and Signs

Neonatal congenital toxoplasmosis is acquired transplacentally, the mother presumably having acquired a primary infection shortly before or during pregnancy. Abortion may ensue if infection occurs early in pregnancy. Infection later in pregnancy may result in miscarriage or stillbirth, or in the birth of a living child with clinical disease. The disease may be severe, fulminating, and rapidly fatal, or there may be no symptoms at all. Symptoms of subacute infection may begin shortly after birth, but more often appear months or several years later. Chronic chorioretinitis; severe jaundice; hepatosplenomegaly; maculopapular rash; thrombocytopenic purpura; intracerebral calcification; convulsion, opisthotonos, psychomotor disturbances, or other CNS symptoms; and hydrocephalus or microcephaly are common. Blindness and severe mental retardation may result. Chronic disease, with relapses, occurs in patients who survive the subacute phase. Visceral lesions, aside from those in the liver, are unusual and heal more readily than CNS lesions.

Acquired toxoplasmosis is seldom symptomatic and is usually recognized serologically. However, symptomatic infection may present in any of 3 ways:

1. The more common **mild lymphatic form** resembles infectious mononucleosis. It is characterized by cervical and axillary lymphadenopathy, malaise, muscle pain, and irregular low fever. Mild anemia, hypotension, leukopenia, lymphocytosis, and slightly altered liver function may be present.

2. An acute, **fulminating, disseminated infection** occurs primarily in immunologically incompetent patients, often with a rash, high fever, chills, and prostration. Some patients may develop meningoencephalitis, hepatitis, pneumonitis, or myocarditis.

3. **Chronic toxoplasmosis** causes severe retinochoroiditis (posterior uveitis); muscular weakness, weight loss, headache, and diarrhea may be present. Symptoms are vague and indefinite and diagnosis is difficult. In the USA, uveitis is seldom due to *Toxoplasma* infection.

Diagnosis

The Sabin-Feldman **(SF)** and indirect fluorescent antibody **(IFA)** tests are the most useful serologic tests; SF and IFA titers are comparable. Because *Toxoplasma* antibodies are commonly present in the general population, serologic diagnosis requires a change from a negative to a positive result, a rapidly ascending titer, or maintenance of a high titer.

The CF test becomes positive more slowly than the SF test, and is useful when SF titers are elevated and stable. Active infection is then indicated when the CF test becomes positive or increases in titer. Serologic tests may remain positive long after convalescence.

The parasite has been isolated during the acute phase of the disease by injecting mice with biopsy material from lymph nodes, muscle, or other tissues.

Prognosis

The prognosis is poor in neonatal congenital toxoplasmosis. Affected children die in infancy or suffer chronic destructive CNS lesions. The prognosis in acquired postnatal toxoplasmosis is good for patients who survive the acute phase and for those detected in the subacute phase. The general mildness of postnatally acquired infection is indicated by the large number of persons with latent or cured toxoplasmosis, and by the fact that the disease is rarely fatal in adults.

Treatment

There is no known treatment for the subacute or chronic congenital lesions. The acute and subacute phases of acquired postnatal infection may respond to standard doses of sulfadiazine or triple sulfonamides, supplemented by pyrimethamine 50 mg/day orally for 2 wk and then 25 mg/day. Treatment should be discontinued if there is no response after a month. Since pyrimethamine may cause megaloblastic anemia or leukopenia, periodic blood counts are advised during therapy. Prednisone 20 to 40 mg/day orally, to be reduced as the patient improves, may alleviate acute allergic reactions associated with exacerbations of chronic toxoplasmosis. It has also been useful in recurrent uveitis.

DISEASES CAUSED BY WORMS

INTESTINAL NEMATODES

ENTEROBIASIS
(See TABLE 1-12 in this chapter and PINWORM INFESTATION in §10, Ch. 4)

TRICHURIASIS
(Whipworm Infection)

An infection caused by Trichuris trichiura *and characterized by abdominal pain and diarrhea.*

Etiology, Pathogenesis, and Epidemiology

Infection results from the ingestion of eggs that have incubated in soil for 2 or 3 wk. The larva hatches in the small intestine, migrates to the colon, and embeds its anterior head in the mucosa. Mature females produce about 5000 eggs/day which are passed in the stool.

This parasite is found principally in the tropics where poor sanitation and a warm moist climate provide the necessary conditions for incubation of the eggs in soil. Clinically significant infections are uncommon in the USA.

Symptoms, Signs, and Diagnosis

Only heavy infection causes symptoms—abdominal pain and diarrhea. Very heavy infections may cause intestinal blood loss, anemia, weight loss, appendicitis, and, in children, rectal prolapse.

The characteristic barrel-shaped eggs are usually readily found in the stool.

Prophylaxis and Treatment

Prevention depends upon adequate toilet facilities and good personal hygiene.

The infection is resistant to standard anthelmintic therapy. However, mebendazole 100 mg orally b.i.d. for 3 days has been highly effective and it is now the drug of choice. If mebendazole is not available, patients with severe symptoms are best treated with a hexylresorcinol enema. The bowel is first cleansed with a saline douche and the buttocks and perianal area are protected with a coat of petrolatum. The colon is filled with a 0.3% aqueous solution of hexylresorcinol, which should be retained for 20 to 30 min.

Thiabendazole may be given in milder cases. A minority of cases are cured with 25 mg/kg body wt b.i.d. orally for 2 to 3 days; a single daily dose of 25 mg/kg for 11 to 30 days may be more effective.

ASCARIASIS

An infection caused by Ascaris lumbricoides *and characterized by early pulmonary and later intestinal symptoms.*

Etiology, Epidemiology, and Pathogenesis

The life cycle of the ascarids resembles that of *Trichuris* except for a phase of larval migration through the lungs. Once the larva hatches, it migrates through the wall of the small intestine and is carried by the lymphatics and bloodstream to the lungs. Here it passes into an alveolus, ascends the respiratory tract, and is swallowed. It matures in the jejunum where it remains as an adult worm. Disease may be caused by both the larval migration through the lung and the presence of the adult worm in the intestine.

The disease occurs worldwide but is concentrated in warm, poorly sanitated areas where it is maintained largely by the indiscriminate defecation and ingestion habits of children.

Symptoms, Signs, and Diagnosis

Fever, cough, wheezing, eosinophilic leukocytosis, and migratory pulmonary infiltrates may be present during the phase of larval migration through the lungs. Heavy intestinal infection may cause abdominal cramping and, occasionally, intestinal obstruction. Adult worms may rarely obstruct the appendix, or the biliary or pancreatic ducts.

Infection with the adult worm is usually diagnosed by finding eggs in the stool. Occasionally, adult worms are passed in the stool or vomited. Larvae are occasionally found in the sputum during the pulmonary phase.

Prophylaxis

Prevention requires adequate sanitation. Drug prophylaxis has been successful in endemic areas.

Treatment

Piperazine citrate syrup 75 mg/kg body wt/day (maximum, 4 Gm) is given orally as a single dose on 2 successive days. Pyrantel pamoate 11 mg/kg (maximum, 1 Gm) in a single oral dose, or thiabendazole 25 mg/kg b.i.d. orally for 2 or 3 days is also effective.

HOOKWORM DISEASE

A symptomatic infection caused by Ancylostoma duodenale *or* Necator americanus *and characterized by abdominal pain and iron-deficiency anemia.* Asymptomatic hookworm infection is more common than symptomatic disease.

Etiology, Pathogenesis, and Epidemiology

The life cycles of the 2 worms are similar. Eggs are discharged in the stool and hatch in the soil after a 1- to 2-day incubation period, releasing a free, living larva which molts a few days later and becomes infective to humans. The larvae penetrate human skin, reach the lung via the lymphatics and blood, ascend the respiratory tract, are swallowed, and, about a week after skin penetration, reach the intestine. They attach by their mouths to the mucosa of the upper small intestine and suck blood.

About 25% of the world's population is infected with hookworms. Infection is most common in warm, moist, poorly sanitated areas. *A. duodenale* is found in the Mediterranean basin, India, China, and Japan. *N. americanus* is found primarily in tropical areas of Africa, Asia, and the Americas; it is the more prevalent species in the USA.

Symptoms and Signs

A pruritic maculopapular rash ("ground itch") may develop at the site of larval penetration. Larval pulmonary migration occasionally causes pulmonary symptoms (see ASCARIASIS, above). Adult worms often cause epigastric pain. Whether iron-deficiency anemia and hypoalbuminemia result from intestinal blood loss depends upon whether the gut losses are replaced in the diet; this, in turn, is related to the worm load and to dietary adequacy. Growth retardation, cardiac failure, and anasarca may accompany chronic severe blood loss. In most infections, however, anemia does not develop.

Diagnosis

In symptomatic infections, the typical eggs are usually readily detected in the stool. If the stool is not examined for several hours, the eggs may hatch and release larvae which may be confused with those of *Strongyloides*.

Prophylaxis

Preventing soil pollution and avoiding direct skin contact with the soil are effective but impractical measures in most endemic areas. Periodic mass treatment and dietary iron supplements may be effective.

Treatment

General supportive treatment and correction of anemia take first priority. Anemia usually responds to oral iron therapy, but parenteral iron or blood transfusions may be required in severe cases. Anthelmintic therapy may be given as soon as the patient's condition is stable. Several effective agents are available. Pyrantel pamoate 11 mg/kg (maximum, 1 Gm) orally is given in a single dose for *Ancylostoma* infections and once/day for 3 days in *Necator* infections. Tetrachloroethylene (the USP preparation available to veterinarians is satisfactory) 0.06 ml/kg for children or 0.12 ml/kg (maximum, 5 ml) for adults is given in a single oral AM dose after an overnight fast; abstinence from food for 4 h and from alcohol for 24 h after administration is recommended. If necessary, treatment may be repeated in 1 wk.

Bephenium hydroxynaphthoate 5 Gm orally in a single dose on an empty stomach may be more effective against *A. duodenale*. Thiabendazole 25 mg/kg b.i.d. orally for 2 or 3 days is also effective. Several promising newer drugs are not yet available in the USA.

STRONGYLOIDIASIS
(Threadworm Infection)

An infection caused by Strongyloides stercoralis *and characterized by eosinophilia and epigastric pain.*

Etiology, Pathogenesis, and Epidemiology

The life cycle closely resembles that of the hookworm, except that the eggs hatch while still in the intestine, and larvae rather than ova are passed in the stool. The larvae generally molt in the soil and develop into the infective filariform stage. Occasionally, the larvae molt in the intestine or on the perianal skin, and the filariform larvae then invade the host directly ("autoinfection" or "hyperinfection") without going through a soil phase. This can result in extremely heavy worm infestation.

The disease is endemic in the tropics and is generally found in the same climatic and sanitary conditions favorable to the spread of hookworm. It may also occur in temperate areas in unsanitary crowded institutions.

Symptoms, Signs, and Diagnosis

Transient bouts of linear urticaria and erythema may accompany autoinfection. Pulmonary manifestations similar to those seen in ascariasis (see above) may occur as a result of larval migration through the lungs. Heavy intestinal infection may cause epigastric pain and tenderness, vomiting, and diarrhea. Potentially fatal massive autoinfection and widespread larval migration may occur in immunodepressed patients, often accompanied by severe enterocolitis and gram-negative bacteremia.

Larvae are found in the stool; several specimens should be examined since only a few larvae may be present. Examination of duodenal aspirates or jejunal biopsies may also demonstrate the larvae.

Prophylaxis and Treatment

Prevention is generally as above, for hookworm. Thiabendazole 25 mg/kg body wt b.i.d. orally for 2 or 3 days is effective treatment.

TISSUE NEMATODES

TRICHINOSIS
(Trichiniasis)

A parasitic disease caused by Trichinella spiralis, *characterized initially by GI symptoms, and later by periorbital edema, muscle pains, fever, and eosinophilia.*

Etiology, Pathogenesis, and Epidemiology

Infection with the roundworm *T. spiralis* results from eating raw or inadequately cooked or processed pork or pork products (rarely, meat of bears and some marine mammals) containing encysted larvae (trichinae). The cyst wall is digested in the stomach or duodenum and the liberated larvae penetrate the duodenal and jejunal mucosa. Within 3 or 4 days, the larvae mature sexually and mate, after which the smaller sized males (1.5 mm) die. The females (3 mm) burrow into the intestinal wall and begin to discharge living larvae by the 7th day. Each female may produce over 1000 larvae. Larviposition continues for about 4 to 6 wk, after which the female worm dies and is digested. The minute (0.1 mm) larvae are carried by the lymphatic and portal circulation to the systemic blood stream, thence to various tissues and organs. Only those larvae reaching skeletal muscle survive; they penetrate individual fibers, causing myositis. They grow to 1 mm in length, coil up, encyst, and eventually calcify. Encystment is complete by the end of the 3rd mo. The larvae may remain viable for several years. The diaphragm and tongue, and the pectoral, eye, and intercostal muscles are especially involved. Larvae reaching the myocardium and other nonskeletal muscles are surrounded by a focus of inflammatory reaction and die. In animals, the encysted larvae are the source of infection for the next host.

Trichinosis occurs worldwide but is rare or absent in native populations of the tropics and where swine are fed root vegetables, as in France. In the USA, it has become sporadic and less frequent; outbreaks are usually caused by the consumption of ready-to-eat pork sausages.

Symptoms and Signs

The clinical course is markedly irregular, severity varying with the number of invading larvae, the tissues invaded, and the physiologic condition of the patient. Many patients remain asymptomatic. GI symptoms and slight fever may appear within 1 or 2 days after ingestion of infected meat, but manifestations of systemic larval invasion usually do not appear for 7 to 15 days. Edema of the upper eyelids appears suddenly about the 11th day of infection and is one of the earliest and most characteristic signs. This may be followed by subconjunctival and retinal hemorrhage, pain, and photophobia. Muscle soreness and pain, urticaria, subungual hemorrhage, thirst, profuse sweating, fever, chills, weakness, prostration, and a rapidly rising eosinophilia may develop shortly after the ocular signs. Soreness is especially pronounced in the muscles of respiration, speech, mastication, and swallowing. Severe dyspnea, sometimes causing death, may occur. Fever is generally remittent, rising to 39 C (102 F) or higher, remaining elevated for several days, and then falling gradually. Eosinophilia usually begins in the 2nd wk, reaches its height (20 to 40% or more) in the 3rd or 4th wk, then gradually declines. It may be obscured by concomitant bacterial infection. Lymphadenitis, encephalitis, meningitis, visual or auditory disorders, pneumonitis, pleurisy, and myocarditis may develop in the 3rd to 6th wk, as the widely disseminated larvae outside the skeletal muscles are destroyed by inflammatory reaction; if myocardial failure develops, it occurs between the 4th and 8th wk. Most symptoms disappear by about the 3rd mo, although vague muscular pains and fatigue may persist for months.

Diagnosis

During the intestinal stage of infection, symptoms are nonspecific and no diagnostic laboratory procedures are available. Diarrhea, nausea, vomiting, and other GI disturbances may be recalled later by the patient. A history of ingesting ready-to-eat pork sausage or insufficiently cooked pork or bear meat, followed by an acute gastroenteritis or an acute facial edema (particularly of the upper eyelids) is helpful in diagnosis. Eosinophilic leukocytosis usually appears within 2 wk of infection. Muscle biopsy performed during the 4th wk of infection may demonstrate larvae or cysts. Even when trichinae cannot be demonstrated in the biopsy specimen, a diffuse myositis may indicate active trichinosis. The parasite is rarely found in the infected meat, or in the patient's stool, blood, or CSF.

The intradermal test, using an antigen prepared from larvae, becomes positive during the 3rd wk of infection and may remain so for 20 yr. Available serologic tests include CF, precipitin, indirect fluorescent antibody, and (probably the best) bentonite flocculation. Since these tests may also remain positive for years, they are of most value if they are initially negative and then turn positive.

Skeletal manifestations of trichinosis must be differentiated from acute rheumatic fever, acute arthritis, angioedema, and myositis; **febrile states** from TB, typhoid fever, sepsis, undulant fever; **pulmonary manifestations** from pneumonitis; **neurologic manifestations** from meningitis, encephalitis, and poliomyelitis; and **eosinophilia** from Hodgkin's disease, eosinophilic leukemia, and polyarteritis nodosa.

Prognosis

This is good in most cases. Unfavorable prognostic signs are the absence of an eosinophilic response, or a sudden fall in the eosinophil level to 1% or zero during the acute phase.

Prophylaxis

Trichinosis can be prevented by thoroughly cooking all pork and pork products. Hogs should not be fed raw garbage since it may contain infected pork wastes.

Treatment

Symptomatic and supportive therapy is aimed at assisting the patient to survive the acute toxemia, which terminates when the larvae becomes encysted. Muscular pains are usually relieved by bed rest, but may require analgesics such as aspirin or codeine. Corticosteroids are indicated for patients with severe allergic manifestations or myocardial or CNS involvement. Prednisone 60 mg/day orally in divided doses is given for 3 or 4 days; dosage is then reduced and the drug is discontinued in 10 days.

Thiabendazole, 25 mg/kg body wt b.i.d. orally for 5 to 10 days, is highly effective against the parasite, but the clinical response is variable.

TOXOCARIASIS
(Visceral Larva Migrans)

A widely distributed clinical syndrome resulting from invasion of human viscera by nematode larvae (e.g., Toxocara canis *and* cati, *normally intestinal parasites of dogs and cats), with subsequent prolonged migration of the larvae through the body.* It usually occurs as a relatively benign disease in children aged 2 to 4, but may afflict older patients.

Etiology and Pathogenesis

The source of infection is the fully embryonated egg of the parasite found in soil contaminated by feces of infected dogs and cats. Children's sandboxes are attractive defecating sites for cats and are a potential hazard. The eggs may be transferred directly to the mouth as the child plays in or eats (geophagia) the contaminated soil, or indirectly through contaminated food or other objects. The incubation period varies from weeks to several months, depending on the intensity and number of exposures, and on the sensitivity of the patient.

The eggs hatch in the intestine after ingestion. Liberated larvae penetrate the intestinal wall and are widely disseminated in the body by the systemic circulation. Almost any tissue may be involved, particularly the CNS, eye, liver, lungs, and heart. The larvae may remain alive for many months, causing damage by their wanderings and by tissue sensitization. They produce a focal granulomatous reaction, though the larvae themselves may be difficult to demonstrate in tissue sections. The parasites do not complete their development in the human body.

Symptoms, Signs, and Diagnosis

Clinically, patients present with fever, cough or wheezing, and hepatomegaly. Skin rash, splenomegaly, and recurrent pneumonia occur in some patients. Eye lesions (chorioretinitis) may be mistaken for retinoblastoma.

High eosinophilia (> 60%), hepatomegaly, pneumonitis, fever, and hyperglobulinemia are suggestive. Liver biopsy and demonstration of a larva or its fragments in the typical granulomatous lesion may be helpful in the diagnosis. Reliable skin tests and indirect HA and fluorescent antibody tests have been developed, but are not generally available. The prognosis is good; the disease is self-limited (6 to 18 mo in the absence of reinfection).

Prophylaxis and Treatment

Infected pet dogs and cats should be dewormed regularly (under veterinary direction), and children's sandboxes should be covered when not in use.

No effective treatment is available. Diethylcarbamazine 2 mg/kg t.i.d. orally after meals for 2 to 4 wk is probably the drug of choice; the use of thiabendazole is under study. Prednisone 20 to 40 mg/day orally, with reduced dosage after 3 to 5 days, helps to control symptoms.

FILARIASIS

A group of diseases occurring in tropical and subtropical countries and caused by Filarioidea.

Etiology and Pathogenesis

Wuchereria bancrofti is found only in humans; *Brugia malayi* is often spread to man from animal hosts. The adult filarioidea live in the human lymphatic system. Microfilariae released by gravid females are found in the peripheral blood, usually at night. Infection is spread by many species of mosquitoes; vectors of *W. bancrofti* are *Aëdes, Culex,* and *Anopheles;* of *B. malayi, Anopheles* and *Mansonia.* The microfilariae are ingested by the mosquito, undergo development in the insect's thoracic muscles, and, when mature, migrate to its mouthparts. When the infected mosquito bites a new host, the microfilariae penetrate the bite puncture, and eventually reach the lymphatics where development to the adult stage occurs.

Pathology

Inflammation and fibrosis occur in the vicinity of the adult worms, producing progressive lymphatic obstruction. The microfilariae probably do not contribute directly to the host reaction.

Symptoms and Signs

The incubation period may be as short as 2 mo. The "prepatent" period (from time of infection to appearance of microfilariae in the blood) is at least 8 mo. Clinical manifestations depend on the severity of the infection; they may include lymphangitis, lymphadenitis, orchitis, funiculitis, epididymitis, lymph varices, and chyluria. Chills, fever, headache, and malaise may also be present. Elephantiasis and other late severe sequelae occur with long-time residence in endemic areas and repeated reinfection.

Diagnosis

Microfilariae may be found in blood or lymph fluid. An intradermal antigen (prepared from *Dirofilaria immitis*) is useful when microfilariae cannot be demonstrated, but is not completely reliable.

Prophylaxis and Treatment

Promising results have been obtained in controlling filariasis by combining mass treatment and mosquito control.

Diethylcarbamazine 2 mg/kg body wt orally t.i.d. after meals for 2 to 4 wk eliminates microfilariae from the bloodstream. In many patients it also kills adult worms or impairs their reproductive capacity, resulting in permanent clearing of the microfilariae. Severe allergic reactions and abscess formation may follow its use, but may be controlled by antihistamines or corticosteroids.

Surgical intervention is indicated only to alleviate certain types of elephantiasis, especially of the scrotum. Elephantiasis of the legs is treated by elevation and elastic bandages.

ONCHOCERCIASIS
(River Blindness)

A disease resulting from infection by Onchocerca volvulus *and characterized by fibrous nodules in the skin and subcutaneous tissues.* Ocular findings are common; blindness may result. The disease, spread by the bite of black flies *(Simuliidae),* occurs in southern Mexico, Guatemala, Venezuela, Colombia, Yemen, and central Africa. **Diagnosis** depends on demonstration of microfilariae in skin snips or nodules.

Treatment

Microfilariae, but not adult worms, are destroyed by diethylcarbamazine, given orally after meals. Since an allergic reaction to the dead microfilariae can result in ocular damage if the eye is involved in the infection, initial dosage is limited to 0.1 to 0.2 mg/kg body wt/day. Dosage is gradually increased to 2 to 3 mg/kg t.i.d. and then maintained at this level for 1 wk. An antihistamine and prednisone 20 to 40 mg/day orally may be necessary to prevent the acute allergic inflammation in and around the eye which follows the rapid destruction of numerous microfilariae.

Adult worms are eliminated by surgically removing the nodules; suramin (CAUTION: *Toxicity*) in a test dose of 100 mg IV, followed by 5 weekly injections of 1 Gm IV, is also effective.

LOIASIS
(Calabar Swellings)

A form of filariasis found in west and central Africa, caused by Loa loa *and transmitted by the bite of flies of the genus* Chrysops. The disease is characterized by localized transient swellings (calabar swellings) caused by migration of adult worms in the subcutaneous tissues. The worms may also migrate across the eye beneath the conjunctiva. Microfilariae are found in the calabar swellings and peripheral blood; eosinophilia is common.

Treatment

Diethylcarbamazine 2 mg/kg body wt orally t.i.d. after meals for 14 days kills both the microfilariae and adult worms. Since allergic reactions are common during the first part of treatment, an antihistamine and prednisone 10 to 30 mg/day orally should be given concurrently during the first 4 days of treatment.

DRACUNCULIASIS
(Dracontiasis; "Fiery Serpent")

A disease caused by the presence of the guinea worm (Dracunculus medinensis) *in subcutaneous tissues.* It is endemic in India, Pakistan, the Near East, tropical Africa, certain West Indies islands, and the Guianas. Infection follows ingestion of water containing infected crustacea *(Cyclops).* The larvae penetrate the intestinal wall, mature in the retroperitoneal space, and migrate to the subcutaneous tissue, producing skin ulcers through which the female discharges larvae. Intense local itching and burning may result. **Diagnosis** is possible only after the adult worm reaches its destination under the skin, at which time its head may be seen in the base of the ulcer, or larvae may be demonstrated in the discharge.

Treatment consists of slow extraction of the adult worm by gradual traction on its head over a period of 10 days. Niridazole (see SCHISTOSOMIASIS, below) causes worms to be eliminated spontaneously, or eases their manual removal. Thiabendazole 50 to 100 mg/kg orally in divided doses for 1 to 3 days is also reported to be effective. Surgical removal is not recommended. Septic and foreign-body reactions should be treated appropriately.

TREMATODES

SCHISTOSOMIASIS
(Bilharziasis)

A visceral parasitic disease caused by blood flukes of the genus Schistosoma.

Etiology, Pathogenesis, and Epidemiology

The schistosomes that affect man are trematodes. Fresh-water snails are the intermediate hosts. Human infection follows contact (by bathing, wading, etc.)

with the free-swimming cercariae of the parasite which penetrate the skin and are carried to the intrahepatic portal circulation, where they mature in 1 to 3 mo. The adult worms then migrate to the venules of the bladder or intestines. Three species cause clinical disease: *S. haematobium* causes symptoms in the GU system or the lower colon and rectum; *S. mansoni* and *S. japonicum* cause disturbances in the small intestine, colon, and rectum.

The disease is endemic in Africa, the Middle East, and Cyprus *(S. haematobium);* Egypt, areas of northern and southern Africa, certain West Indies islands, and the northern ⅔ of South America *(S. mansoni);* and Japan, central and south China, the Philippines, the Celebes, Thailand, and Laos *(S. japonicum)*. *S. mansoni* is frequently encountered in Puerto Ricans residing in the USA.

Several schistosome species do not dwell in man, but are capable of causing dermatitis **("swimmer's itch")**, seen in the USA as well as elsewhere. The definitive hosts are usually migratory birds; both fresh and salt water mollusks serve as intermediate hosts.

Symptoms and Signs

Initially, a pruritic papular dermatitis appears where the cercariae entered the skin. In "swimmer's itch" the disease never progresses beyond this point. In other forms, the adult worm develops in the liver, causing fever, eosinophilia, and often urticaria, hepatosplenomegaly, and lymphadenopathy. When the adults migrate to the viscera, the damage caused by the reaction to their eggs produces symptoms referable to the affected visceral structures (cystitis, chronic diarrhea). Hepatic cirrhosis, splenomegaly, ascites, and esophageal varices may occur from inflammation and fibrosis around eggs, especially in *S. mansoni* and *S. japonicum* infections. Eggs of *S. haematobium* and *S. mansoni* may cause pulmonary damage; those of *S. japonicum* and *S. mansoni* may cause CNS damage.

Diagnosis

Eggs are found in the stool *(S. japonicum* and *mansoni)* or urine *(S. haematobium)*, or in rectal or bladder biopsies. Repeated stool examinations using concentration technics may be necessary. Positive skin and serologic tests are not sufficient basis for therapy, but should lead to a vigorous search for eggs. Only the demonstration of living eggs in a patient warrants initiation of treatment.

Prophylaxis

Control of the disease is difficult and depends upon proper disposal of urine and feces, use of molluscacides, provision of a pure water supply, and treatment with anthelmintics.

Treatment

Since the severity of schistosomiasis depends on the intensity of infection, the aim of therapy is to reduce the worm load. Prolonged or repeated courses of antischistosomal agents in an attempt to effect a cure are unwarranted because of the toxicity of available agents. The trivalent antimony compounds tartar emetic (antimony potassium tartrate), stibophen, and stibocaptate (sodium antimony dimercaptosuccinate) are effective and should be used in *S. japonicum* infections, the most resistant of the infections to therapy. These drugs, however, are **contraindicated** in liver, kidney, and cardiac disease.

Tartar emetic is the most toxic, but most effective, of the trivalent antimonials and is probably the drug of choice in *S. japonicum* infections. It is given slowly IV as a 0.5% solution 2 or 3 h after a light meal. The needle should be wiped with a sterile sponge; extravasation of fluid should be **avoided** since the solution irritates tissues and may cause sloughing. The patient should remain recumbent for at least an hour after treatment. The drug is given on alternate days. The initial dose is 40 mg (8 ml). If tolerated, the dose is increased by 20 mg (4 ml) every other day, to a maximum dose of 140 mg (28 ml). This last dose is continued until a total of 15 injections has been given.

Toxic effects of tartar emetic include coughing immediately upon injection (which is not important), nausea, vomiting, stiff joints and muscles, a sense of constriction of the chest, upper abdominal pain, cardiac arrhythmias, dizziness, and collapse. Hepatitis, nephritis, or hemolytic anemia may occasionally occur. The drug should be stopped at once if critical toxic reactions occur during injection. Following any major toxic effect, subsequent doses should be reduced, or administration of the drug temporarily or permanently discontinued, according to the circumstances. Severe coughing can be controlled or avoided by giving future doses in 2 portions 1 h apart.

Stibophen and stibocaptate are very effective against *S. haematobium* and are the drugs of choice for *S. mansoni*. They should be used in *S. japonicum* infections only when tartar emetic cannot be tolerated. Stibophen is given slowly IM as a 6.3% solution; 4 ml is given every other day, to a total of 80 to 100 ml. Nausea and vomiting are the only expected toxic symptoms; rarely, joint and muscle pains may appear. If severe toxic symptoms occur, subsequent doses should be reduced or administration temporarily or permanently discontinued. Stibocaptate is given IM as a 10% solution twice weekly for 5 doses. The total dose should be 35 to 50 mg/kg (maximum, 2 Gm).

Niridazole 25 mg/kg/day orally in 2 divided doses for 5 to 7 days is effective against *S. mansoni* and is the drug of choice for *S. haematobium* infections. Mental confusion, psychosis, and, less commonly, convulsions may occur during treatment but disappear when the drug is discontinued. Stibocaptate at a total dosage of 40 mg/kg, given IM in 5 divided doses once or twice/wk, is effective against *S. mansoni* infections. Hycanthone, a thioxanthene given as a single IM injection, is also effective against *S. mansoni* and *S. haematobium,* but its mutagenic and hepatotoxic properties limit its usefulness.

Patients should be examined for the presence of living eggs 3 and 6 mo after treatment. Retreatment is indicated if egg excretion has not decreased markedly.

CESTODES

BEEF TAPEWORM INFECTION
(*Taenia saginata* Infection; Taeniasis Saginata)

A usually asymptomatic infection of the intestinal tract caused by the cestode Taenia saginata.

Etiology, Pathogenesis, and Epidemiology

The adult worm inhabits the human intestinal tract and is composed of a small head (scolex) 1 to 2 mm in diameter, and up to 1000 hermaphroditic proglottids which give the worm its characteristic ribbon-like shape. The worm measures 4.5 to 9 m (15 to 30 ft). Egg-bearing proglottids are passed in the stool and ingested by cattle. The eggs hatch in the cattle, invade the intestinal wall, and are carried by the bloodstream to striated muscle, where they encyst (cysticercus stage). Humans are infected by ingesting the cysticercus in raw or undercooked beef.

The infection is particularly common in Africa, the Middle East, Eastern Europe, Mexico, and South America. Infection in the USA is uncommon, but still occurs in California and New England.

Symptoms, Signs, and Diagnosis

The infection is usually asymptomatic, although epigastric pain, diarrhea, and weight loss may occur. Occasionally, the patient may feel an active proglottid crawling through the anus.

The diagnosis is usually made by finding the characteristic proglottids or, more rarely, the scolex in the stool. The perianal area may also be examined by pressing the sticky side of cellophane tape against the area, placing the tape on a glass slide, and microscopically examining it for eggs deposited by ruptured proglottids.

Prophylaxis

Infection may be prevented by thoroughly cooking beef at a minimum of 56 C (133 F) for 5 min. Meat inspection and adequate toilet facilities also help to control infection.

Treatment

A single dose of 2 Gm niclosamide is given as 4 tablets (500 mg each) which are chewed and swallowed with a small amount of water. The worm is then usually digested by the time it is passed. The stool should be rechecked in 3 mo to make certain a cure has been obtained.

Quinacrine is an alternative, but it is less convenient than niclosamide and causes more side effects. The patient is given a purgative the day before treatment. Following an overnight fast, 4 doses of 200 mg quinacrine are given orally every 10 min (total, 800 mg). The nausea and vomiting that accompanies ingestion of quinacrine may be alleviated by giving sodium bicarbonate 600 mg with each dose of quinacrine, or by giving the quinacrine by duodenal tube. A second purgative is given 2 h after completing therapy, and the stool is searched for the scolex. Bithionol 1 Gm orally, repeated in 1 h, is also very effective.

PORK TAPEWORM INFECTION
(*Taenia solium* Infection; Cysticercosis)

An intestinal infection caused by the adult cestode Taenia solium. *Infection with the larvae (cysticerci) causes* **cysticercosis,** *an occasional occurrence in man.*

Etiology, Pathogenesis, and Epidemiology

The adult *T. solium* measures 2.5 to 3 m (8 to 10 ft) in length, and is composed of a scolex armed with several hooklets and a body composed of 1000 proglottids. The gravid proglottids have fewer uterine branches than gravid *T. saginata* proglottids have. The life cycle resembles that of *T. saginata* except that hogs rather than cattle serve as the normal intermediate hosts. Humans may also act as intermediate hosts either by ingesting the eggs directly, or by regurgitating gravid proglottids from the intestine to the stomach where the embryos are released, penetrate the intestinal wall, and are carried to the subcutaneous tissue, muscle, viscera, and CNS. Viable cysticerci cause only a mild tissue reaction; dead larvae, however, provoke a vigorous reaction.

T. solium infections are frequent in Asia, Russia, Eastern Europe, and Latin America; infection in the USA is rare.

Symptoms and Signs

Infection with the adult worm is usually asymptomatic. Heavy larval infection (cysticercosis) may cause muscle pains, weakness, fever, or, if the CNS is involved, meningoencephalitis or epilepsy.

Diagnosis

In adult worm infections, eggs may be found in the perianal area or stool. The proglottids or scolex must be recovered from the stool and examined in order to differentiate *T. solium* from *T. saginata.* Cysticercosis should be suspected in any patient who lives in an endemic area and develops neurologic findings. Calcified cysticerci may be seen on x-ray. Encysted larvae may occasionally be recovered in biopsied subcutaneous nodules. A hemagglutination test has been developed, but its usefulness is uncertain.

Prophylaxis and Treatment

Infection may be prevented by thoroughly cooking pork.

Niclosamide is therapeutically effective, but it results in digestion of the worm and release of eggs, and might cause cysticercosis. For this reason, quinacrine (see BEEF TAPEWORM INFECTION, above) is the preferred treatment. An antiemetic should be given prior to treatment in order to prevent vomiting with return of proglottids to the stomach. Surgery may be necessary in CNS cysticercosis.

FISH TAPEWORM INFECTION
(Diphyllobothriasis)

An intestinal infection caused by the adult cestode Diphyllobothrium latum.

Etiology, Pathogenesis, and Epidemiology

The adult worm possesses several thousand proglottids, and measures 4.5 to 9 m (15 to 30 ft) in length. Operculated ova are released from the proglottid in the intestinal lumen and are passed in the stool. The egg hatches in fresh water, releasing the embryo which is eaten by small crustaceans that may, in turn, be ingested by a fish. Humans are infected by eating raw or undercooked infected fish.

The infection occurs in Europe (particularly Scandinavia), Japan, Africa, South America, Canada, and, in the USA, in Florida and the North Central States. Uncooked "ludefish" or "gefilte fish" may harbor infection.

Symptoms, Signs, and Diagnosis

Infection is usually asymptomatic, although mild GI symptoms may be noted. Rarely, an anemia that resembles pernicious anemia may develop, presumably because of host-tapeworm competition for vitamin B_{12}.

Operculated eggs are easily found in the stool.

Prophylaxis and Treatment

All fresh-water fish should be thoroughly cooked, or frozen at -10 C (14 F) for 48 h. Treatment requires niclosamide (see BEEF TAPEWORM INFECTION, above).

---

9. DISEASES OF UNCERTAIN ETIOLOGY

SARCOIDOSIS

A multisystem granulomatous disorder of unknown etiology characterized histologically by epithelioid tubercles involving various organs or tissues, with symptoms dependent on the site and degree of involvement.

Etiology and Incidence

The cause is unknown. A single provoking agent (e.g., a slow virus) or a disordered defense reaction triggered by a variety of insults may be responsible; genetic factors may be important. Sarcoidosis occurs predominantly between ages

20 and 40 and is most common among northern Europeans and American Negroes. The incidence in some advanced countries exceeds that of tuberculosis.

Pathology

The characteristic histopathologic findings are multiple noncaseating epithelioid granulomas, with little or no necrosis, which may resolve completely or proceed to fibrosis. They occur commonly in mediastinal and peripheral lymph nodes, lungs, liver, eyes, and skin, and less often in the spleen, bones, joints, skeletal muscle, heart, and CNS.

Symptoms and Signs

Symptoms may be absent, slight, or severe and depend on the site of involvement. Impairment of function may be due to the active granulomatous disease or to secondary fibrosis. Fever, weight loss, and arthralgias may be initial manifestations. Persistent fever is especially common with hepatic involvement.

Peripheral lymphadenopathy is common and usually asymptomatic. Even insignificant nodes may contain characteristic tubercles. Mediastinal adenopathy is often discovered by routine chest x-ray. X-ray findings of bilateral hilar and right paratracheal adenopathy are virtually pathognomonic; adenopathy is occasionally unilateral. Diffuse **pulmonary infiltration** may accompany or follow the adenopathy and may have a diffuse fine ground-glass appearance on x-ray or occur as reticular or miliary lesions, or as multiple confluent infiltrations producing large nodules that resemble metastatic tumors. Pulmonary involvement may also occur without visible adenopathy. It is usually accompanied by cough and dyspnea, but symptoms may be minimal or absent. Pulmonary fibrosis, cystic changes, and cor pulmonale are the end results of longstanding progressive disease.

Skin lesions (plaques, papules, and subcutaneous nodules) are frequently present in patients with severe chronic sarcoidosis. Nasal and conjunctival mucosal granulomas may occur. **Erythema nodosum** with fever and arthralgias is a frequent manifestation in Europe, but less common in the USA.

Hepatic granulomas are found in 70% of patients examined by percutaneous biopsy, even if patients are asymptomatic with normal liver function tests. Hepatomegaly is noted in fewer than 20% of patients; progressive and severe hepatic dysfunction with portal hypertension and esophageal varices is rare.

Granulomatous uveitis occurs in 15% of cases; it is usually bilateral, and may cause severe loss of vision from secondary glaucoma if untreated. Retinal periphlebitis, lacrimal gland enlargement, conjunctival infiltrations, and keratitis sicca are occasionally present. **Myocardial involvement** may cause angina, congestive failure, or fatal conduction abnormalities. Acute **polyarthritis** may be prominent; chronic periarticular swelling and tenderness may be associated with osseous changes in the phalanges. **CNS involvement** is of almost any type, but cranial nerve palsies (especially facial paralysis) are most common. **Diabetes insipidus** may occur. **Hypercalcemia** and **hypercalciuria** may cause renal calculi or nephrocalcinosis with consequent renal failure, but prednisone therapy has reduced the frequency and importance of disordered calcium metabolism.

Laboratory Findings

Leukopenia is frequently present. Hyperglobulinemia is common among Negroes. Elevated serum uric acid is not uncommon, but gout is rare. Serum alkaline phosphatase may be elevated as a result of hepatic involvement. Depression of delayed hypersensitivity is characteristic, but a negative second-strength tuberculin reaction reliably excludes a complicating tuberculosis.

Pulmonary function tests show restriction, decreased compliance, and impaired diffusing capacity. CO_2 retention is uncommon since ventilation is rarely obstructed except in patients with endobronchial disease or in late stages with severe pulmonary fibrosis. Serial measurements of pulmonary function are a guide to treatment and to the course of the disease.

Diagnosis

A clinical diagnosis may be made in asymptomatic patients with typical chest x-ray findings. Tissue biopsy, with microbiologic as well as histologic examination, is essential if symptoms are present and corticosteroid therapy seems indicated. When superficial or palpable lesions (e.g., in skin, lymph nodes, palpebral conjunctiva) are present, biopsy is positive in 87% of specimens. Liver biopsies show granulomas in 70% of cases. Biopsy of nodes in the scalene fat pad is positive in about 75%, but mediastinoscopy is preferred since it is positive in more than 95% of patients. Lungs, skeletal muscle, and lacrimal and parotid glands are other possible biopsy sites, depending on clinical indications. Local sarcoid reactions in a single organ and granulomas due to infection or hypersensitivity must be excluded. In questionable cases, histologic changes should be demonstrated in several sites.

The Kveim reaction (a granulomatous reaction appearing 4 wk after intradermal injection of sarcoid spleen or lymph node tissue) is positive in 50 to 85% of patients, but reactions occur in other diseases as well.

Tuberculosis and fungus infection, particularly histoplasmosis and coccidioidomycosis, must be excluded. Tuberculosis has become a declining problem, and aspergillosis and cryptococcosis are now more frequent complications. Hodgkin's disease must also be excluded. Typical sarcoid granulomas are found in 5% of liver biopsies done for staging of Hodgkin's disease; it is uncertain whether they indicate concurrence of the two diseases or a sarcoid reaction to the neoplasm.

Course and Prognosis

Evaluation of treatment is difficult since spontaneous improvement or clearing is common. Massive hilar adenopathy and extensive infiltrates may disappear in a few months or years. Mediastinal adenopathy persists without change for many years in about 10% of cases. Complete clearing of the disease occurs in ⅓ of the patients; recovery with minor residua in another ⅓; and progressive disease requiring treatment in the remaining ⅓. Mortality is 5 to 8%. Gradual pulmonary fibrosis, leading to pulmonary insufficiency, pulmonary hypertension, and cor pulmonale, is the leading cause of disability and death; pulmonary hemorrhage from aspergillosis is the second most common cause of death.

Treatment

The aim of treatment is to prevent progressive tissue damage and irreversible fibrosis, but no available therapeutic agents have been shown to accomplish this in the lungs. Asymptomatic hilar or peripheral adenopathy needs no treatment. Corticosteroid therapy is indicated for suppression of the active inflammatory reaction and for troublesome or disabling symptoms, such as dyspnea, severe arthralgia, or fever. It should be started promptly if active ocular disease, respiratory failure, hepatic insufficiency, cardiac arrhythmia, CNS involvement, or hypercalcemia is present.

Prednisone 40 to 60 mg/day orally may be given when a prompt effect is desired, but 15 mg/day orally is usually adequate to control the inflammatory reaction. Prolonged therapy with doses exceeding 15 mg/day should be given on an alternate-day schedule. Treatment may be needed for weeks, for years, or indefinitely. Maintenance doses of 5 to 10 mg/day control symptoms and radiologic changes in many chronic cases. Clinical examination, x-rays, and pulmonary function studies should be made at frequent intervals when dosage is reduced or medication terminated. Serious complications of corticosteroid therapy have been infrequent. Concomitant isoniazid therapy (300 mg/day for a year) is indicated only for patients with positive tuberculin skin tests.

Disfiguring skin lesions may respond to hydroxychloroquine 400 to 800 mg/day orally; remission may be maintained with 200 to 400 mg/day. Hydroxychloroquine is not given for longer than 6 mo because of the danger of ocular damage; relapse is common following discontinuance. Chlorambucil and methotrexate have been tried experimentally and may be useful when corticosteroids are not tolerated, although they must be used with caution.

REYE'S SYNDROME

The syndrome of acute encephalopathy and fatty degeneration of the viscera **(AEFDV)** *of unknown etiology, which tends to follow some acute viral infections.*

Reye's syndrome was first characterized as a distinct clinical and pathologic entity in 1963. While the etiology is unknown, viral agents such as influenza B and varicella virus, exogenous toxins such as *Aspergillus flavus* aflatoxin, and intrinsic metabolic defects in urea-cycle enzymes such as ornithine transcarbamylase have been implicated as associated or contributory factors.

Epidemiology

The syndrome is seen in children under 18 yr of age. In the USA, most cases occur in late fall and winter. Both geographic and temporal clusters of the disease, as well as sporadic cases, have been described. Widespread outbreaks have occurred in association with regional influenza B epidemics. Varicella virus, the enteroviruses, Epstein-Barr virus, and the myxoviruses have been associated with sporadic cases. In Thailand, AEFDV has been associated with aflatoxin ingestion. An increased incidence among siblings has been noted, but whether environmental factors (e.g., common exposure to exogenous toxins or viruses) or genetic predispositions (e.g., an inherited enzyme deficiency) account for the familial clustering is unknown.

Pathology

With light microscopy, uniform intracytoplasmic panlobular microvesicular fatty infiltration of the liver is seen, which stains with oil red O, a Sudan dye, on frozen section. Fatty accumulation in the pancreas, heart, kidney, spleen, and lymph nodes, and pulmonary histiocytes have also been described. Fatty infiltration is thought to be neutral lipid (probably triglyceride) and hepatic inflammation is generally absent or slight. An occasional patient, especially one who has had significant hypotension, may show zonal hepatic necrosis that is typically central in the hepatic lobule. Electron microscopic sections of liver show mitochondrial injury which varies with the severity of the disease but includes glycogen depletion, smooth endoplasmic reticulum proliferation, peroxisome damage, and swelling of the mitochondrial matrix. Histologic abnormalities of the liver usually return to normal by 8 to 12 wk after the onset of the disease.

CNS findings are generally nonspecific and include cerebral edema, gyral flattening, swollen white matter, and ventricular compression. On microscopy, perineuronal and perivascular clear spaces with swollen astrocytes are seen.

Symptoms and Signs

Severity of the disease varies greatly, but the syndrome is characterized by a biphasic illness: initially a viral infection, usually a URI, occasionally exanthematous, followed on about the 6th day by the onset of pernicious nausea and vomiting and by a sudden change in mental status. When associated with varicella, the encephalopathy usually develops on the 4th to 5th day of the rash. The changes in mental status may vary from a mild amnesia and noticeable lethargy to intermittent episodes of disorientation and agitation which often progress rapidly to deepening stages of coma manifested by progressive unresponsiveness, decorticate and decerebrate posturing, seizures, flaccidity, fixed dilated pupils, and respiratory arrest. Focal neurologic findings are usually not present. Hepatomegaly occurs in about 40% of cases, but jaundice is rare.

Complications include electrolyte and fluid disturbances, diabetes insipidus, inappropriate ADH syndrome, hypotension, cardiac arrhythmias, bleeding diatheses (especially gastrointestinal), pancreatitis, respiratory insufficiency, and aspiration pneumonia. In fatal cases, the mean time from hospitalization to death is 4 days.

Diagnosis and Laboratory Findings

Reye's syndrome should be suspected in any child exhibiting the acute onset of an encephalopathy without known heavy metal or toxin exposure, associated with hepatic dysfunction. Liver biopsy provides the definitive diagnosis and is especially useful in sporadic cases and in young children. The diagnosis may also be made when the typical clinical findings and the history are associated with a constellation of laboratory findings consisting of increased liver transaminases (SGOT, SGPT > 3 times normal), bilirubin < 2.5 mg/100 ml, increased blood ammonia level, a prothrombin time < 60% of normal, and a noninflammatory CSF. CSF examination usually shows increased pressure, < 8 to 10 WBC/cu mm, and normal protein; the glutamine level may be elevated. Hypoglycemia and hypoglycorrachia are seen in 15% of cases, and especially in children under age 4 yr.

Signs of widespread metabolic derangements also may be present and include elevated serum levels of the amino acids glutamine, alanine, lysine, and α-amino-N-butyrate, and of the medium-chain free fatty acids; acid-base disturbances, usually hyperventilation with mixed respiratory alkalosis and metabolic acidosis; and other electrolyte abnormalities such as hyper- and hypo-osmolality, hypernatremia, hypokalemia, and hypophosphatemia. Elevated amylase and CPK levels reflect widespread organ involvement.

Differential diagnosis includes other causes of dehydration, shock, and coma such as sepsis or enteritis (especially in infants); phosphorus or carbon tetrachloride intoxication; acute encephalopathy caused by salicylism or other drugs or poisons; viral encephalitis or meningitis; and acute hepatitis. Similar light-microscopy findings on liver biopsy may be seen with idiopathic steatosis of pregnancy and tetracycline liver toxicity.

Prognosis

Outcome is related to the severity and rate of progression of coma, severity of the increased intracranial pressure, and degree of blood ammonia elevation. Fatality rates average 42% but may vary from 20% in patients with only mild neurologic abnormalities to above 80% in patients who have seizures, flaccidity, and respiratory arrest. Prognosis for survivors is usually good. Recurrences are uncommon. The incidence of neurologic sequelae (mental retardation, cranial nerve palsies, motor dysfunction) is unknown but may be related to the severity of coma.

Treatment

As the cause of the syndrome is unknown, and as widespread metabolic derangements are present, no universally accepted therapy exists. Intensive supportive care is the mainstay of treatment. Meticulous and constant attention to the neurologic, electrolyte, metabolic, cardiovascular, respiratory, and fluid status is essential to cope with rapid changes. Treatment includes the use of IV fluid and electrolyte solutions containing glucose, usually 5 to 10% but occasionally up to 50%, small doses of insulin, judicious use of cathartics and nonabsorbable antibiotics (e.g., neomycin 100 mg/kg body wt/day orally in divided doses q 6 h), and vitamin K 5 mg/day IV or IM. Increased intracranial pressure must be controlled with such agents as mannitol 0.5 to 1.5 mg/kg body wt given IV over 45 min, dexamethasone 0.5 mg/kg/day IV, and glycerol 3 to 6 Gm/kg/day by gastric tube; continuous monitoring of intracranial pressure may help to guide this therapy. Monitoring of blood gases, blood pH, and blood pressure by arterial catheters, and endotracheal intubation and controlled ventilation, are commonly employed. Exchange transfusion, peritoneal dialysis, hemodialysis, "total body washout" (i.e., the procedure in which a patient's entire blood volume is removed and life is supported transiently with substitutes before blood is replaced), and therapy with citrulline or nicotinic acid are under evaluation.

§2. IMMUNOLOGY; ALLERGIC DISORDERS

1. INTRODUCTION

The science of immunology began with an attempt to understand resistance to infection, which was initially thought to be the only function of the immune system. Its relationship to hypersensitivity (allergy) was recognized early in this century and led to elucidation of the general biologic functions of the immune system, including a role in immunity to cancer, prevention of tissue transplantation from one individual to another, and the capability of *causing* diseases by injuring normal tissue.

These functions are accomplished in man by a complex immune system that has emerged through the phylogenetic scale, retaining elements of all the immune responses noted in other vertebrate species (see TABLE 2-1). When operating normally, several immunologic processes result in very precise functions: (1) recognition and memory of, (2) specific response to, and (3) clearance of, foreign substances (chemical and cellular antigens) which either penetrate the protective body barriers of skin and mucosal surfaces (microorganisms, transplanted tissue) or arise *de novo* (malignant transformation). These processes depend upon (1) the development of T and B cell lymphocytes; (2) clonal proliferation of immunologically committed T and B lymphocytes; (3) plasma cell differentiation and antibody production; (4) T cell differentiation into memory, activated, helper, and suppressor cells; (5) macrophages, required for processing antigen; (6) phagocytosis by polymorphonucleocytes and by macrophages and other cells of the reticuloendothelial system; and (7) amplification of the immune response by lymphokines, the complement system, lysosomal enzymes, and vasoactive amines. These same protective processes may, under special circumstances, result in injury. When the immune system becomes hyperactive, the result is a hypersensitivity disorder or an autoimmune disease; when the system is underactive, the result is an immunodeficiency disease or the growth of malignant cells.

GLOSSARY OF IMMUNOLOGIC TERMS

Activated lymphocyte: A T cell that has become stimulated by contact with antigen and is therefore able to induce a cell-mediated immune reaction.

Afferent phase (limb): The stages of the immune response concerned with the way in which foreign substances come in contact with T and B lymphocytes, are recognized, are processed, and stimulate the immune response.

Allergen: An antigen responsible for a hypersensitivity reaction, especially an atopic reaction.

Allergy: Synonymous with hypersensitivity, but often restricted to immediate-type IgE-mediated reactions (atopic diseases).

Allogeneic: Denoting tissues that are antigenically distinct, but from the same species (said of tumors and transplants).

Allograft (homograft): Transfer of tissue between members of the same species.

Amplification: Originally, the various processes of the immune system which augmented the phylogenetically primitive mechanisms of phagocytosis and the inflammatory response. Now often used to refer to any processes which are capable of increasing the effects of activated T cells or antibody molecules. *Examples:* The effects of opsonization by antibody, complement activation, mast cell release of vasoactive amines, and the production of lymphokines by activated T cells.

Anamnestic response: See Immune response, secondary.

Anergy: Inability to react to specific antigens; it may be either humoral or cell-mediated.

Antibody: An immunoglobulin molecule with a specific amino acid sequence and tertiary surface configuration which enables it to react specifically with a matching site on the surface of a homologous antigen. Antibodies are produced by plasma cells in response to stimulation by antigen.

Antigen: A substance capable both of combining with antibody and of eliciting a specific immune response, either humoral (antibody production) or cell-medi-

TABLE 2-1. IMMUNOLOGIC FUNCTION ACCORDING TO PHYLOGENETIC SCALE*

Class	Humoral Antibody	Graft Rejection	Lympho-cytes	Plasma Cells	Thymus	Spleen	Gut-Associated Lymphoid Tissue	Lymph Nodes	Lymphoid Bone Marrow	Bursa
Cyclostomes										
Hagfish	+	+	+	–	–	–	–	–	–	–
Lampreys	+	+	+	–	primitive?**	primitive	–	–	–	–
Elasmobranchs										
Stingrays	+	+	+	–	+	+	primitive?	–	–	–
Sharks	+	+	+	+	+	+	primitive?	–	–	–
Teleosts										
Bony fish	+	+	+	+	+	+	+	–	–	–
Amphibians	+	+	+	+	+	+	+	+	+	primitive?
Reptiles	+	+	+	+	+	+	+	+	+	primitive?
Birds	+	+	+	+	+	+	+	+	+	+
Mammals	+	+	+	+	+	+	+	+	+	equivalent

* Plus (+) = present; minus (–) = absent.
** Not clearly identified by structure.

ated. Sometimes used to mean a substance which can combine with an antibody but cannot by itself elicit an immune response, but such a substance is more properly called a **hapten**. (See Hapten, Immunogen.)

Antigenic determinant: The specific configuration on the surface of an antigen that determines its ability to react with a corresponding configuration on an antibody. (*Synonyms*: Epitope, Combining site, Antigenic grouping.) Sometimes used to mean the combining site on the surface of an antibody.

Antiglobulin (anti-immunoglobulin): Antibody produced in one individual against an immunoglobulin from another individual, the immunoglobulin here acting as an antigen.

Arthus reaction: The development of an inflammatory lesion due to the action of precipitating antibodies **(precipitins)**, and characterized by induration, edema, hemorrhage, and necrosis within hours after intradermal injection of antigen to which the individual has been sensitized. It is caused by complement-dependent antigen-antibody complexes, which precipitate in and around blood vessels, plugging the vessels and causing exudation of fluid rich in polymorphonuclear neutrophils.

Atopy: An inherited tendency to develop asthma, hay fever, and other IgE-mediated hypersensitivity to allergens that provoke no immune reactions in most persons. (*Adjective*: Atopic.)

Autoantigen: An endogenous tissue component that stimulates an immune reaction (e.g., **autoantibody** production) in the person in whom it exists.

Autochthonous tumors: Tumors arising in the same host.

Autograft: Transfer of tissue from one location to another in the same individual.

Autoimmune disease: A clinical disorder resulting from an immune response against an autoantigen. The term does not refer to diseases in which there are autoantibodies of no pathologic significance.

B cell: A lymphocyte, probably derived from bone marrow in man, which is responsible for the production of humoral antibodies. (*Synonyms*: B lymphocyte, Thymus-independent lymphocyte; when used adjectivally, synonymous with Humoral.)

Blastogenic factor: A lymphokine that is capable of inducing other lymphocytes to undergo transformation into lymphoblasts. (*Synonyms*: Lymphocyte transforming factor, Mitogenic factor.)

Blocking antibody: An antibody that can block the combination of an antigen with another antibody (e.g., in IgE-mediated hypersensitivity, antibody which combines with antigen and inhibits the effect of further antigen-antibody reaction); or an antibody that can prevent T cell—antigen reactions. (*Synonym*: In tumor immunology, Enhancing antibody. See that term; see also Immunologic enhancement.)

Bradykinin: A basic nonapeptide which is one of the vasoactive plasma kinins. It is detectable in the serum in experimental anaphylaxis and may play a role in IgE-mediated reactions.

Bursa of Fabricius: A gut-associated (juxta-cloacal) lymphoepithelial organ in birds, responsible for B cell formation and subsequent antibody production. The bone marrow is the presumed equivalent in man.

Carcinoembryonic antigen (CEA): A protein-polysaccharide complex found in colon carcinomas, and in normal fetal gut, pancreas, and liver. It may also be detected in the serum of patients with colon carcinoma and inflammatory disease of the small intestine, colon, and liver.

Carrier protein: Protein to which a hapten can become attached, enabling the hapten to induce an immune response (either cell-mediated or humoral).

Cell-mediated (cellular): Pertaining to those aspects of the immune response that are under the control of thymus-dependent (T) cells. (See Immune response, cell-mediated.)

Central phase: The stage of the immune response concerned with the formation of antibody.

Chemotaxis: Enhanced migration of cells in the presence of chemical substances, usually toward the substance. Leukocyte chemotaxis, which occurs in response to substances released during an immune reaction, is a part of the inflammatory response.

Clonal inhibition factor: See Lymphotoxin.

Clonal proliferation: Asexual division of a single cell (first into 2 cells, then into 4 cells, etc.), resulting in a large number of progeny cells (the **clone**) that are genetically identical to the original cell.

Combining site: On an antigen, the antigenic determinant (epitope); on an antibody, the corresponding surface configuration (paratope, antigen-binding site) that controls the specificity of the antibody to link only with a matching (or very similar) antigenic configuration. The antibody configuration and specificity are determined by the amino acid sequence at the combining site.

Committed lymphocyte: Originally, a lymphocyte that was able to respond only to a specific antigen as a result of prior contact with that antigen. Now, a lymphocyte that has been "programmed," by passage through the thymus (T cell) or bone marrow (B cell), to react against a single (or very similar) antigen (i.e., committed even before the first contact) and to develop along a particular line— i.e., into T or B memory cells, helper or suppressor T cells, or antibody-producing plasma cells. (*Synonyms:* Immunologically competent cell, Small lymphocyte, Immunocyte.)

Complement: A complex series of 11 distinct enzymatic proteins, acting as 9 functioning **components** designated C1 through C9 (C1 has 3 subunits, C1q, C1r, and C1s), which are activated sequentially in a manner similar to the coagulation factors. **Complement activation** by the **classic pathway** takes place when antibody of the IgM or IgG class combines with antigen and activates C1, stimulating the full cascade of sequential events. An **alternate pathway** exists whereby properdin activates C3, bypassing the initial components (C1, C4, and C2). As the components are activated (**fixed**), they participate in a variety of immunobiologic activities, including anaphylatoxin production, leukocyte chemotaxis, opsonization, phagocytosis, and antibody-mediated cytolysis.

Complement-dependent: Requiring the activation of complement components.

Cross-reaction: The reaction between an antibody and an antigen with a nonhomologous but very similar combining site.

Cytotoxic antibodies: IgG or IgM antibodies which can fix complement and then react with antigens on the surface of a cell to produce cell injury.

Cytotoxic factor: A lymphokine which causes the destruction of human tissue culture cells.

Delayed hypersensitivity: A T-cell-mediated hypersensitivity reaction manifested as an inflammatory reaction to the intradermal injection or topical administration of an appropriate antigen, which becomes manifest only after several hours, takes 24 to 48 h to reach maximum, and slowly subsides. Since it is one of the major indicators of **cell-mediated immunity,** it is often used as a synonym for that term.

Derepression: In genetic theory, the inactivation of a repressor substance with the result that normally inactivated genetic material is able to exert an effect; hence, in tumor immunology, the activation (by a carcinogen) of genetic material that is normally suppressed during fetal development, giving rise to antigens with a specificity for certain tumors.

Efferent phase (limb): The stages of the immune response during which immune reactions are brought about by the interactions of antibodies or T cells with antigen.

Enhancing antibody: In tumor immunology, an antibody which complexes with tumor-specific antigens present on the tumor surface, preventing (blocking) destruction of the tumor by T cells, thus favoring (enhancing) the growth of the tumor. (See Blocking antibody; Immunologic enhancement.)

Epitope: The region on the surface of an antigen that is responsible for its specific interaction with an antibody having a matching (or very similar) site. (*Synonyms*: Antigenic determinant, Combining site. See also Specific.)

Fetoproteins: Proteins found in fetal tissue and in a number of malignant diseases. (*Synonym:* Fetoglobulins.)

Graft rejection: The immunologic reaction between the graft recipient and antigens present in the graft which results in necrotic destruction of the graft. The reaction may be of the immediate (antibody-mediated) type, but is more often a delayed (cell-mediated) reaction (the latter is sometimes called a **host-vs.-graft reaction**).

Graft-vs.-host reaction: Reaction of a graft containing immunologically competent T cells against antigens in the tissues of a graft recipient whose immunologic competence is defective or has been reduced by irradiation or immunosuppressive drugs.

Hapten: A substance which reacts specifically with antibody, but which is unable to induce antibody formation unless attached to other "carrier" molecules, usually proteins.

Helper cell: A T cell that is able to augment antibody production by plasma cells.

Heterograft: See Xenograft.

Heterotopic: Situated in an abnormal location (said of grafts placed in an abnormal site in the recipient—e.g., a kidney transplant placed in the iliac fossa).

Histocompatibility antigens: Genetically determined isoantigens, carried on the surface of most nucleated cells, which are important in transplantation because they elicit the immune reactions responsible for rejection of the graft when donor and recipient are histoincompatible. (Often used synonymously with Transplantation antigens; HLA antigens.)

HLA (Human Leukocyte Antigen; Histocompatibility Locus A) system; complex; loci; antigens: A term referring to a chromosome region having a complex of genetic loci with a multiplicity of alleles which govern a number of human tissue antigens. Originally of greatest importance in transplantation as the major mediators of graft rejection, the HLA antigens have become highly significant of late because of the newly discovered statistical associations between certain HLA alleles and a number of otherwise unrelated disorders.

Homograft: See Allograft.

Homologous: Having matching parts. Said of antigens and antibodies that have matching combining sites and are therefore specific for one another.

Host-vs.-graft reaction: See Graft rejection.

Humoral: Pertaining to bodily fluids (as opposed to formed elements); hence, those aspects of the immune response that are associated with circulating antibody. (See also Immune response, humoral.)

Hypersensitivity: An exaggerated response to an antigen that occurs after a prior exposure to the antigen, with consequent tissue damage. The four types of hypersensitivity reactions are discussed in §2, Ch. 4. (See also Allergy.)

Immune: Properly, resistant to a disease because of the formation of antibodies or the development of cellular immunity; now often used to refer to any aspect of the immunologic system and its functions.

Immune adherence: A complement-dependent adherence of antigen-antibody complexes or antibody-coated antigens (e.g., bacteria) to particulate material such as RBCs.

Immune response (strictly, **Specific immune response**): The changes which occur in the immune system in response to antigen.

Immune response, cell-mediated (or **cellular**): The development, proliferation, and differentiation of T cells after exposure to antigen, and the consequent phenomena of delayed hypersensitivity, graft rejection, and defense against malignant cells and certain viral, fungal, and bacterial infections.

Immune response, humoral: The development, proliferation, and differentiation of B cells after exposure to antigen, resulting in antibody production and consequent immunity or hypersensitivity.

Immune response, nonspecific: The various responses of the immune system which do not depend on the specific recognition of and reaction to antigen.

Immune response, primary: The response of immunologically competent cells on first exposure to an antigen. B cells, after a short lag period, produce a small amount of antibody (chiefly IgM) and differentiate into B memory cells and cells capable of becoming plasma cells. The response in T cells is undetectable, but they differentiate into T memory cells and helper or suppressor cells.

Immune response, secondary: The accelerated response which ensues on subsequent exposure to an antigen by B and T cells that have undergone a primary response to that antigen. B cells rapidly develop into plasma cells which produce large amounts of antibody (chiefly IgG). T cells transform into activated lymphocytes and induce such reactions as delayed hypersensitivity and graft rejection. (*Synonyms*: Anamnestic response, Booster response.)

Immunity: Properly, the state of being highly resistant to a disease, especially an infectious disease, because of the presence of antibodies (or activated T cells). **Active immunity** results from antigenic stimulation (either through natural infection or inoculation), is manifested by the prompt production of antibodies (or delayed skin test) in response to antigenic challenge, and is long-lasting or permanent. **Passive immunity** results from administration of exogenous antibodies (or T cells or transfer factor), does not induce antibody formation because no antigenic stimulation takes place, and therefore is not lasting. (Delayed sensitivity passively transferred with lymphocytes or transfer factor is longer lasting.) The term immunity is now often used more broadly to mean the ability to react to an antigenic substance. (*Verb*: **Immunize**.)

Immunization: The administration of antigen, antibodies, sensitized T cells, or transfer factor in order to induce reactivity to antigenic substances.

Immunocyte: See Committed lymphocyte.

Immunogen: A substance that is capable of inducing an immune response. Usage is confusing. Some limit the term to mean a substance capable of inducing a cellular immune response. Others use it to mean an antigen that is capable of inducing an antibody response, in contrast to an antigen (hapten) that is only capable of combining with antibody.

Immunoglobulin: A protein produced by plasma cells, usually having antibody activity. Each immunoglobulin is composed of one or more molecules, each molecule being made up of two light and two heavy polypeptide chains linked by disulfide bonds. The nature of the heavy chains determines whether the immunoglobulin is IgG, IgM, IgA, IgD, or IgE, the **five major classes** in man. Most myeloma globulins are immunoglobulins in structure but appear to have no antibody activity. (See Antibody.)

Immunologic enhancement: In tumor immunology, the enhancement of tumor growth by substances (enhancing or blocking antibodies) which inhibit the antitumor activity of T cells.

Immunologic tolerance: Failure to respond to a substance which normally induces an immune response. It may result from fetal or postnatal contact with antigen (when the immature immune system is unable to distinguish foreign substances from "self"), or may result from initial contact later in life with very low amounts of antigen **(low-zone tolerance)** or very large amounts **(high-zone tolerance; immunologic paralysis).**

Immunologically competent cell: A cell that is capable of responding to antigen and engaging in an immune response—i.e., a B cell or T cell. Most commonly used in reference to cells that have had prior contact with antigen.

Immunotherapy: Originally, passive immunization with antibody. Now extended to mean any treatment for the purpose of altering the immune system.

Isoantigen: An antigen that occurs in different allelic forms in a species; one allelic form induces an immune response in an individual with a different allele. *Examples:* Blood group antigens, histocompatibility antigens. (*Synonym*: Allotypic antigen.)

Isogeneic: See Syngeneic.

Isograft: Transfer of tissue between identical twins.

Kinins: Peptides having the ability to produce vasodilation and smooth muscle contraction, formed from kininogens in the plasma by the action of esterases known as kallikreins. (See also Bradykinin.)

Lymphocyte transformation: An in vitro test of T cell function in which lymphocytes in short-term tissue culture transform into lymphoblasts as a result of contact with specific antigen. Also, the in vitro transformation of lymphocytes into lymphoblasts by blastogenic factor released from activated lymphocytes after contact with antigen. (*Synonym*: T cell transformation.) Plant mitogens (phytohemagglutinin [PHA], pokeweed, concanavallin A) transform both T and B cells.

Lymphoid tissue, central (primary): Thymus, bone marrow (and, in birds, bursa of Fabricius); the sites at which stem-cell–derived lymphoid cells take on the properties that later characterize them as T cells and B cells.

Lymphoid tissue, peripheral (secondary): Lymph nodes, spleen, and blood; the sites at which lymphocytes are found in large numbers. T cells are found in **thymus-dependent areas**—around the central arterioles in the white pulp of the spleen and in the paracortical and deep cortical regions of lymph nodes. B cells are found in **thymus-independent areas**—the germinal follicles and perifollicular regions of the spleen, and the germinal centers, far cortical areas, and medullary cortex of lymph nodes. Of the circulating lymphocytes, 30% are B cells and 70% are T cells.

Lymphokines: Soluble factors released by activated T lymphocytes which induce the changes noted in cellular immunity, delayed hypersensitivity, and tissue rejection. (*Synonyms*: T cell mediators, T cell effectors.)

Lymphotoxin: A lymphokine which injures lymphocytes and prevents clonal proliferation of lymphocytes. (*Synonym*: Clonal inhibition factor.)

Lysosome: A cytoplasmic vacuole containing various hydrolytic enzymes important in phagocytosis.

Macrophage: A cell of the reticuloendothelial system characterized by its capacity to phagocytose both foreign and endogenous particulate substances; it may also play a role in making antigens recognizable to lymphocytes. **Fixed macrophages** (fixed phagocytes, resting wandering cells), the most common, are present in subcutaneous and connective tissue, lymph nodes, bone marrow, spleen, liver, and brain; those stimulated by inflammation to become **free macrophages** (wandering histiocytes) are mobile and highly phagocytic. **Angry macrophages** are unusually phagocytic; this activity is thought to be an effect of a lymphokine, migration inhibition factor.

Mast cell: A connective tissue cell containing strongly basophilic cytoplasmic granules which release pharmacologically active agents such as heparin, histamine, eosinophilic chemotactic factor, and slow reactive substance—all important mediators of immediate-type hypersensitivity reactions—when antigen reacts with IgE bound to the mast cell surface, disrupting the cell and causing its degranulation.

Memory cell: A T cell or B cell that has encountered a specific antigen and is therefore committed to respond on subsequent encounter with the same antigen.

Migration inhibition factor (MIF): A lymphokine which causes macrophages to agglutinate and thereby prevents their migration from the area of a T cell that has been stimulated by antigen.

Mitogenic factor: See Blastogenic factor.

Opsonins: Substances that can adhere to bacteria and other cells, enhancing their phagocytosis. Some are heat-stable antibodies; others are heat-labile components of complement.

Opsonization (opsonification): The facilitation of phagocytosis by opsonins; e.g., the increase in phagocytosis that occurs after the attachment of antibody or complement component, especially C3, to cells.

Orthotopic: Located in the normal anatomic site; said of tissue transferred from a donor to a similar site in a recipient (e.g., a heart transplant).

Paralysis, immune: See Immunologic tolerance.

Paratope: See Combining site.

Phytohemagglutinin (PHA): A hemagglutinin derived from bean plants which is capable of inducing lymphoblast transformation and mitosis of both T and B lymphocytes in man.

PK (Prausnitz-Küstner) reaction: A passive transfer test for identifying allergens in a highly atopic individual. Serum from the atopic individual is injected intradermally into a nonatopic individual, and an allergen is applied to the site by scratch or intradermally 48 h later. A typical wheal-and-flare reaction occurs in 15 to 20 min at the test site if the test is positive.

Plasma cell (plasmacyte): The antibody-producing progeny of the B cell. A mononuclear cell with abundant, strongly basophilic **(pyroninophilic)** cytoplasm, it is highly motile and is prevalent in the extracellular plasma of lymphoid tissue but relatively uncommon in peripheral blood.

Primary immune response: See Immune response, primary.

Properdin: A globulin present in normal serum which plays a part in lysis of gram-negative bacteria by activation of the complement cascade beginning at complement component C3.

Properdin system: Originally (before properdin was identified), the combination of properdin, complement, and magnesium ions that acts nonspecifically against viruses and gram-negative bacteria. Now, the combination of properdin and two or more proteins **(Factors A and B)** that can initiate the alternate pathway of complement activation.

Reaginic antibody: See Skin-sensitizing antibody.

Rosette formation: The rose-like clustering of RBCs around lymphocytes seen during in vitro tests using various reagents to detect T or B cells. Most commonly, sheep RBCs are used to detect T cells.

Secondary immune response: See Immune response, secondary.

Sensitized lymphocyte: A lymphocyte that has participated in a primary immune response and can therefore act as an effector of immunologic reactions on another encounter with its homologous antigen.

Skin reactive factor: A lymphokine which causes an inflammatory process in the skin of animals, including an increase in vascular permeability.

Skin-sensitizing antibody: Antibody which is capable of producing a PK reaction, especially IgE; more recently, IgM and IgG skin-sensitizing antibodies have been demonstrated. (*Synonyms for IgE*: Reaginic, atopic, anaphylactic, or PK antibody.)

Slow reacting substance [of anaphylaxis] **(SRS-A):** A substance released during mast cell degranulation that appears later and persists longer than histamine; it causes slow, prolonged smooth muscle contraction.

Specific: (1) With respect to antibodies (or T cells) and their corresponding antigens—reacting only with one another because of identical combining sites; hence (2) pertaining to those aspects of the immune system having to do with the recognition of, remembrance of, and reaction to, a particular antigen by B cells, T cells, their progeny cells, and their products. The **specificity** of an antibody (and presumably of a T cell), and of a protein antigen, is determined by the amino acid sequence at the combining site; the specificity of a polysaccharide antigen, by its sugar side chains.

Suppressor cell: A T cell that can inhibit antibody production by plasma cells.

Syngeneic: Having identical genotypes (said of individuals or tissues—e.g., identical twins or grafts between them). (*Synonym*: Isogeneic.)

T cell: A lymphocyte altered by passage through the thymus, which becomes responsible for the phenomena of cellular immunity. (*Synonyms*: Thymus-dependent lymphocyte; when used adjectivally, synonymous with Cell-mediated, Cellular.)

Thymus-dependent (T-cell–dependent): Requiring the participation (in an immune response) or presence (in tissue) of T cells. (See also Lymphoid tissue, peripheral.)

Thymus-independent: See B cell; Lymphoid tissue, peripheral.

Tolerance: See Immunologic tolerance.

Transfer factor: An extract derived from the lymphocytes of an individual with delayed hypersensitivity which, when injected into a previously nonreactive individual, will induce delayed hypersensitivity in the recipient. The reaction is specific; i.e., the recipient will show delayed hypersensitivity only to the antigen that originally induced the reaction in the donor.

Transplantation antigens: The genetically determined antigens that cause the immunologic reactions which occur when blood cells or tissues are transplanted from a donor into a non-syngeneic recipient. Included are the histocompatibility antigens and the blood group antigens.

Tumor-associated transplantation antigens: Antigens present on tumor cells which, when injected into normal syngeneic animals, protect the recipient from developing a tumor by causing a graft rejection reaction if cells from the same type of tumor are injected. They may be tumor-specific (present on tumor cells but not on normal cells), or may be antigens normally present but intracellular, released through some effect of the neoplastic process on the cell membrane. (*Synonym*: Tumor-specific transplantation antigens, TSTA.)

Unblocking factors: In tumor immunology, substances present in the serum which decrease (unblock) the action of enhancing or blocking antibody. These substances may be antibody, antigen-antibody complexes, or circulating antigen.

Uncommitted lymphocyte: A lymphocyte (either T or B) which has not yet had its initial encounter with antigen. Since progenitors of lymphocytes are now thought to become programmed for (committed to) their specific antigens at the time when they pass through the thymus or bone marrow and develop into T or B cells, the concept of an uncommitted lymphocyte no longer holds true; however, the term is still used in the above sense.

Xenograft (heterograft): A graft between members of different species.

---

2. BIOLOGY OF THE IMMUNE SYSTEM

The immune response in humans is divided into humoral (antibody) and cellular or cell-mediated (delayed immunity) components. **Humoral** processes involve the interactions between antigens and antibodies; **cellular** processes involve the interactions between antigens and certain specialized (thymus influenced) lymphocytes, which act both directly and through the elaboration of substances other than antibody. The humoral and cell-mediated processes are thought of as specific for two reasons: (1) The lymphocytes and antibodies recognize, remember, and respond to unique pattern configurations on the surfaces of antigens; and (2) each lymphocyte and each antibody responds only to one specific antigenic configuration.

Other mechanisms of the immune system, such as phagocytosis and complement activation, are **nonspecific** since they do not involve such pattern recognition. However, these nonspecific processes often act in concert with antibodies and lymphocytes in reactions against antigenic substances.

Current concepts have evolved from study of animal models and humans and are depicted in FIG. 2-1. A primitive stem cell originates in the yolk sac, migrates through the liver and spleen, and settles in the bone marrow. These stem cells are thought to be multipotential and to develop into precursors of the lymphoid, myeloid, erythroid, and megakaryocytoid series. There is evidence to suggest that the stem-cell–derived lymphoid cells in the bone marrow are already committed

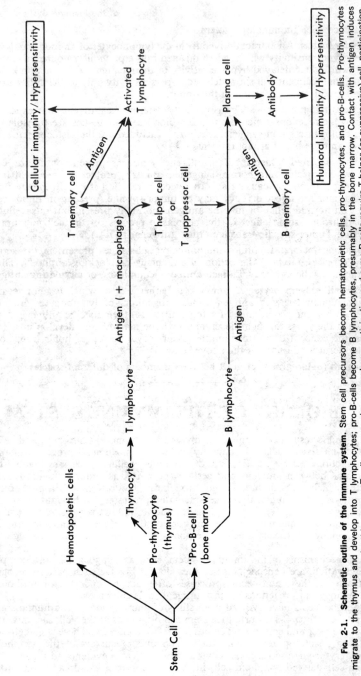

Fig. 2-1. Schematic outline of the immune system. Stem cell precursors become hematopoietic cells, pro-thymocytes, and pro-B-cells. Pro-thymocytes migrate to the thymus and develop into T lymphocytes; pro-B-cells become B lymphocytes, presumably in the bone marrow. Contact with antigen induces lymphocytic differentiation; for this process, T cells may require macrophage participation and some B cells require T helper (or suppressive) cell participation. Both first and later contacts with antigen result in activated T cells or plasma cells, the mediators, respectively, of cellular and of humoral immunity and hypersensitivity.

to become T and B cells, and are called pro-thymocytes and pro-B cells. The pro-thymocyte migrates to the thymus where it develops the characteristics of a T cell. The pro-B cell becomes a B cell probably in the bone marrow, possibly also in the spleen. The two types of cells are identical in appearance at this time in their development and are already programmed for the antigens to which they will respond.

CELLULAR IMMUNE SYSTEM
(Delayed Sensitivity; Cell-Mediated Immunity)

That portion of the immune system mediated by T cells and which is responsible for delayed skin tests, delayed hypersensitivity, graft rejection, and an important defense against malignant cells, viral infection, fungal infection, and some bacteria. The specific type of immune response is mediated by *small* lymphocytes in man, and in most animals is dependent upon the presence of the thymus at birth.

In man, the thymus anlage is differentiated into a compact epithelial structure which can participate in the immune response by the 12th wk of gestation. The pro-thymocyte migrates from the bone marrow to the thymus where it proliferates and differentiates into thymic lymphoid cells **(T cells)**. Each cell is programmed for the number of antigens to which it will react. These cells leave the thymus to circulate in the blood as "long-lived" small and medium-sized lymphocytes with a life span up to 5 yr. Some settle in lymph nodes and the spleen, specifically the corticomedullary junction of lymph nodes and cuffing the penicilliary arteries in the spleen.

In the blood, T cells comprise 70% of circulating lymphocytes and can be distinguished by two surface markers: (1) receptors for normal sheep RBCs (SRBC), which can be detected by observing rosette formation (collection of RBCs around lymphocytes) when SRBCs are mixed with lymphocyte preparations; (2) specific T cell antigen, detected by immunofluorescence using antiserum prepared in animals immunized with human thymus cells (thoracic duct cells) and rendered specific for T cells by absorption with B cell lymphocytes derived from patients with chronic lymphatic leukemia.

Some antigens, such as proteins from bacteria, viruses, fungi, and protozoa, can induce a cellular immune response directly. Haptens such as nickel, rhus antigen (poison ivy), and paraphenylenediamine (hair dye) are capable of inducing a cellular immune response after combining with tissue proteins (carrier protein).

As discussed later, macrophages are considered to be necessary for processing and presenting all antigens to T cells. On initial contact with antigen, the T cell undergoes clonal proliferation and differentiates into sensitized lymphocytes or **committed** T cells with various functions. Some cells become **activated** and are responsible for mediating cellular immunity or resulting in injury to host tissue (hypersensitivity reactions). Others become T **memory cells,** thereby increasing the number of cells with the ability to react to specific antigen. Still others are presumed to become **helper** or **suppressor cells** and regulate the production of antibody by B cells by concentrating antigen on their surfaces or releasing a local humoral factor responsible for stimulating B cells to produce antibody. These are important because of data suggesting that autoimmune diseases and some immunologic deficiency disorders may be due to defects of suppressor T cells, autoimmune disease representing a decrease in suppressor activity and immunologic deficiency representing a result of excessive suppressor activity of T cells.

The activated T lymphocyte mediates cellular immunity by a direct toxic effect, reacting directly with cell-membrane–associated antigens, or by releasing various soluble factors called lymphokines. **Lymphokines** are referred to as the chemical mediators of cellular immunity and several factors have now been defined: Migration inhibition factor **(MIF)** causes macrophages to become sticky and agglutinate in the area of delayed sensitivity. It also augments the bactericidal activity of macrophages **(macrophage activation).** Blastogenic factor **(BF,** lymphocyte transforming factor [LTF], mitogenic factor) is capable of inducing other lymphocytes to undergo transformation into lymphoblasts. Cytotoxic factor causes the destruction of human tissue culture cells. Lymphotoxin **(LT,** cloning inhibitor factor [CIF]) prevents clonal proliferation of lymphocytes and damages lymphocytes. Skin reactive factor produces vasodilation and an inflammatory response in the skin of animals. Interferon has an antiviral effect within the cells.

HUMORAL IMMUNE SYSTEM

That portion of the immune system mediated by antibodies produced by B cells.

In birds, it is quite clear that the bursa of Fabricius (a gut-associated lymphoepithelial organ) is the site at which a pro-B cell becomes a B cell capable of producing immunoglobulins. The bursal equivalent in man has not been established, but the bone marrow is considered the most likely site. Other possible areas include gut-associated lymphoid tissue (such as that found in the appendix, the cecum, and Peyer's patches), liver, and spleen. B cell maturation is thought to take place in two stages. The pro-B cell is first converted into a B cell capable of producing immunoglobulin of the IgM class. Some of these cells migrate to the blood, spleen, and peripheral lymph nodes and continue to produce IgM. Others differentiate to cells producing IgG, some of which migrate to peripheral tissues while others remain in the bone marrow to later become IgA-producing cells. The sequence of development of IgD- and IgE-producing cells has not been established.

B cells, which comprise 30% of blood lymphocytes, are "short-lived," having a life span of 15 days. Though morphologically indistinguishable from T cells, they can be distinguished by technics that detect surface markers: (1) immunoglobulins of the major classes can be detected on the surface with fluorescein-labeled anti-immunoglobulin (immunofluorescent technic); (2) receptors for the 3rd component of complement (C3 receptors) can be detected by the adherence of complement-coated RBCs to the surface of B cells, forming "rosettes;" (3) receptors for immunoglobulins can be detected by adherence of antigen-antibody complexes or aggregated γ-globulin to B cells. B cells can also be evaluated by histologic examination: in the lymph node they make up the outer cortical area containing germinal centers and medullary cord; in the spleen they compose the germinal follicles and perifollicular areas.

The B cells in peripheral tissues are precommitted to respond to a limited number of antigens. The first interaction between antigen and antibody is known as the **primary immune response,** and the B cells committed to respond to this antigen undergo differentiation and clonal proliferation. Some of these become **memory cells** and others differentiate into mature antibody-synthesizing **plasma cells.** The principal characteristics of the primary immune response are a latent period before the appearance of antibody, the production of only a small amount of antibody, chiefly IgM, and, most importantly, the creation of a large number of cells that are capable of responding to the same antigen in the future.

The **secondary (anamnestic** or **booster) immune response** takes place on subsequent encounters with the same antigen. Its principal characteristics are a rapid proliferation of B cells, a rapid differentiation into mature plasma cells, and the prompt production of large quantities of antibody. This antibody, which is chiefly of the IgG class, is released into the blood and other body tissues where it can effectively encounter and react with the antigen.

T and B Cell Cooperation

Cooperation between T and B cells appears to be important in the immune response, but the phenomenon leaves much to be elucidated. For example, a secondary (humoral) immune response to a hapten will not occur unless there are T cells present that are capable of interacting with the hapten's carrier protein. In the humoral immune response to antigens, the need for T cell cooperation varies according to the nature of the antigen. Polymeric antigens such as *Salmonella* flagella protein, pneumococcal polysaccharide, *Escherichia coli* lipopolysaccharide, and povidone (polyvinylpyrrolidone) are T-cell-independent antigens—they are capable of inducing antibody formation (predominantly IgM) in T-cell-deprived animals. Other antigens are T-cell-dependent (e.g., the monomeric form of flagellar *Salmonella* antigen)—they require the presence of T cells to induce production of large amounts of IgM and IgG antibodies, although small amounts of both can be produced without T cells. The need for T cell cooperation also depends on the class of immunoglobulin produced. IgG production seems to be more T-cell-dependent than IgM, while IgA is still more dependent on the presence of T cells.

Humoral Immunity

Immunity can be active or passive. In **active immunization**, antibody production is stimulated by administration of antigen or by exposure to naturally occurring antigens such as bacteria, viruses, or fungi. In **passive immunization**, preformed antibodies actively produced in another person or animal are given to the recipient in the form of serum or γ-globulin. The protection offered by humoral antibody may be direct, such as toxin or viral neutralization by serum IgG or viral neutralization by secretory IgA, or may depend upon activation of the complement system.

ANTIGENS

Antigen Structure and Antigenicity

Antibodies combine with antigens by virtue of matching combining sites on the two molecules, which fit together much like the pieces of a jigsaw puzzle. The antigenic combining sites that are recognized by antibody molecules are specific configurations, known as **epitopes** or **antigenic determinants,** which are present on the surfaces of large molecules of high mol wt such as proteins, polysaccharides, and nucleic acids. It is the presence of at least one such epitope that makes a molecule an **antigen.**

In fact, two essentials are required for a substance to be antigenic (immunogenic); i.e., capable of both binding to antibody and inducing an immune response. (1) The sum of the antigenic determinants on its surface must make up a configuration that differs from configurations recognized by the immune system as "self," and (2) the substance must be of sufficient mol wt (about 10,000 as a minimum). Plausibly, the larger the molecule, the more room on its surface for antigenic determinants; and the greater the number of "foreign"-looking antigenic determinants present on its surface, the greater will be its antigenicity.

A **hapten** is a substance of lower mol wt than an antigen that can *react* specifically with antibody, but which is unable to *induce* antibody formation unless attached to another molecule, usually a protein (the **carrier protein**). Examples of haptens are the allergenic substances in penicillin and numerous other drugs; and nickel, rhus antigen (poison ivy), and paraphenylenediamine (hair dye). The former are capable of inducing a humoral immune response, and the latter a cellular immune response, when they combine with carrier protein.

The combining sites of antibody and the antigen to which it is committed fit avidly together, with a strong force of attraction, because the matching areas on the surface of each molecule are relatively large. The same antibody molecule can also combine **(cross-react)** with related antigens if their surface determinants are similar enough to the determinants on the homologous (original) antigen. However, the antigen-antibody binding in such cross-reactions is weaker because smaller surface areas are in close contact, due to the differences in configuration.

The processing of an antigen by initial phagocytosis appears to be important to its antigenicity, although the role of the macrophage in the initial recognition of a substance as antigen is unclear. The lymph nodes and spleen are rich in phagocytic cells as well as in lymphocytes. When antigen first enters the body it is trapped and largely metabolized by these phagocytes. A small proportion of the antigen, localized on the surface of the macrophage, comes into contact with nearby T cells. These T cells will participate in either the production of cellular immunity or the production of humoral antibody by T-dependent B cells. T-cell-independent antigens do not require macrophages to stimulate antibody production. Cytoplasmic bridges between macrophages and lymphocytes have been observed, suggesting that the macrophage transfers genetic information to the lymphocyte by attaching messenger RNA to the antigen, and that the RNA of the antigen-RNA complex genetically "instructs" the lymphocyte to recognize the attached antigen. Or it may be that the RNA or lysosomal enzymes within the macrophage alter the structure of the foreign molecule to produce or enhance its antigenicity. This processing of antigen appears to be most important in the primary immune response. In the secondary immune response, antigen interacts with antibody fixed to the dendritic macrophages of cortical lymphoid follicles before it can be ingested by the macrophage.

IMMUNOGLOBULINS
(Antibodies)

The antibodies (immunoglobulins [Ig]) offer humoral protection against viruses and bacterial pathogens such as pneumococci, *Haemophilus influenzae,* streptococci, and staphylococci. IgM is the predominant antibody in the primary immune response and IgG in the secondary immune response. Other special biologic properties of the different Ig classes are described below.

Immunoglobulin Structure

Immunoglobulins are a family of serum proteins with antibody activity which are remarkably heterogeneous but which have a number of common properties. The γ-globulin fraction of serum is rich in antibody activity, but other globulin fractions also contain antibody.

The molecular subunits of the immunoglobulins all have the same structure: each is composed of 4 polypeptide chains—2 identical **heavy chains** and 2 identical **light chains** (so called because of their relative mol wt)—joined into a Y shape by disulfide bonds. There are 5 major types of heavy chains, which give their name to the **5 major Ig classes** in man: IgM, IgG, IgA, IgD, and IgE (see TABLE 2-2). There are 2 types of light chains, called κ and λ; a single molecule has only 1 type of light chain, but molecules of both types are found in all 5 of the major classes. Thus, there are 10 different types of Ig molecules. IgG, IgD, and IgE are each monomers; i.e., made up of 1 molecule (2 heavy and 2 light chains). IgM is a polymer of 5 molecules (10 heavy chains, 10 light chains), while IgA occurs in 3 forms—as a monomer and as polymers of 2 and 3 molecules.

Additional chains have been identified. Joining (J) chains link the 5 subunits of IgM and the 2 or 3 subunits of IgA; and secretory IgA has an additional polypeptide chain, secretory component (SC, secretory piece, transport piece), which is produced in epithelial cells and added to the IgA molecule.

TABLE 2-2. CHARACTERISTICS OF THE IMMUNOGLOBULINS

Immuno-globulin Class	Heavy Chains	Light Chains	Additional Chains	No. of Basic Molecules	Sub-classes	Molecular Weight	Sedimen-tation Coefficient	Mean Survival T½ (days)	Mean Serum Conc. (Adult; mg/100 ml)	Biologic Properties
IgM	μ	κ, λ	J	5	IgM_1 IgM_2	900,000	19S	1	45–150	Appears early in immune response; efficient agglutinator & opsonizer; fixes complement; major antibody for polysaccharides, gram-neg. bacteria
IgG	γ	κ, λ		1	IgG_1 IgG_2 IgG_3 IgG_4	150,000	7S	23	720–1500	Most abundant; found esp. in extravascular fluids; crosses placenta; subclasses 1, 2, & 3 fix complement (1 & 3 > 2); major antibody for antitoxins, viruses, bacteria
IgA	α	κ, λ	J SC	1–3	IgA_1 IgA_2	170,000	7–15S	6	90–325	Major immunoglobulin in seromucous secretions at body surfaces
IgD	δ	κ, λ		1		180,000	7S	3	3	Not yet identified
IgE	ϵ	κ, λ		1		200,000	8S	2	0.03	Found in seromucous secretions; levels increased in parasitic infections; mediator of atopic allergies

J = joining chain; SC = secretory component

Antibody Structure and Specificity

The Y-shaped Ig molecule is divided into a **variable region,** located at the distal ends of the Y arms, in which the amino acid sequence differs for the various antibody molecules, and a **constant region,** where the amino acid sequence is relatively constant for each Ig class. Electron microscopy has shown that the variable regions hold the concave **combining sites (antigen-binding sites)** of the antibody molecules. It is the great variety of possible amino acid sequences in the variable regions that confers **specificity** on the antibodies, since each clone of B cells can produce its own specific amino acid sequence, and thus its own antibody configuration that is specific for a particular antigen.

The structure-function relationships of the antibody molecule were originally studied by fragmentation with proteolytic enzymes. Papain splits the molecule into two univalent **Fab** (antigen-binding) **fragments,** which contain the variable regions and thus the combining sites, and one **Fc** (crystallizable) **fragment** that contains most of the constant region. Pepsin produces a fragment designated **F(ab')₂,** which retains divalent antibody activity.

Both B and T cells are capable of recognizing and responding to antigen, but the way in which this occurs is still unclear. B cells (but not T cells) carry small amounts of Ig bound to the cell surface, and it is assumed that this surface Ig serves as a specific recognition antibody in the initiation of an immune response. The T cell recognition site has not been defined. Antibodies of the IgM, IgG, and IgA classes are all capable of responding to the same antigen. One hypothesis to explain this assumes that the B cells derived from a single pro-B cell may differentiate (during the process of B cell maturation described above) into a family of B cells genetically programmed to synthesize antibodies of a single antigenic specificity, while having representative cells committed to the production of each antibody class. The cells undergoing this differentiation from IgM- to IgG- to IgA-producing cells are not yet plasma cells—the development of B cells is independent of antigenic stimulation, but differentiation into plasma cells capable of synthesizing goodly amounts of antibody does require antigenic stimulation.

By use of the ultracentrifuge, sedimentation coefficients can be determined for each Ig protein. IgM has the highest sedimentation coefficient—19S, while IgG is 7S. In addition to these broad classes, it is now recognized that there are Ig subclasses, termed IgG$_{1,2,3,4}$, IgA$_{1,2}$, and IgM$_{1,2}$. These distinctions may be important since specific biologic functions are beginning to be associated with various subclasses. For example, IgG$_4$ does not fix complement, whereas the other three IgG subclasses do; IgG$_3$ has a half-life significantly shorter than the other three.

Biologic Properties of Antibodies

The amino acid structure in the constant region of the heavy chain in the antibody molecule appears to determine certain biologic properties of the immunoglobulins. Each class of Ig has its own characteristics.

IgG, the most prevalent type of serum Ig, diffuses readily into the extravascular spaces, and is the only Ig that crosses the placenta. As the prime mediator of the secondary immune response, it provides the body's chief serologic defenses against bacteria, viruses, and toxins. Different subclasses of IgG neutralize bacterial toxins, fix complement, and enhance phagocytosis by opsonization. Commercial γ-globulin is almost entirely IgG. IgG can also inhibit the immune response, and one suggested mechanism for desensitization in atopic allergies is the development of **blocking IgG antibodies,** which prevent IgE-antigen interactions.

IgM (macroglobulin) is largely confined to the bloodstream. It is the earliest globulin to appear after antigenic challenge, but if IgM is the only antibody to respond to the antigen, immunologic memory is not achieved. The large IgM molecules also fix complement and are active opsonizers, agglutinators, and cytolytics that assist the reticuloendothelial system in eliminating many kinds of microorganisms. Most antibodies to gram-negative organisms are IgM globulins.

IgA (secretory antibody) is found in the seromucous secretions of body tracts exposed to the external environment (saliva, tears, respiratory and gastrointestinal tract secretions, colostrum), where it provides an early antibacterial and antiviral defense. Secretory IgA is synthesized in the subepithelial regions of the gastrointestinal and respiratory tracts and is present in combination with locally produced secretory component. Few IgA-producing cells are noted in the lymph node and spleen. Serum IgA may derive from secretory IgA and, if this is so, both should have the same antibody specificities despite structural differences between the two forms, serum IgA not containing secretory component. Serum IgA contains antibodies against brucella, diphtheria, and poliomyelitis.

The biologic activity of **IgD** is not yet known. **IgE (reaginic, skin-sensitizing,** or **anaphylactic antibody),** like IgA, is secreted chiefly in the respiratory and gastrointestinal subepithelium. Only small amounts are found in serum. IgE is the mediator of atopic allergies; its beneficial role is not established, though it may be active against parasitic and respiratory infections.

MEASUREMENT OF CELLULAR AND HUMORAL IMMUNITY

A number of in vivo and in vitro technics are available to evaluate the presence and functional competence of T and B cells. Since these procedures are often used in the evaluation of suspected immunodeficiency disorders, they are discussed in §2, Ch. 3. The cell-mediated phenomenon of delayed hypersensitivity is also discussed under TYPE IV HYPERSENSITIVITY REACTIONS in §2, Ch. 4.

Delayed sensitivity can be passively transferred from one individual to another with an extract prepared from immune lymphocytes **(transfer factor).** A successful transfer is demonstrated when the recipient is converted from skin-test–negative to skin-test–positive. The conversion only applies to those antigens to which the donor has a positive delayed skin test.

The **complement fixation (CF) test** is most commonly used in the diagnosis of viral diseases by detecting the presence of specific antibody to viruses in a patient's serum. The serum is first heated to destroy its complement activity. Subsequently, antigen (such as a virus particle) and a known amount of complement are added to the mixture. The presence of antigen and antibody in the mixture will utilize complement, thus reducing its activity. Any remaining free complement is detected by adding antibody-sensitized RBCs, which will undergo lysis in the presence of free complement. The absence of hemolysis indicates that the antigen-antibody complex has fixed all the available complement.

THE COMPLEMENT SYSTEM

An important process by which antibody production leads to immunity or hypersensitivity occurs when antibody combines with antigen and initiates complement activity. The complement system consists of 11 proteins comprising 9 distinct components that react sequentially and mediate a number of biologically significant consequences. Phenomena which have been described in vitro include immune adherence (adherence of antigen-antibody complexes or antibody-coated bacteria to macrophages or RBCs); production of anaphylatoxin (a protein which causes release of histamine from mast cells or basophils); chemotaxis (causing the migration of cells toward the area where complement activity is present); phagocytosis; and lysis of cells (RBCs, nucleated cells, and many bacteria).

For historic reasons the first 4 components to react are numbered out of order as C1, C4, C2, and C3; but the remaining 5 components are numbered sequentially C5 through C9. The first component of human complement is composed of 3 distinct protein molecules called C1q, C1r, and C1s. In general the activation of the components of the complement system involves enzymatic cleavage of each component into 2 fragments, the larger of which joins the preceding activated component to generate a new enzymatic activity capable of cleaving the next component.

The classic pathway of complement activation (see FIG. 2-2) begins when C1 comes in contact in vivo with antigen-antibody complexes or, in vitro, with aggregated IgG or IgM. If the antigen is a virus, viral neutralization occurs in the course of activation when the first 2 components of complement (C1´ and C4) have been activated. This may be an important defense mechanism during the early phases of a viral infection when limited amounts of antibody are present.

In guinea pigs when C2 is activated, a kinin-like factor (distinct from bradykinin) is generated; it is similar to a kinin-like activity noted in patients with hereditary angioedema during the active phase of the disease. In activating C3, C3a and C3b are produced. When the antigen is a cell, C3b attaches to a cell membrane receptor that is separate from the site of attachment of C142, resulting in immune

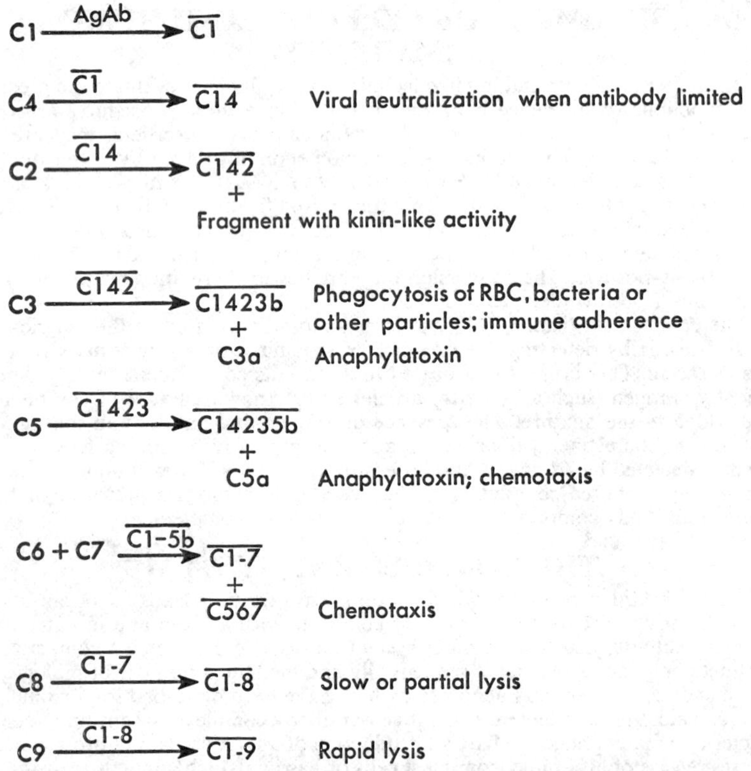

$$C1 \xrightarrow{\text{AgAb}} \overline{C1}$$

$$C4 \xrightarrow{\overline{C1}} \overline{C14} \qquad \text{Viral neutralization when antibody limited}$$

$$C2 \xrightarrow{\overline{C14}} \overline{C142}$$
$$+$$
Fragment with kinin-like activity

$$C3 \xrightarrow{\overline{C142}} \overline{C1423b} \qquad \text{Phagocytosis of RBC, bacteria or}$$
$$+ \qquad\qquad \text{other particles; immune adherence}$$
$$C3a \qquad \text{Anaphylatoxin}$$

$$C5 \xrightarrow{\overline{C1423}} \overline{C14235b}$$
$$+$$
$$C5a \qquad \text{Anaphylatoxin; chemotaxis}$$

$$C6 + C7 \xrightarrow{\overline{C1-5b}} \overline{C1-7}$$
$$+$$
$$\overline{C567} \qquad \text{Chemotaxis}$$

$$C8 \xrightarrow{\overline{C1-7}} \overline{C1-8} \qquad \text{Slow or partial lysis}$$

$$C9 \xrightarrow{\overline{C1-8}} \overline{C1-9} \qquad \text{Rapid lysis}$$

FIG. 2-2. **Classic pathway of complement activation.** The initiating antigen (Ag) can be erythrocyte, bacteria, virus, other cell, or any other antigen; the antibody (Ab) can be IgG$_1$, IgG$_3$, IgG$_2$, or IgM. A bar over the component indicates that the component has acquired enzymatic or other biologic activity.

adherence and phagocytosis. The fragment C3a is also called anaphylatoxin and is capable of releasing histamine from mast cells. C5a, which has anaphylatoxin and chemotactic properties, is generated in binding C5. Subsequently, when C6 and C7 are activated a trimolecular complex, C567, is formed; it either fixes on the cell membrane or remains in solution and is chemotactic for leukocytes, macrophages, and probably eosinophils. When RBCs, bacteria, or nucleated target cells in tissue culture have reacted with complement components from 1 through 8, slow or partial lysis occurs. When all 9 components of complement have reacted, rapid lysis of cells occurs.

An alternate pathway (see Fig. 2-3) for the activation of the terminal complement components from C3 to C9 has also been described in which activation of C3 by certain bacterial polysaccharides and IgA is accomplished without prior activation of C1, C4, and C2. Another name for the alternate pathway is the **properdin system.** The diagram is only an outline since there are many unanswered questions concerning the exact steps in this pathway.

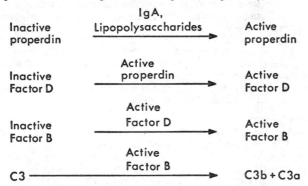

Fig. 2-3. Alternate pathway of complement activation. The initiating substance may be endotoxin, yeast cell wall, bacterial capsules, or IgA.

Inhibition occurs at 2 points in the complement cascade. There is an inhibitor present for the activated first component, and one for the C3b fraction of the third component which also inhibits the alternate pathway. There may also be a C6 inactivator.

Activation of this same complement system, which is so important for host defense, can also result in **injury of normal tissue** by several mechanisms: (1) The generation of anaphylatoxins which produce increased vascular permeability, edema, and smooth muscle contraction. (2) The generation of chemotactic factors which result in migration of polymorphonuclear cells into an area of inflammation. When these cells break down they release lysosomal enzymes which are proteolytic and destroy tissue. (3) Destruction of RBCs in autoimmune hemolytic anemia. (4) Activation of the kinin system which results in vasodilation, increased vascular permeability, and pain. The clinical counterparts of these processes are the hypersensitivity reactions Types II and III elaborated by Coombs and Gell (see §2, Ch. 4).

IMMUNOLOGIC STATUS OF THE FETUS AND NEWBORN

The fetus in utero is in a sterile environment, protected from contact with most microorganisms and other antigens. Abrupt entry into a world of antigens provides a powerful stimulus to the development of the specific immune mechanisms, but these, and nonspecific mechanisms as well, are still relatively deficient in the neonate and the young infant.

Cellular Immunity

In man, the thymus anlage is generated from the epithelium of the 3rd and 4th pharyngeal pouches at about the 6th wk of gestation; by the 12th wk it can participate in the immune response. The thymus is most active during fetal development and in early postnatal life. It increases in size rapidly in utero, then more gradually until puberty, then involutes during adult life. The same pattern of change occurs in all lymphoid tissue, and parallels the sequential appearance of immunoglobulins during maturation. The thymus is considered to be the mediator of the tolerance to "self" antigens that develops during fetal and perinatal life, possibly by the elimination of potential "self"-reactive T cells or production of "self" suppressor cells. It also appears to be essential to the development and maturation of peripheral lymphoid tissue. The epithelial elements in the thymus produce humoral substances which are thought to control the activities of T cells in the peripheral lymphoid tissue.

The capacity of fetal T cells to respond to antigenic stimulation is present by the end of the first trimester of gestation. The ability of the neonate to exhibit a delayed hypersensitivity reaction is difficult to elicit, however (although neonates can reject skin grafts normally), perhaps because the T cells are not yet fully capable of elaborating lymphokines that can recruit local lymphocytes to participate in the delayed hypersensitivity response.

The Immunoglobulins

In the fetus, IgM, IgG, and IgA cell surface markers on lymphocytes can be demonstrated in the bone marrow, blood, liver, and spleen by 11½ wk of gestation. However, IgM and IgG synthesis by plasma cells cannot be demonstrated until about 20 wk of gestation. IgA synthesis occurs at about 30 wk. Moreover, since the fetus normally is in an antigen-free environment, it produces only small amounts of immunoglobulins, although capable of producing larger amounts if stimulated antigenically. The neonate's immunity to various diseases therefore depends on the kinds of IgG antibodies that the fetus has received from the mother transplacentally. Placental transfer of IgG occurs largely in the third trimester, so that the infant born before 34 wk of gestation can have a severe IgG deficiency. Only IgG crosses the placenta, so that the full-term neonate is relatively deficient in IgM and IgA.

Serum IgG levels fall after birth, reaching their lowest levels between age 3 and 6 mo when the catabolism of maternally derived IgG exceeds the synthesizing ability of the infant. This is the time of greatest susceptibility to many serious infections, such as *Haemophilus influenzae* and pneumococcal meningitis. The duration of maternally derived IgG antibodies varies—for measles, they may persist as long as 1 yr; for pertussis, as little as 1 mo. The newborn infant also has a less vigorous and more short-lived antibody response to initial antigenic stimulation than does the adult. In addition, maternally derived diphtheria and measles antibodies may interfere with the newborn's ability to respond to antigenic stimulation. These considerations are important in the scheduling of routine childhood immunizations.

Adult Ig levels are achieved at varying ages—IgM at about 1 yr; IgG at about 8 yr; IgA at about 11 yr.

Nonspecific Immaturity

Susceptibility of the newborn and infant to infection with low-virulence enteric bacteria and to transcutaneous infection with certain strains of staphylococci (e.g., the scalded skin syndrome) suggests a deficit of immune function at the portals of entry of microorganisms. In addition to this evidence of deficiencies in barrier defenses, chemotaxis and phagocytosis are depressed. This is probably due to a combination of relative deficiencies. Phagocytosis may be suppressed in part because of the IgM deficiency. Levels of total complement are also low (resulting especially from deficiency of C3, C4, and C5), as are levels of properdin Factor B. These both affect chemotaxis and opsonization by the classic and alternate pathways of complement activation. Complement levels are, however, sufficient to support normal bacteriolysis and immune adherence.

---

3.   IMMUNODEFICIENCY DISEASES

A diverse group of conditions, characterized chiefly by an increased susceptibility to various infections with consequent severe acute, recurrent, and chronic disease, which result from one or more defects in the specific or nonspecific immune systems.

The primary immunodeficiencies are divisible into **specific** and **nonspecific** groups. The former result from failure to manifest efficient humoral (B cell, plasma cell, immunoglobulin [Ig], antibody) responses or cellular (T cell) responses, or from a combined deficiency in both humoral and cellular functions. Complement deficiencies (opsonic defect) and disorders of phagocytosis and intracellular bacteriolysis make up the latter group.

Genetic features distinguish the primary immunodeficiency disorders from **secondary immunodeficiency,** such as (1) hypogammaglobulinemia secondary to hypercatabolism (nephrotic syndrome—which causes renal loss of γ-globulins; protein-losing enteropathy—gastrointestinal loss); (2) certain lymphopenic states (intestinal lymphangiectasia—gastrointestinal loss; radiation, cytotoxic drugs—bone marrow and lymphoid tissue suppression); (3) immunodeficiencies associated with malignancy, malnutrition, aging, and debilitation; and (4) the impaired phagocytosis that results from the neutropenia or pancytopenia caused by toxic drug reactions, radiation, antimetabolite therapy, and leukemia and other malignancies.

An immunodeficiency state also exists **perinatally,** because the immune system of the fetus and neonate is still immature. Although it is physiologic, the immunodeficiency puts the fetus and infant at risk of susceptibility to infection. Infection during early gestation can result in multiple congenital anomalies (congenital rubella); infection at or near term can cause multiple organ involvement and persistence of the organism (herpes simplex, cytomegalovirus); while postnatal infection can range in severity from localized oral candidiasis (thrush) to overwhelming gram-negative septicemia and meningitis. The prolonged shedding of contagious virus that occurs in infants after intrauterine infection indicates a complex impairment of both specific and nonspecific immune mechanisms.

PRIMARY SPECIFIC IMMUNODEFICIENCY DISORDERS

These diseases, recognized only since 1952, were formerly classified as either congenital or acquired, based on age at the time of recognition. It is now known that most primary specific immunodeficiency disorders are genetically determined, even though the time of clinical onset is variable, being dependent upon both the nature and severity of the immunologic defect and upon chance exposure to infectious agents.

Although most of these disorders appear to be genetically determined, intrauterine stress (e.g., viral infection such as rubella) may play a necessary role in some cases. Thus, for example, selective IgA deficiency is a complication of congenital rubella, but it is also known to occur familially. No genetic influence is known in DiGeorge syndrome, and the intrauterine events which lead, in this condition, to nondevelopment of the 3rd and 4th pharyngeal pouches also remain unexplained.

Advances in immunochemistry and immunobiology have made it possible to distill the basis of classification, from clinical description alone, to functional deficits, to cellular deficiencies, and finally to the molecular and genetic origins of disease (see TABLE 2-3). Therapy has paralleled this understanding. Use of γ-globulin to replace a functional deficit has been supplanted by "engineering" (cellular, molecular, and genetic) to correct some immunodeficiencies more specifically, using bone marrow transplants, fetal thymic implants, and transfer factor for "immunoreconstitution."

Pathology

The pathologic changes seen in lymphoid tissue depend on the type of defect. Acellular T-cell–dependent areas in spleen and lymph nodes are found in pure T cell defects (e.g., DiGeorge syndrome); absence of germinal follicles in pure B cell deficiencies (e.g., infantile X-linked agammaglobulinemia); and rudimentary reticular structures in both central and peripheral lymphoid tissue in combined (T and B cell) immunodeficiency. In selective IgA deficiency (with or without ataxia telangiectasia), in X-linked immunodeficiency with hyper-IgM, and in some variable immunodeficiencies, patients possess lymphoid tissue with evident T and B cell areas. They have both T and B cells, but some or all of the latter are unable to differentiate into plasma cells and produce immunoglobulins. It appears that excessive inhibition of B cells by suppressor T cells or the absence of helper T cells underlies the Ig deficiency. In some of the disorders this deficiency is total; in others, only certain immunoglobulins are lacking. At times follicular hyperplasia occurs, which may be clinically expressed as lymphadenopathy, nodular intestinal lymphoid hyperplasia, and splenomegaly.

Clinical Features

The nature and the degree of the specific immunologic defect determine the age of onset, clinical expression, severity, and types of infections to which the patient is susceptible. When considered with genetic data (family history and sex), these clinical clues are diagnostically helpful in pinpointing the specific defect. Patients with severe combined T and B immunodeficiency develop viral, bacterial *(Staphylococcus, Escherichia coli, Enterobacter, Klebsiella)*, fungal, or *Pneumocystis carinii* infections in early life, most frequently before age 6 mo, and rarely survive beyond age 12 to 18 mo. Patients with pure T cell deficiency have similar infections and early onset of disease. Those with pure B cell defects usually become symptomatic at age 6 to 12 mo when placentally transferred IgG antibodies have reached low levels. Infections with extracellular pyogenic bacteria (staphylococci, streptococci, pneumococci, *Pseudomonas, Haemophilus influenzae,* meningococci) are the rule.

Evaluation of Suspected Immunologic Deficiency

Immunodeficiency is suspected when the clinical picture is one of severe acute, acute recurrent, or chronic infection. The following discussion suggests routes to the diagnosis of immunodeficiency and delineation of the immunologic defect. It must be remembered that defects may exist singly or in combinations, and may be partial or complete.

History: The time of onset of **infections** and the **causative organisms** give important clues. Onset before age 6 mo suggests a cell-mediated defect; onset after age 6 mo, a humoral defect. Recurrent staphylococcal infections with granuloma formation suggest chronic granulomatous disease; recurrent pneumococcal infections suggest splenic disorders (sickle cell [SS] disease or splenic aplasia); and other gram-positive infections suggest a defect in complement-associated antibodies. Salmonella infections may be a sign of sickle cell disease; pseudomonas infections suggest a deficiency of IgM; and other gram-negative infections, a defect in T-cell–associated complement components. Fungal infections point to a T cell defect that may involve complement, a lymphokine released from T cells, or both. Generalized vaccinia may be the result of a cell-mediated defect or, rarely, a humoral defect; cytomegalovirus, *P. carinii,* and *Giardia lamblia* infections occur with either T cell or B cell defects.

In evaluating recurrent infections in children, it must be remembered that recurrent otitis media, a few bouts of pneumonia, sequential viral diseases, or frequent tonsillitis is more likely to represent one end of the spectrum of ordinary childhood susceptibility to infection than to be a sign of immunodeficiency. Moreover, respiratory allergies may resemble recurrent URIs and at first be misconstrued. When chronic and recurrent pulmonary disease occurs in children and young adults, not only immunodeficiency disorders but also congenital anomalies, cystic fibrosis, and α_1-antitrypsin deficiency should be included in the differential diagnosis.

Family history: Points to be noted include the occurrence of early deaths or failure to thrive, recurrent infections, collagen vascular diseases, and malignancies, as well as the occurrence of specific hereditary disorders such as ataxia telangiectasia or the Wiskott-Aldrich syndrome. If possible, a pedigree chart should be constructed to determine any hereditary patterns.

Physical examination: The size of lymphoid and reticuloendothelial organs should be noted. Lymph nodes, tonsils, and adenoids are enlarged in some humoral defects, especially in some immunodeficiencies with variable onset and expression where there is a defect in the conversion of B cells to Ig-secreting plasma cells. They may be small in either cellular (combined immunodeficiency) or humoral (X-linked agammaglobulinemia) defects. Posteroanterior and lateral chest x-rays should be obtained for neonates, to determine the presence or absence of the thymus; abdominal x-rays and a radioisotope scan may be helpful in visualizing the spleen, or establishing its absence. The spleen is absent in congenital aplasia, may be enlarged or small and fibrotic in sickle cell disease, and is enlarged in some humoral and cellular defects. Since the liver is also a reticuloendothelial organ, it may also become enlarged, presumably as a compensatory phenomenon.

Eczema is common in the Wiskott-Aldrich syndrome; a nonspecific dermatitis is often present in chronic granulomatous disease. Certain physical signs are specific: the child's appearance is typical in the DiGeorge syndrome, adenosine deaminase deficiency, and short-limbed dwarfism. Telangiectasias, especially conjunctival, occur in ataxia telangiectasia; neonatal hypocalcemic tetany in the DiGeorge syndrome; and albinism in the Chédiak-Higashi syndrome.

Laboratory studies and tests: Laboratory confirmation of immunodeficiency can be quite extensive and can require sophisticated procedures available only at a large hospital or academic laboratory. However, certain laboratory tests are widely available, and some can be performed as office procedures. Persistent or periodic lymphopenia below 1000 or 2000 cells/cu mm suggests a cell-mediated defect; cyclic or persistent neutropenia may be either cell-mediated or humoral. Coombs-positive hemolytic anemia occurs in certain humoral defects; thrombocytopenia in the Wiskott-Aldrich syndrome. Serum calcium is low in the DiGeorge syndrome.

TABLE 2-3. PRIMARY SPECIFIC IMMUNODEFICIENCY DISORDERS

Type	Genetics	Cellular Defect	Clinical Features	Therapy‡
Pure B cell defects				
Selective immunoglobulin (IgA) deficiency (Janeway Type 3 dysgammaglobulinemia)	Autosomal recessive	B*	Most common disorder. Bronchitis, sinusitis, malabsorption, steatorrhea; or asymptomatic	Fresh-frozen plasma
Infantile X-linked (Bruton's) agammaglobulinemia	X-linked recessive	B	Recurrent infection with extracellular pyogenic pathogens	Gamma globulin; fresh-frozen plasma
Transient hypogammaglobulinemia of infancy	Familial	B	Recurrent infection with extracellular pyogenic pathogens	Gamma globulin
X-linked immunodeficiency with hyper-IgM (Janeway Type 1 dysgammaglobulinemia)	X-linked recessive	B*	Recurrent infection, thrombocytopenia, aplastic and hemolytic anemia	Immunotherapy under study
Pure T cell defects				
Thymic hypoplasia (DiGeorge syndrome)	No evidence	T	Usually fatal in infancy; frequent viral, fungal, or pneumocystis infection	Human fetal thymus implantation
Episodic lymphopenia with lymphocytotoxin	?	T	Recurrent infection, lymphopenia	Immunotherapy under study
Combined immunodeficiency diseases				
Immunodeficiency with variable onset and expression	Autosomal recessive or dominant	BT†	2nd most common disorder. Recurrent infection, both viral and bacterial	Gamma globulin; fresh-frozen plasma

Condition	Inheritance	Cells	Clinical features	Immunotherapy‡
Immunodeficiency with normal globulinemia or hyperimmunoglobulinemia	?	B T†	Recurrent pneumonia	Immunotherapy under study
Ataxia telangiectasia	Autosomal recessive	B T	Cerebellar ataxia; telangiectasias (esp. conjunctival); frequent sinopulmonary infection in cases with low IgA	Fresh-frozen plasma
Immunodeficiency with thrombocytopenia and eczema (Wiskott-Aldrich syndrome)	X-linked recessive	B T	Frequent infection with viruses, fungi, and pyogens	Transfer factor; fresh-frozen plasma
Immunodeficiency with thymoma	?	B T	Recurrent infections with pyogens, sometimes with viruses, fungi	Thymectomy (thymic transplant usually not indicated)
Immunodeficiency with short limbed dwarfism	Autosomal recessive ?	B T	Short-limbed dwarfism; lymphopenia	Immunotherapy under study
Severe combined immunodeficiency (a) Autosomal recessive (b) X-linked (c) Sporadic		B T S / B T S / B T S	Recurrent infection; failure to thrive	Bone marrow transplantation; gamma globulin; fresh-frozen plasma; transfer factor
Immunodeficiency with hematopoietic hypoplasia (reticular dysgenesis)		B T S	Rarely survive beyond first few weeks of life	Bone marrow transplantation

B = B cells; T = T cells; S = Stem cells.
* Involves some, but not all, B cells.
† Encountered in some, but not all, patients.
‡ Therapy also includes appropriate antibiotic and antiviral therapy for all conditions.

Tests of humoral immunity: Many laboratories are now able to determine **serum Ig levels.** Immunoelectrophoresis may be used to identify agammaglobulinemia, a deficiency of IgG, IgM, or IgA, or the presence of immunoglobulins of limited mobility. The technic is not quantitative, however, and in order to obtain specific levels of IgG, IgM, IgA, or IgD, radiodiffusion is used; IgE is determined by radioimmunoassay. (These procedures are described in §24, Ch. 2.)

The presence of normal serum Ig levels (see TABLE 2-4) does not necessarily mean that antibody synthesis is intact: determining the presence or amount of Ig does not identify its antibody specificity. To determine **antibody content,** the most commonly used technics are gel precipitation (a known antigen is combined with serum in a liquid gel medium; if antibody to that antigen is present in the serum a solid sediment forms) and agglutination (the antigen is a cell or a particulate substance—bacteria, RBCs, latex particles—to which antigen is attached; in the presence of the specific antibody, agglutination occurs).

Specific antibody assays are significant in children who have had or have been immunized against measles, rubella, mumps, influenza A or B, tetanus, diphtheria, or poliomyelitis. A positive Schick test in an immunized person indicates an IgG defect; except in patients of blood group AB, A and B isohemagglutinin titers indicate an IgM defect. If no specific antibodies are found on assay, antibody responsiveness to diphtheria, tetanus, typhoid, poliomyelitis, mumps, measles, or blood group substances can be tested by vaccine or antigen injection. (CAUTION: *Not with live or attenuated vaccines.*) Antibody stimulation by other antigenic substances (bacterial, viral, carbohydrate) can also be tested.

To determine **local immune function,** the IgA level in saliva, bronchial washings, and nasal secretions may be determined; tissue obtained by biopsy of respiratory or gastrointestinal mucosa may be examined for immunoglobulins by fluorescent microscopy; or tetanus toxoid may be applied to the nasal mucosa, which is then examined for the presence of toxoid-induced antibody. Positive skin tests for immediate-type (atopic) hypersensitivity indicate the presence of IgE in the skin; skin tests for fixed IgE may also be performed with anti-IgE antigen.

Since B cells have identifiable surface markers, the number of peripheral **circulating B cells** can be determined. Surface immunoglobulins can be detected with fluorescein-labeled anti-immunoglobulin (immunofluorescence—see TYPE II HY-

TABLE 2-4. IMMUNOGLOBULIN LEVELS IN NORMAL CHILDREN
EXPRESSED AS PERCENT OF NORMAL ADULT LEVELS

Immunoglobulin	IgG	IgM	IgA
Adult	1158 ± 305 mg/100 ml	99 ± 27 mg/100 ml	200 ± 61 mg/100 ml
Newborn	89% ± 17%	11% ± 5%	1% ± 2%
1 − 3 mo	37 ± 10	30 ± 11	11 ± 7
4 − 6 mo	37 ± 16	43 ± 17	14 ± 9
7 − 12 mo	58 ± 19	55 ± 23	19 ± 9
13 − 24 mo	66 ± 18	59 ± 23	25 ± 12
25 − 36 mo	77 ± 16	62 ± 19	36 ± 19
3 − 5 yr	80 ± 20	57 ± 18	47 ± 14
6 − 8 yr	80 ± 22	66 ± 25	62 ± 23
9 − 11 yr	97 ± 20	80 ± 33	66 ± 30
12 − 16 yr	82 ± 11	60 ± 20	74 ± 32

Values represent mean ± 1 S.D. *Above* **percentages** *can be applied when local laboratories determine their own normal adult values.*

Adapted from E.R. Stiehm and H.H. Fudenberg, Pediatrics Vol. 37, pp. 715–727, May 1966. Used with permission.

PERSENSITIVITY REACTIONS in §2, Ch. 4); a B cell receptor for the 3rd component of complement (C3 receptor) can be detected by the adherence of complement-coated RBCs to the B cells, forming rosettes; and a receptor on the Fc portion of the antibody molecule can be detected with antigen-antibody complexes or aggregated γ-globulin. A bone marrow biopsy will detect signs of maturation or arrest of cells in the neutrophil series and will determine the presence or absence of **plasma cells;** architectural changes in a lymph node, determined by biopsies performed before and after local immunization (e.g., DTP in the thigh, with inguinal node biopsy), will enable determination of **B cell and plasma cell function.** Rectal biopsy tissue may also be examined for lymphoid tissue, B cells, and plasma cells.

Tests of cell-mediated immunity: A lymphocyte count above 2000/cu mm suggests that the cell-mediated immune system is normal. However, repeated blood counts may be necessary to detect periodic or progressive lymphopenia, which occurs with partial deficiencies of the cell-mediated immune system.

A number of antigens are now commercially available for specific **delayed-hypersensitivity skin tests** (see TABLE 2-5). These tests are usually performed by injecting 0.1-ml amounts of the antigen into the skin. If T memory cells for the test antigen are present, induration and erythema become apparent at the test site at about 24 h, peak at 48 h, and then resolve over the next day or two. In order to test a patient's ability to *develop* cell-mediated immunity, a test must be performed with an antigen that he has not previously encountered. The antigens most commonly used are dinitrochlorobenzene (DNCB) and dinitrofluorobenzene (DNFB). These are applied to the skin as in a patch test (see TYPE IV HYPERSENSITIVITY REACTIONS in §2, Ch. 4), but first in a sensitizing dose and then in a test dose. If the patient's T cells are immunologically competent, a contact dermatitis will follow the test dose. These tests are more reliable in children and adults than in neonates: delayed hypersensitivity reactions are more difficult to induce and to elicit in neonates because their immune system is still immature. A positive delayed skin test to *Candida albicans* can usually be elicited in a normal 1-yr-old.

The patient's ability to reject a skin graft from an unrelated (and hence incompatible) donor also indicates his cell-mediated immunologic competence, but the procedure is seldom used in humans as a diagnostic test.

A number of sophisticated **in vitro tests** can be performed to evaluate cellular immunity and the presence of T memory cells. The occurrence of rosette formation when sheep RBCs (SRBC) are mixed with lymphocyte preparations indicates the presence of T cells but not their functional capacity. For this purpose, a

TABLE 2-5. COMMERCIALLY AVAILABLE ANTIGENS FOR EVALUATING DELAYED HYPERSENSITIVITY

Antigen*	Concentration	
	Initial	Final
Candida albicans, 500 PNU/ml	1:1,000	1:10
Trichophyton, 500 PNU/ml	1:1,000	1:10
Mumps	1:1	—
Diphtheria-tetanus fluid toxoid	1:10	1:1
Streptokinase-streptodornase	1:1,000	—
PPD (tuberculin)	Intermediate strength	Second strength
Histoplasmin	1:1	—
1–Chloro–2,4–dinitrobenzene (DNCB)	1% in acetone (Sensitizing dose)	0.1% in acetone (Test dose)

* DNCB 0.25 ml is applied to intact skin as in patch testing (see TYPE IV HYPERSENSITIVITY REACTIONS in §2, Ch. 4); other antigens are given intradermally in 0.1-ml doses.

specimen of the patient's lymphocytes may be placed into short-term culture and their response to the addition of antigen observed. T memory cells will transform into lymphoblasts **(lymphocyte transformation)** which can be counted directly. Alternatively, the amount of radioactive thymidine incorporated by the lymphocytes (indicating protein synthesis) may be used as a measure of transformation. It is also possible to measure the supernatant for lymphokines after antigen has been added to the lymphocytes; the **MIF (migration inhibition factor) assay** is the one most commonly used and indicates the presence of activated T cells.

Phytohemagglutinin **(PHA)**, an extract from the seeds of a bean plant, stimulates lymphocyte transformation or thymidine incorporation in both T and B memory cells and although it cannot be used as a measure of cellular immunity alone, testing with this mitogen is useful when humoral immunity is known to be normal.

Principles of Treatment

Precautions: Patients with either T or B cell defects should be protected from exposure to infectious disease, and should not be immunized with live virus vaccines. Use of corticosteroids and immunosuppressive drugs is also **contraindicated** in these patients, and they should not be subjected to splenectomy, since these therapeutic measures will compromise the remaining immunologic defenses. In addition, patients with T cell deficiency should not be given fresh blood or plasma transfusions, since these may induce a graft-vs.-host reaction. Those with selective IgA deficiency should not be given γ-globulin, blood, or plasma in any form, because production of anti-IgA antibodies may result in an anaphylactic reaction. Surgery should be avoided in patients with thrombocytopenia; and patients with splenomegaly should avoid contact sports and other activities which increase the risk of splenic rupture.

Infections: When a patient with an immunodeficiency disorder develops an infection, it is safest to assume that it is bacterial and to begin ampicillin therapy as soon as specimens have been taken for culture, later changing the therapy as indicated by the culture results. The possibility of viral, fungal, or *P. carinii* superinfection must be borne in mind. The therapy of choice for *P. carinii* infections is pentamidine (see PNEUMONIA CAUSED BY *Pneumocystis carinii* in §5, Ch. 9); for cytomegalovirus, idoxuridine **(IDU)**, floxuridine, or cytarabine **(Ara-C)**; for generalized herpes simplex infection, IDU or Ara-C; and for severe *Candida* or *Aspergillus* infection, amphotericin B (see General Therapeutic Principles in §1, Ch. 6). Some patients may need continuous antibiotic and γ-globulin therapy to minimize recurrent infections.

γ-Globulin provides mostly IgG, and cannot effectively replace IgA or IgM. However, it is the treatment of choice in panhypogammaglobulinemia. γ-Globulin will not correct cell-mediated, phagocytic, or complement deficiencies. It is **contraindicated** in selective IgA deficiency (because of a tendency to anaphylaxis) and in thrombocytopenic states (risk of bleeding at the injection site). The usual dose is 0.6 ml/kg IM of 16.5% γ-globulin. Initially, a loading dose of 1.8 ml/kg (as 3 separate injections) is given; then 0.6 ml/kg every 3 to 4 wk, to maintain IgG serum levels at 200 mg/100 ml. The maximum tolerable dose is about 20 to 30 ml. It is given only IM; intravascular injection must be avoided. Aged preparations may contain aggregated γ-globulin and should not be used because they may cause local, toxic, or anaphylactic reactions.

Fresh-frozen plasma infusion provides the three major immunoglobulins, IgG, IgA, and IgM. If obtained from specifically immunized donors, it provides specific antibodies. It can be used in place of the large initial loading dose of γ-globulin, and is also useful in patients with disorders causing large renal or gastrointestinal losses of γ-globulin and in patients with thrombocytopenia. It has been used with some success in certain complement defects, particularly C5 dysfunction and C1-esterase deficiency. Fresh-frozen plasma is **contraindicated** in selective IgA deficiency since, like γ-globulin, it may cause anaphylaxis. In T cell deficiencies, it may cause a graft-vs.-host reaction, but the risk can be reduced by allowing the plasma to age for 2 wk and by irradiation with 3000 R, which eliminates the T cells in the plasma. The usual dose is 15 to 20 ml/kg, given every 3 to 4 wk in hypogammaglobulinemia, and weekly or biweekly in opsonic and complement deficiencies. The plasma should be tested for syphilis and hepatitis before use.

Transfer factor, a nonviable dialyzable extract of activated lymphocytes, given subcutaneously, has shown promise in treatment of the Wiskott-Aldrich syndrome and chronic mucocutaneous candidiasis. When taken from a donor who responds strongly to delayed hypersensitivity skin tests, it has induced conversion of T cell anergy in patients for 6 to 12 mo, though more frequent doses may be necessary. Transfer factor does not induce graft-vs.-host reactions or cause hepatitis, but local and febrile reactions may occur.

Lymphocyte infusions are useful in T cell disorders, but donors must be HLA-identical or a graft-vs.-host reaction may occur. **Bone marrow transplantation** has been effective in severe combined immunodeficiency, but again the donor must be HLA-identical. **Thymus implantation** has been effective in restoring T cell immunity in the DiGeorge syndrome. The thymus from a 12- to 20-wk-old fetus is implanted IM, subcutaneously, or intraperitoneally. Although the risk of a graft-vs.-host reaction is minimal, the thymus graft is usually rejected and the procedure may need to be repeated to maintain T cell function. Lymphocyte infusions, bone marrow transplants, and thymus implants are performed only at specialized centers.

SELECTIVE IgA DEFICIENCY

This is the most common Ig deficiency. Occurring in 1:600 to 1:800 persons, it is 10 times more common than panhypogammaglobulinemia. Both autosomal dominant and autosomal recessive modes of inheritance have been described. Some people with IgA deficiency have no problems and are healthy, possibly because they can substitute low mol wt IgM for the deficient IgA and are thus able to maintain immunologic defense at the levels of the gastrointestinal and sinopulmonary epithelium. Other patients have recurrent sinopulmonary infections. Incidence of selective IgA deficiency is increased in patients with respiratory allergy, chronic urticaria, celiac disease, rheumatoid arthritis, SLE, and ataxia telangiectasia, and in families of patients with agammaglobulinemia. IgA-deficient children with recurrent viral respiratory disease and chronic serous otitis media have been observed to synthesize IgA spontaneously as their infections become less frequent and their clinical conditions improve. Therefore, their serum IgA levels should be determined yearly. In addition, although prospective studies of individuals with selective IgA deficiency have not been done, the association of this deficiency with other diseases should be kept in mind.

Treatment is symptomatic. IgA cannot be replaced with γ-globulin or plasma, as anaphylactic reactions are likely to occur. Prognosis is good to excellent with symptomatic management, especially if the defect is not accompanied by associated conditions.

DiGEORGE SYNDROME
(Thymic Hypoplasia)

A congenital syndrome characterized by neonatal hypocalcemic tetany and recurrent candidal and pneumocystis infections caused by combined thymus and parathy-

roid hypoplasia or aplasia due to abnormal fetal development of the 3rd and 4th pharyngeal pouches. Associated somatic features include hypertelorism, notched low-set ears, small mouth, and downward-slanting eyes. Bifid uvula, esophageal atresia, right-sided aortic arch, and tetralogy of Fallot may occur.

B cell function and therefore Ig levels are normal. Peripheral lymphocyte counts may be normal. However, in addition to the thymic hypoplasia, depletion of T-cell-dependent areas is seen in lymphoid tissue. Infants who survive neonatal tetany develop chronic rhinitis, diarrhea, oral candidiasis, and *P. carinii* pneumonia. Death usually occurs before age 2 yr unless the thymus defect is only partial, or unless T cell function can be restored by implantation of a human fetal (12- to 20-wk) thymus. Reimplantation may be necessary to maintain T cell function.

CHRONIC MUCOCUTANEOUS CANDIDIASIS

An uncommon form of candidiasis, characterized by chronic infection of the skin, nails, scalp, and mucous membranes, usually developing in infancy, and apparently caused by inability of T lymphocytes to react to Candida *antigen.* The occurrence in siblings and some mother-child pairs suggests a genetic factor. One of the hallmarks is that topical antifungal agents and even systemic amphotericin B therapy produce only transient and partial clearing of infections. Besides *Candida,* chronic *Trichophyton, Epidermophyton,* and *Mycobacterium* infection may also occur. The severity of the condition is quite variable. Candidal involvement of the mouth, nose, and palate may lead to nasal speech and difficulty in eating. Esophageal involvement may lead to chronic esophagitis and esophageal stricture.

The immunologic picture is also variable. Most, but *not* all, patients lack delayed skin reactivity to *Candida* antigens. Some patients who do not react to *Candida* do react to other delayed hypersensitivity antigens. Again, some but not all patients have a decreased number of circulating T cells. Since the production of **MIF** on exposure of patients' lymphocytes to *Candida* antigen is diminished or absent in some (though not all) cases, these patients are thought to have an **efferent limb defect** (i.e., one in which the products of immunoresponsiveness are not synthesized). B cell function is usually normal; however, isolated IgA deficiency and an IgG inhibitor directed against *Candida* clumping factor (an opsonin found in normal serum) have been described.

Besides topical and systemic antifungal therapy, immunoreconstitution with **transfer factor** has been attempted in a small number of cases, about half of whom have benefited clinically and have shown in vitro and in vivo evidence of restored reactivity to *Candida.* Oral and IM iron therapy has been helpful in some cases.

ATAXIA TELANGIECTASIA

An autosomal recessive hereditary progressive multisystem disease characterized by cerebellar ataxia, telangiectasias, recurrent sinopulmonary infections, and variable immunologic defects.

Serum IgA is low to absent in 60 to 80% of cases; less common B cell defects include low to absent secretory IgA, increased catabolism of serum IgA, development of anti-IgA, and deficiency of serum IgE. Evidence of impaired T cell function includes periodic lymphopenia, a decreased response to delayed hypersensitivity tests and to in vitro tests of lymphocyte function, and thymus abnormalities (small gland; decreased lymphocytes; absence of Hassall's corpuscles).

Both neurologic symptoms and evidence of immunodeficiency are variable in onset. Ataxia usually develops at about the time when patients begin to walk but may be delayed until age 4 yr. Its progression leads to severe disability. Speech becomes slurred, choreoathetoid movements and ophthalmoplegia occur, and muscle weakness usually progresses to muscle atrophy. Progressive mental retardation may occur. Telangiectasias develop between 1 and 6 yr of age, most prominently on the bulbar conjunctiva, ears, antecubital and popliteal fossas, and sides of the nose. The recurrent sinopulmonary infections, which result from the immunologic deficits, lead to recurrent pneumonia, bronchiectasis, and chronic obstructive and restrictive lung disease.

Endocrine abnormalities may occur, including gonadal dysgenesis, testicular atrophy, and an unusual form of diabetes mellitus characterized by marked hyperglycemia, resistance to ketosis, absence of glycosuria, and a marked plasma insulin response to glucose or tolbutamide.

The incidence of cancer is increased, most often as lymphosarcoma but also including Hodgkin's disease, leukemia, gastric adenocarcinoma, cerebellar medulloblastoma, reticulum cell carcinoma, and frontal lobe glioma.

Prognosis is generally poor, with death occurring from chronic sinopulmonary infections or malignancy. However, the progressively and severely handicapped patients may survive into their 30s.

WISKOTT-ALDRICH SYNDROME

A sex-linked recessive disorder with a defect in both T and B cell function, characterized by eczema, thrombocytopenia, and absence of isohemagglutinins (anti-A, anti-B, or both). Total serum γ-globulin level is normal. IgA, IgG, and albumin levels are also normal but their serum half-life is shortened and the levels are maintained by increased synthesis. Some patients have moderately elevated IgE levels. IgM levels may be low, reflecting its defective ability to be stimulated by antigen, especially polysaccharides (blood group substances, bacterial capsular antigens). The poor response to polysaccharide antigens has been called an **afferent limb defect** (i.e., an inability to recognize certain antigens, in contrast to efferent limb defects, such as chronic mucocutaneous candidiasis, above). The defects in T cell function, which are usually progressive, result in lymphopenia of variable degree and a depletion of T-cell-dependent areas in lymph nodes and spleen. Because of the combined deficiency in both B and T cell function, infections occur with pyogenic bacteria, viruses, fungi, and *P. carinii.* The thrombocytopenia is due to decreased platelet synthesis, and causes petechiae, purpura, and life-threatening gastrointestinal hemorrhage. As with other primary immunodeficiencies, the incidence of cancer seems to be increased. Malignancies are usually lymphoreticular (lymphoma, leukemia), but sarcoma and astrocytoma also occur.

Early mortality is likely, but the disease is variable in severity and some patients survive to the early teens. **Treatment** is with appropriate antibiotics (bearing in mind the likelihood of fungal, viral, and pneumocystis superinfections). The administration of **transfer factor,** obtained from activated lymphocytes, has been effective in about half the cases, producing resistance to infections, clearing of the eczema, and regression of splenomegaly and the bleeding diathesis. The return of immunologic function is evidenced by a response to delayed hypersensitivity tests, production of MIF, and the appearance of peripheral T cells.

IMMUNODEFICIENCY WITH THYMOMA

A combined immunodeficiency disorder associated with thymoma (either benign or malignant) occurring in adulthood and characterized by recurrent infections, chronic diarrhea, stomatitis, aplastic anemia, thrombocytopenia, chronic hepatitis, arthritis, and diabetes mellitus. Myasthenia gravis may coexist. The disorder occurs after age 20 and twice as often in women as in men. There is no known inheritance pattern.

Immunologic studies have shown deficiency of IgG, IgA, and IgM, impaired antibody response to injected antigens, lymphopenia, negative skin tests to delayed hypersensitivity antigens, and lack of lymphocyte transformation on in vitro testing.

Onset of symptoms is gradual. Infections become recurrent, especially affecting the respiratory tract and skin. Both bacterial and viral infections occur. Septicemia may ensue. Chronic diarrhea suggests intestinal *Giardia* infection. The thymoma (usually spindle-cell) is diagnosed by finding a mass in the anterior mediastinum on x-ray. Tracheal compression by the mass may cause wheezing. The appearance of the thymoma may precede or follow by years the clinical and laboratory signs of immunodeficiency. Therefore, adults with "acquired" immunodeficiency should be examined for this complication.

Prognosis is generally poor, the progressive immunologic deterioration eventually leading to fatal infection. Death is often from cytomegalovirus or *P. carinii* infection. **Treatment** consists of γ-globulin and antibiotics to control the recurrent infections; γ-globulin therapy may also control chronic diarrhea in some cases. Excision of the thymoma is indicated, but this does not improve immunologic function.

IMMUNODEFICIENCY WITH SHORT-LIMBED DWARFISM

A spectrum of immunodeficiency disorders with achondroplasia-like features. The syndrome is inherited as an autosomal recessive condition, with most cases to date described in an Amish kindred with histories of fatal or severe varicella. X-rays show metaphyseal dysostosis but, usually, a normal skull and spine, unlike the findings in achondroplasia. Some children also have hypoplasia of cartilage and hair, and some with Type II have congenital (aganglionic) megacolon. Three types have been classified. Type I shows combined B and T cell immunodeficiency; Type II, the commonest form, only T cell deficiency; and Type III, only B cell deficiency. Types I and II have the poorest prognosis, vaccinia and varicella being the commonest cause of death; Type I is fatal before age 1 yr. The prognosis is better in Type III because patients can be treated with γ-globulin replacement therapy.

ADENOSINE DEAMINASE DEFICIENCY AND IMMUNODEFICIENCY

A deficiency of adenosine deaminase **(ADA)** has been found in about half the children with combined immunodeficiency disease **(CID)**. This erythrocyte enzyme converts adenosine to inosine and provides a reutilization pathway for purine metabolites, which are important in nucleic acid synthesis. It is normally present in high concentrations in lymphoid tissue. Parents may have half-normal ADA levels, suggesting an autosomal recessive mode of inheritance. However, the relationship of CID to ADA deficiency is not clear. ADA and CID may only share a chromosomal locus, or ADA, since it is active in purine metabolism, may be necessary for proper lymphocyte function. Patients with ADA deficiency also show complete or incompletely formed thymic Hassall's corpuscles, in contrast to those with CID but with normal ADA, who show a complete absence of Hassall's corpuscles.

There appear to be two clinical types. Children in the first group are less severely affected, having some residual T and/or B cell function. Those in the second group are more severely impaired and, besides an undue susceptibility to bacterial and viral infections, have unusual bone lesions, with flaring and cupping of the costochondral junction of the ribs, radiolucent bands in the metaphyses of the long bones, and abnormalities of the spine, pelvis, and scapulas.

The treatment of choice is bone marrow transplantation, but graft-vs.-host disease and overwhelming infection present formidable problems in these immunologically compromised patients.

PRIMARY NONSPECIFIC IMMUNODEFICIENCY DISORDERS

The **phagocytic system** is impaired in congenital neutropenia or pancytopenia because the number of phagocytic cells is reduced. Primary nonspecific immunodeficiency syndromes involving functional deficits of phagocytic cells may occur as a result of (1) complement deficiencies, which cause impaired chemotaxis and adherence; (2) impaired chemotaxis due to a defect in WBCs; (3) failure to kill phagocytized bacteria because of an intracellular enzyme defect (chronic granulomatous disease); and (4) failure to kill phagocytized bacteria because of a lysosomal defect (Chédiak-Higashi syndrome).

COMPLEMENT DEFICIENCIES

Primary deficiencies of components of the complement system have been described; though case reports are few, they have added to our understanding of the protective role of complement against infection. **Secondary complement deficiency** may be the result of complement consumption, as occurs during serum sickness, the early stages of acute post-streptococcal glomerulonephritis, and acute active SLE.

Complement activation and its biologic effects are described in §2, Ch. 2. Patients with **deficient C3** lack the crucial link for activation of both classic and alternate pathways, and clinically resemble those with agammaglobulinemia, with recurrent pyogenic bacterial infections of the sinuses, ears, and lungs. They require treatment with antibiotics. Inherited **C1q, C1r, and C1s deficiencies** have been described in patients with SLE and their relatives. **C2 and C4 deficiencies** have also been described in collagen vascular disease such as dermatomyositis and SLE. Recurrent infections may be associated with the disease and its treatment with corticosteroids rather than with the complement deficiency. **C5 deficiency** has been described in a patient with SLE and **C7** in a family and patient with scleroderma. The former patient had recurrent infections but had been receiving corticosteroid treatment. A small number of patients have been described with **C6 or C8 deficiency.** They have had gonococcal and meningococcal infections (arthritis, septicemia, and meningitis), suggesting that the late components of complement are important in the bodily defense against *Neisseria.*

In addition to the above, **familial dysfunction of C5** has been described. It occurs in infants and is similar to Leiner's disease, with failure to thrive, widespread refractory seborrheic dermatitis, chronic diarrhea, and recurrent sepsis. Total hemolytic complement and immunoquantitation of C5 are normal, but there is a defect in phagocytosis of yeast particles which is corrected by the addition of normal C5. Patients have responded to the infusion of fresh plasma. However, the syndrome resembles the symptoms of combined immunodeficiency, and prior to plasma therapy normal cell-mediated immunity should be demonstrated in order to avoid the risk of graft-vs.-host reactions.

HYPERIMMUNOGLOBULINEMIA-E

This was first reported in two unrelated boys with recurrent pyogenic cutaneous, pulmonary, and joint infections (chiefly from *S. aureus*), growth retardation, coarse facies, chronic dermatitis, exquisite immediate hypersensitivity, and eosinophilia. Some features are similar to the Job syndrome in which recurrent "cold" abscesses occur in red-haired, fair-skinned females. Each has been associated with a defect in leukocyte chemotaxis, but with normal serum complement component activities. Besides the hyperimmunoglobulinemia-E and defective neutrophil chemotaxis, there may be T lymphocyte dysfunction and depressed antibody formation in other immunoglobulin classes. The chemotaxis defect may be intrinsic to the neutrophil or an inhibition of chemotaxis by histamine, the release of which is IgE-mediated. Long-term antistaphylococcal therapy has been partially successful.

THE "LAZY LEUKOCYTE" SYNDROME

This syndrome, reported in two unrelated children with recurrences of stomatitis, gingivitis, otitis media, and low-grade fever, is thought to reflect an abnormality in chemotaxis. Humoral and cellular immunity were normal, but severe peripheral neutropenia occurred, despite normal numbers of mature, morphologically normal neutrophils in the bone marrow. Neutrophils from peripheral blood or bone marrow showed normal phagocytic and bactericidal activities but lacked chemotactic activity, and random mobility of leukocytes was defective. The Rebuck skin window test (abraded skin is covered repeatedly with cover slips, which are then examined for the presence of neutrophils followed later by monocytes) failed to yield a typical inflammatory response. Fresh plasma transfusions did not correct the defect, indicating a primary defect in neutrophil function rather than a deficiency of plasma chemotactic factors.

Impaired chemotaxis and leukotaxis have also been described in a young boy with chronic granulomatous disease. The defect in leukocyte function was attributable, in part, to a circulating serum inhibitor of leukotactic function, and normal human serum restored the patient's leukotactive responsiveness.

CHRONIC GRANULOMATOUS DISEASE

A disorder characterized by repeated infections with granuloma and abscess formation, resulting from the inability of phagocytes to destroy certain microorganisms after normal phagocytosis. The disease occurs primarily in boys as an X-linked trait; in a few boys and in affected girls, inheritance appears to be autosomal recessive. Both circulating phagocytes and macrophages of the reticuloendothelial system (RES) are affected. The defect is due to the inability of phagocytes to generate hydrogen peroxide which, in conjunction with iodide ions and peroxidase (released from lysosomal granules), normally induces intracellular bacterial (and fungal) killing after phagocytosis. Patients do not become infected with the catalase-negative streptococci, pneumococci, or lactobacilli because these organisms produce hydrogen peroxide and therefore are able to "self-destruct." Viruses are also handled normally. Catalase-positive organisms, which are not destroyed by the deficient phagocytic cells, include *Staphylococcus aureus* and *albus, Klebsiella, Aerobacter, Escherichia coli, Pseudomonas, Aspergillus, Proteus, Serratia, Salmonella,* and *Candida.* Prolonged intracellular residence of these organisms occurs, resulting in granuloma and abscess formation throughout the RES.

Laboratory tests can be performed which demonstrate the defect: no significant killing of catalase-positive bacteria; normal killing of catalase-negative bacteria; no increase in glucose oxidation, O_2 consumption, or hydrogen-peroxide–dependent formate oxidation during phagocytosis; and lack of iodide fixation during phagocytosis.

A test which is useful in diagnosis is to demonstrate the failure of the patient's leukocytes to transform nitroblue tetrazolium (NBT) from colorless to deep blue during phagocytosis. In the sex-linked variety, mothers of patients have a partial defect which can be detected by the NBT test. Mothers are usually asymptomatic, but a few have chronic dermatitis and chronic infection.

Symptoms, Signs, and Course

Onset of clinical disease usually occurs in early childhood, but has been delayed until the early teens in a few patients. The clinical picture is characterized by suppurative lymphadenitis, hepatosplenomegaly, pneumonia, and hematologic evidence of chronic infection. Persistent rhinitis, dermatitis, persistent diarrhea, perianal abscess, ulcerative stomatitis, osteomyelitis, brain abscess, laryngeal destruction, and bronchial stenosis (from the granulation formation) also occur. Nonspecific laboratory findings include leukocytosis, normochromic-normocytic or mildly hypochromic-microcytic anemia, and hypergammaglobulinemia. Antibody formation is normal, although one patient has shown an isolated IgA deficiency. Studies suggest that mechanisms of cellular immunity may be secondarily impaired.

Prognosis and Treatment

Prognosis is generally poor. The disease in boys usually ends fatally before adolescence; survival to the late teens or early adulthood is rare. Life expectancy in girls seems longer than in boys.

No specific treatment has been found. Long-term therapy with antibiotics directed against the specific organisms (e.g., cephalexin; trimethoprim and sulfamethoxazole) is given to help prevent infections. Attempts at in vivo activation of deficient intracellular enzymes have been unsuccessful. Bone marrow transplantation is being investigated. Acutely ill patients may benefit from leukocyte transfusions, but these provide only circulating phagocytic cells, and the disease also affects phagocytes of the reticuloendothelial system.

CHEDIAK-HIGASHI SYNDROME

A progressive autosomal recessive disorder characterized clinically by partial albinism, severe recurrent pyogenic infections, and development of pancytopenia; and pathologically by giant intracytoplasmic granules in peripheral leukocytes. The defect is at the lysosomal level: phagocytosis occurs at a normal rate but the intracytoplasmic granules are unable to discharge their enzymes into phagocytic vacuoles and consequently intracellular bacterial killing cannot be accomplished. In contrast to chronic granulomatous disease, the hexose monophosphate shunt, O_2 consumption, and hydrogen peroxide formation are normal or even exaggerated. Abnormal granulocyte chemotaxis has been reported. The incidence of lymphoreticular malignancy is high.

Diagnosis is based on the familial pattern, the occurrence of partial albinism, and examination of the peripheral blood smear for large intracytoplasmic granules in both circulating neutrophils and lymphocytes. **Treatment** is unsatisfactory; antibiotics and leukocyte transfusions are used as emergency measures.

SPLENIC DEFICIENCY SYNDROMES

The spleen has two important functions in resistance to infection: it is the site of specific antibody production by B cells, and it acts as part of the reticuloendothelial system **(RES)**, clearing microorganisms from the plasma. The first is most important in early childhood, when most specific antibodies are being formed; the second function becomes most important when disorders occur that impair the RES function of the liver, such as thalassemia major and certain immunodeficiency states (e.g., Wiskott-Aldrich syndrome).

In **congenital splenic aplasia** and following **splenectomy** before age 2, both functions of the spleen are lost. Septicemia and meningitis from encapsulated pathogens (pneumococci, meningococci, *H. influenzae, E. coli*) may occur within 2 yr, and the child may remain susceptible to overwhelming infection. Splenectomy may be performed for rupture of the spleen and in the management of hereditary spherocytosis, acquired hemolytic anemia, idiopathic thrombocytopenic purpura, and thalassemia major. In sickle cell anemia, **functional hyposplenism** occurs because plugging of splenic vessels causes bypass of the splenic macrophage clearance of organisms; in addition, pneumococcal opsonins may not be produced, further complicating the process of phagocytosis.

The **diagnosis** of congenital aplasia of the spleen can be suspected when severe septicemia or meningitis recurs and other immunodeficiency syndromes are ruled out. Finding Heinz and Howell-Jolly bodies in peripheral RBCs supports the diagnosis, but these may also be found with certain congenital heart lesions. The spleen may or may not be visible on x-ray; it will not be visible on radioisotope scanning when there is either hypofunction or aplasia.

In **prevention and treatment,** elective splenectomy is postponed until after infancy, and multiple immunizations to a variety of pneumococcal antigens and other microorganisms are given before splenectomy to induce antibody formation. Penicillin is given prophylactically after splenectomy in childhood, and to children with congenital splenic aplasia. Some clinicians recommend prophylactic antibiotics for all post-splenectomy patients regardless of age.

---

4.   HYPERSENSITIVITY REACTIONS

At the present stage of knowledge it is difficult to formulate a classification that adequately categorizes the gamut of diseases in which hypersensitivity phenomena are felt to play a role—diseases which range from hay fever, which results from hypersensitivity to an exogenous antigen, is limited to the respiratory and ocular mucosal surfaces, and lacks systemic morbidity; to SLE, a multisystem disease with significant morbidity, and which results from hypersensitivity to antigens in one's own body tissues. There are, moreover, those diseases in which antibodies to host tissues can be demonstrated even though their pathologic significance is unknown; for example, the antibody to heart tissue that appears following heart surgery or myocardial infarction.

Various classifications have been proposed, based on the time required for the appearance of symptoms or skin test reactions after exposure to antigen (such as immediate and delayed hypersensitivity), on the type of antigen (such as drug reactions), or on the nature of organ involvement. These, however, have not taken into account that more than one type of immune response may be occurring or that more than one type may be necessary to produce immunologic injury. While this is also true of the classification of hypersensitivity reactions into four types devised by Coombs and Gell, theirs has proved to be clinically and conceptually helpful and has come to be widely used. It is based on animal experiments in which the four types of reaction can be clearly distinguished. Although the processes involved are often more complex in the clinical setting, the Coombs and Gell classification does allow one to plan a diagnostic and therapeutic approach to a clinical problem. It should be emphasized that in order to be classed as a hypersensitivity reaction a pathologic process must be the result of a specific interaction between antigen (exogenous or endogenous) and either humoral antibodies or sensitized lymphocytes. This definition therefore excludes those diseases in which antibodies are demonstrated but have no known pathophysiologic significance, even though their presence may have diagnostic value.

TYPE I REACTIONS

(Immediate-Type, Atopic, Reaginic, Anaphylactic, or IgE-Mediated
Hypersensitivity Reactions)

Reactions resulting from the release of pharmacologically active substances such as histamine, slow-reactive substance of anaphylaxis (SRS-A), and eosinophilic chemotactic factor (ECF) from IgE-sensitized basophils and mast cells after contact with specific antigen. The released substances cause vasodilation, increased capillary permeability, smooth muscle contraction, and eosinophilia. The consequent clinical manifestations include urticaria, angioedema, hypotension, and spasm of bronchial, gastrointestinal, or uterine musculature.

The clinical conditions in which Type I reactions play a role include allergic extrinsic asthma, seasonal allergic rhinitis, systemic anaphylaxis, reactions to stinging insects, some reactions to foods and drugs, and some cases of urticaria.

Diagnostic Tests

The most convenient test for the detection of IgE-sensitized mast cells is the **direct skin test.** Solutions for direct skin tests are made from extracts of materials which are inhaled, ingested, or injected, such as wind-borne pollens from certain trees, grasses, and weeds; house dust; animal danders; molds; foods; insect venoms; horse serum; and certain drugs. The tests are performed either by applying the test solutions to scratches or shallow punctures of the skin or by injecting them intradermally. The former is usually safer because less antigen is introduced, and is often done initially to identify materials which may cause a systemic reaction if injected intradermally. Scratches about 1 cm long and 2.5 cm apart are made with a needle on the forearm or back and a drop of concentrated (1:20) test extract is placed on each scratch. Alternatively, the skin is punctured through a drop of test extract with commercially available scarifiers or with a darning needle (prick technic). Control tests are performed simultaneously, using the diluent and either histamine (0.01 mg histamine base/ml) or morphine sulfate (0.1 mg/ml), which is a mast cell degranulator. The diluent should give a negative test result and the latter two substances should produce a wheal measuring 1 cm or less. The histamine and morphine tests determine the reactivity of the capillaries in the skin and the presence of mast cells, and are especially important as controls when the patient has been taking drugs, such as antihistamines and hydroxyzine, that are known to inhibit skin tests.

A positive wheal-and-flare reaction is usually obvious by 15 to 20 min after the test extract is applied. If the diameter of the wheal is more than 0.5 cm larger than the diluent control wheal, the test is positive and an intradermal test should not be performed. An intradermal test can be done if the reaction is smaller than this or if the patient has dermographism so that there is a question whether the wheal and flare are immunologically mediated.

In the intradermal test, a tuberculin syringe and short-bevel No. 26 needle are used to inject 0.02 ml of a 1:500 or 1:1000 concentration of the test extract into the skin; again, control tests are performed with diluent and histamine or morphine. A wheal more than 0.5 cm larger than the diluent control wheal, appearing in 15 min, is a positive reaction. The size of the skin test reaction shows a rough correlation with clinical symptoms, although some patients with large reactions do not have symptoms and some patients with small intradermal skin test reactions do have symptoms. Therefore, most physicians monitor the patient with periodic clinical reevaluations to determine the significance of skin tests.

Occasionally, direct skin testing is not possible because of generalized dermatitis, extreme dermographism, or the patient's anxiety. A **radioallergosorbent test (RAST)** or a **passive transfer test** (the **PK** [Prausnitz-Küstner] reaction) may be performed instead. The **RAST** detects the presence of antigen-specific serum IgE. In this test, a known antigen, in the form of an insoluble polymer-antigen conjugate, is mixed with the serum to be tested. Any IgE in the serum that is specific for the antigen will attach to the conjugate. Adding ^{125}I-labeled anti-IgE antibody and measuring the amount of radioactivity taken up by the conjugate determines the quantity of antigen-specific IgE in the patient's circulation.

Many commercial laboratories are now able to perform the RAST, but if a laboratory cannot test for antigens of interest to the physician, a **PK test** may be performed. (Since serum from the patient is injected into another individual in this test, the patient should first be tested for syphilis and hepatitis-associated antigen, and SGOT, SGPT, alkaline phosphatase, and bilirubin levels should be obtained.) Serum from the patient is obtained under sterile precautions or sterilized by filtration and 0.1-ml amounts are injected intradermally into several sites in a nonallergic subject (usually a relative). After 48 h, these sites are tested with antigen as in the direct skin test. Indirect skin testing is possible because IgE antibody in the patient's serum can adhere to the recipient's mast cells.

Another in vitro test is measurement of antigen-induced histamine release from the patient's leukocytes (**leukocyte histamine release**), which detects antigen-specific IgE on sensitized basophils. Though not widely used diagnostically, this test has given valuable insight into the kinetics of histamine release and has been useful in evaluating drugs for their ability to inhibit histamine release.

A positive skin test sometimes raises a question concerning the role of the particular antigen in the production of symptoms. In such cases, **provocative challenge** may be performed by applying the antigen to the eyes, nose, or lungs. Ophthalmic testing offers no advantage over skin testing and is rarely positive when skin tests are negative. However, it is sometimes used in testing hypersensitivity to pollens in suspected atopic conjunctivitis. A small amount of antigen (e.g., dried pollen or an aqueous extract of pollen in the same concentration as used for intradermal testing) is applied to the lower conjunctival sac. An appropriate control (e.g., the diluent or dried pine pollen), is used in the other eye. A positive response is characterized by burning, smarting, itching, or redness of the bulbar conjunctiva exceeding that in the control eye. Edema often follows. If a positive reaction occurs the eye should be irrigated with isotonic saline, then a drop of epinephrine 1:1000 instilled.

Nasal challenge is occasionally performed. There are numerous methods for introducing the antigen—insufflating dried pollen into the nose, spraying aqueous extract from a squeeze bottle or by nebulizer, or inserting a cotton pledget soaked in aqueous extract. Response is positive if itching, sneezing, and rhinorrhea occur, accompanied by a change in the appearance of the mucosa.

Bronchial inhalation challenge has long been used by European allergists to select the antigens to be used for immunotherapy. Although it remains predominantly an investigative tool in this country, some allergists use bronchial challenge when the clinical significance of a positive skin test is unclear.

Provocative food testing may be performed when symptoms are suspected of being food-related and skin tests are of doubtful clinical significance. Food elimination and challenge may be tried: The patient is put on a limited diet (see ELIMINATION DIETS in §11, Ch. 1); if symptoms are relieved, one new food is added to the diet and eaten regularly for 3 to 7 days or until symptoms recur. Alternatively, small amounts of the food to be tested are eaten in the physician's presence and the patient's reactions are observed. A positive response reproduces the patient's symptoms.

The determination of **total IgE level** has also been used in evaluating patients with Type I reactions. Serum IgE levels can be elevated in allergic asthma, allergic bronchopulmonary aspergillosis, parasitic infections, and eczema; they are normal in allergic alveolitis. Very high IgE levels are seen in allergic bronchopulmonary aspergillosis and can therefore be used to distinguish this form of allergic lung disease from asthma induced by pollen, dust, and mold and from nonallergic forms of asthma. The normally wide range of IgE levels, however, limits its usefulness in separating allergic from nonallergic asthma.

TYPE II REACTIONS
(Cytotoxic Reactions; Cytolytic Complement-Dependent Cytotoxicity; Cell-Stimulating Reactions)

Reactions which result when antibody reacts with antigenic components of a cell or tissue elements or with an antigen or hapten which has become intimately coupled to cells or tissue. The antigen-antibody reaction may cause opsonic adherence, through coating of the cell with antibody; immune adherence through activation of complement component C3, with consequent phagocytosis of the cell; or activation of the full complement system with consequent cytolysis of tissue damage. In some situations stimulation of secretory organs such as the thyroid may occur.

Clinical examples of cell injury in which antibody reacts with antigenic components of a cell are Coombs-positive hemolytic anemias, antibody-induced thrombocytopenic purpura, and leukopenia. These reactions occur in patients receiving incompatible transfusions, in hemolytic disease of the newborn, and in neonatal thrombocytopenia. They may also play a part in multisystem hypersensitivity diseases such as SLE.

The mechanism of injury is best exemplified by the effect on RBCs. In hemolytic anemias the RBCs are destroyed either by intravascular hemolysis or by macrophage phagocytosis, predominantly within the spleen. In vitro studies have demonstrated that in the presence of complement some complement-binding antibodies such as the blood group antibodies anti-A and anti-B cause rapid hemolysis; others such as anti-Le cause a slow lysis of cells; and still others do not damage cells directly but cause their adherence to and phagocytosis by phagocytes. By contrast, Rh antibodies do not activate complement, and they destroy cells predominantly by extravascular phagocytosis.

Examples of Type II reactions in which the antigen is a component of tissue include *early acute* (hyperacute) graft rejection of a transplanted kidney, which is due to the presence of antibody to vascular endothelium, and Goodpasture's syndrome, which is due to antibody reacting with glomerular and alveolar basement membrane endothelium. In experimental Goodpasture's syndrome complement is an important mediator of injury, but the role of complement has not been clearly determined in the early acute graft rejection.

Examples of reactions that are due to haptenic coupling with cells or tissue include many of the drug hypersensitivity reactions, such as penicillin-induced hemolytic anemia and purpura.

Cell-dependent cytotoxicity is a newly described form of Type II immunologic injury which has been observed in mice; its role in human disease has not been defined. In this reaction cells which have been coated with antibody are destroyed by lymphocyte-like cells which are neither T nor B cells. Whether complement plays a role in the reaction is not yet known.

Another effect of antibody is to stimulate cell function, as occurs with long-acting thyroid stimulator **(LATS)**. LATS is found in the IgG fraction of serum and is considered to be an autoantibody directed against some determinant on the thyroid cell membrane, causing excessive hormone secretion.

Diagnostic Tests

A Type II reaction is tested (1) by detecting the presence of antibody or complement on the cell or on tissue, or (2) by detecting the presence, in serum, of antibody to a cell surface antigen, a tissue antigen, or an exogenous antigen. Although complement is often required for Type II cell injury and may be detected on the cell or in the tissue, total serum hemolytic complement activity is not depressed as it is in Type III hypersensitivity reactions.

The direct antiglobulin and anti-non-γ-globulin tests detect antibody and complement on cells, respectively. These tests use rabbit antiserums, one to immunoglobulin and the other to complement. When these reagents are mixed with RBCs coated with immunoglobulin or complement, agglutination occurs. Antibodies eluted from these cells have demonstrated both a specificity for RBC blood group antigens and an ability to fix complement, thus demonstrating that they are true autoantibodies and account for the complement present on the RBCs in the direct non-γ-globulin tests.

The indirect antiglobulin test is used to detect the presence of a circulating antibody to RBC antigens. The patient's serum is incubated with RBCs of the same blood group (to preclude false results due to incompatibility) and the antiglobulin test is then performed on these RBCs. Agglutination confirms the presence of antibody to RBC antigens. In penicillin-induced hemolytic anemia the patient has a positive direct Coombs test while receiving penicillin but has a negative indirect antiglobulin test. The patient's serum, however, will agglutinate the indirect-test RBCs if they are coated with penicillin.

Fluorescent microscopy is most commonly used to detect the presence of immunoglobulin or complement in tissue (by the direct technic) and can also be used to determine the specificity of a circulating antibody (by the indirect technic). In the **direct immunofluorescent technic,** animal antibody that is specific for human immunoglobulin or complement is labeled with a fluorescent dye (usually fluorescein) and then layered on tissue. When the tissue is examined under the fluorescent microscope, a typical fluorescent color (green for fluorescein) indicates the presence of human immunoglobulin or complement in the tissue. Direct immunofluorescence can also be used to detect the presence of other serum proteins, tissue components, or exogenous antigen as long as specific animal antibodies to them can be produced. The technic itself does not indicate a Type II reaction unless the antibody can be eluted from the tissue and its specificity for tissue antigens determined.

In Goodpasture's syndrome the immunofluorescent pattern is seen as a linear fluorescence on kidney and lung basement membrane. When antibody is eluted from the kidney of patients with Goodpasture's syndrome and layered on normal kidney or lung, it attaches to the basement membrane and gives the same linear fluorescent pattern when tested with fluorescein-labeled antibody to human γ-globulin **(indirect immunofluorescence).**

The indirect immunofluorescence technic can also be used to detect tissue-specific circulating antibodies in many disorders, such as thyroiditis (antithyroid antibodies), SLE (anti-nuclear antibodies, anti-cytoplasmic antibodies), and pemphigoid (anti-skin-basement-membrane antibodies).

TYPE III REACTIONS
(Toxic Complex Reactions; Soluble Complex or Immune Complex
Hypersensitivity Reactions)

Reactions which result from deposition of soluble circulating antigen-antibody (immune) complexes in vessels or tissue. The antigen-antibody complexes activate complement and thereby initiate a sequence of events that results in polymorphonuclear cell migration and release of lysosomal proteolytic enzymes and permeability factors in tissues, thereby producing an acute inflammatory reaction. The consequences of immune complex formation depend in part on the relative proportions of antigen and antibody; with an excess of antibody, the complexes rapidly precipitate near the site of the antigen (e.g., within the joints in rheumatoid arthritis) or are phagocytosed by macrophages and are therefore not toxic; an antigen excess tends to cause soluble complexes which may cause systemic reactions or be widely deposited in various tissues.

Examples of clinical conditions in which Type III reactions appear to play some role are serum sickness due to serum, drugs, or viral hepatitis antigen, SLE, rheumatoid arthritis, polyarteritis, cryoglobulinemia, hypersensitivity pneumonitis, bronchopulmonary aspergillosis, acute glomerulonephritis, chronic membranoproliferative glomerulonephritis, and renal disease associated with bacterial endocarditis, malaria, and leprosy. In bronchopulmonary aspergillosis, drug- or serum-induced serum sickness, and some forms of renal disease, a Type I reaction is thought to precede the Type III reaction.

The classic laboratory examples of Type III reactions are the Arthus reaction and experimental serum sickness.

In the **Arthus reaction,** animals are first hyperimmunized to induce large amounts of circulating IgG antibodies and are then given a small amount of antigen intradermally. The antigen precipitates with the excess IgG and activates complement, so that a highly inflammatory, edematous, painful local lesion rapidly appears, which may progress to a sterile abscess containing many polymorphonuclear cells, and then to gangrene. A necrotizing vasculitis with occluded arteriolar lumens can be seen microscopically. No lag period precedes the reaction because antibody is already present.

In **experimental serum sickness,** a large amount of antigen is injected into a nonimmunized animal. After a lag period, antibody is produced; when this reaches a critical level, antigen-antibody complexes form which are deposited in endothelial vessels (particularly in glomeruli), where they produce widespread vascular injury that is characterized by polymorphonuclear leukocytes. During the appearance of the vasculitis a fall in serum complement can be detected, and antigen, antibody, and complement can be found in the areas of vasculitis. The antigen-antibody complexes are not capable of inducing injury by themselves, however, but require the presence of a Type I reaction to enhance vascular deposition.

Diagnostic Tests

Type III reactions can be suspected in human disease when a vasculitis occurs that is similar to the conditions observed in experimentally induced Arthus reaction and serum sickness. In polyarteritis this is the only clinical evidence to support a presumed Type III reaction. Further support to document a Type III reaction may be obtained by direct immunofluorescence tests (as described above for Type II reactions), which may indicate the presence of antigen, immunoglobulin, and complement in the area of vasculitis.

In experimental studies, fluorescent microscopy shows a coarse granular deposit ("lumpy bumps") along the basement membrane when animal glomeruli are stained for the presence of immunoglobulin and complement. A similar distribution can be seen in Type III human renal diseases. The electron microscope can also be used to detect electron-dense deposits (similar to those seen in experimental serum sickness), which are felt to be the antigen-antibody complexes. Rarely, the presence of both antigen and antibody can be detected by immunofluorescence in the inflamed tissue—this has been demonstrated in the renal disease of SLE and the vasculitic lesions of hepatitis-antigen–associated serum sickness.

Further evidence in support of a Type III reaction is obtained by demonstrating the presence of circulating antibody to antigens such as horse serum, hepatitis antigen, DNA, RF, and mold spores. In SLE, for example, a rise in antibody to native undenatured, double-stranded DNA and a fall in serum complement occur during exacerbations of renal disease. If the antigen is unknown, levels of total serum complement and of the early components (C1, C4, or C2) can be tested; a depressed level indicates classic complement activation and therefore that a Type III reaction is occurring. The C4 assay is the one most readily available.

In allergic pulmonary aspergillosis an intradermal skin test with aspergillus antigen may produce a Type I wheal-and-flare reaction followed by a Type III (painful edematous) reaction.

TYPE IV REACTIONS
(Cellular, Cell-Mediated, Delayed, or Tuberculin-Type Hypersensitivity Reactions)

Reactions caused by sensitized lymphocytes (T cells) after contact with antigen, which result from direct cytotoxicity or from the release of lymphokines. Delayed hypersensitivity differs from the other immune reactions in that it is mediated by sensitized lymphocytes and not by antibody. Thus, transfer of delayed hypersensitivity from sensitized to normal persons can be demonstrated with peripheral blood leukocytes or with an extract of these cells (transfer factor), but not with serum.

The T lymphocyte that has been sensitized (activated) by contact with antigen may cause immunologic injury by a direct toxic effect or through the release of soluble substances (lymphokines). In tissue culture, activated T lymphocytes have been demonstrated to destroy "target" cells to which they have been sensitized, when they are brought into direct contact with the target cells. The lymphokines released from activated T lymphocytes include several factors affecting the activity of macrophages, skin reactive factor, and a lymphotoxin.

Examples of clinical conditions in which Type IV reactions are felt to be important are contact dermatitis, allograft rejection, granulomas due to intracellular organisms, some forms of drug sensitivity, thyroiditis, and encephalomyelitis following rabies vaccination. The evidence for the last two is based on experimental models and, in human disease, on the appearance of lymphocytes in the inflammatory exudate of the thyroid and the brain.

Diagnostic Tests

A Type IV reaction can be suspected when an inflammatory reaction is characterized histologically by perivascular lymphocytes and macrophages. Delayed-hypersensitivity skin tests (see Tests of cell-mediated immunity in §2, Ch. 3) and patch tests are the most readily available methods of testing for delayed hypersensitivity.

Patch tests are performed to identify allergens causing a contact dermatitis. The suspected material (in appropriate concentration) is applied to the skin under a nonabsorbent adhesive patch and left for 48 h. If burning or itching develops earlier, the patch is removed. A positive test consists of erythema with some induration and, occasionally, vesicle formation. Because some reactions do not appear until after the patches are removed, the sites are reinspected at 72 h. Patch testing is done after the patient's contact dermatitis has cleared in order to prevent its exacerbation.

When the antigen is known, in vitro tests such as lymphocyte transformation or thymidine incorporation can be performed in a patient with a negative skin test, to determine whether the defect is an inability of the skin to react to lymphokines or an inability of T cells to produce lymphokines. The best correlate with delayed hypersensitivity, however, is the production of migration inhibition factor. (These tests are described in §2, Ch. 3.)

---

5. DISORDERS DUE TO HYPERSENSITIVITY

ATOPIC DISEASES
(Allergic Disorders)

Disorders caused by Type I hypersensitivity, resulting from the release of vasoactive substances by mast cells and basophils that have been sensitized by the interaction of antigen with IgE (**reaginic** or **skin-sensitizing antibody**).

The terms **hypersensitivity** and **allergy** are often used synonymously to mean an exaggerated response to an antigen which leads to various types of tissue damage. However, the term **allergy** is now often restricted to mean an IgE-mediated (atopic) hypersensitivity disorder.

The most common human allergic disorders—hay fever (seasonal allergic rhinitis), asthma (particularly in children), infantile eczema, and some cases of urticaria and gastrointestinal food reactions—are atopic diseases. Patients with atopic diseases have in common an inherited predisposition to develop hypersensitivity to substances (allergens) in the environment which are harmless to 80% of people. Features similar to atopy have been identified in several mammalian species.

Diagnostic Procedures

History: A careful review of the symptoms, their relation to the environment and to seasonal and situational variations, and their clinical course should yield sufficient information to allow classification of the disease as atopic. The history and clinical course are more valuable than tests in determining whether a patient is allergic, and it is inappropriate to subject the patient to extensive skin testing unless there is reasonable clinical evidence for atopy. Age of onset may be an important clue (for example, childhood asthma is much more likely to be atopic than asthma beginning after age 30). Also indicative are symptoms which are seasonal (e.g., correlating with specific pollen seasons), or appear after exposure to animals, hay, or dust, or develop in specific environments (e.g., at home, at work).

It is also helpful, for advising the patient, to investigate the effects of nonspecific contributory factors, such as tobacco smoke and other pollutants, cold air and cold beverages, certain drugs, and life stresses.

Tests: These are used to confirm sensitivity to an antigen when it is suspected that the patient is allergic. For details on direct and passive-transfer skin tests, the radioallergosorbent test (RAST), provocative challenge tests, and leukocyte histamine release, see TYPE I HYPERSENSITIVITY REACTIONS in §2, Ch. 4.

Nonspecific findings: Eosinophilia is associated with some atopic conditions, particularly asthma and eczematous eruptions, but its absence does not rule out allergy. **IgE levels** are of diagnostic significance in eczema, since they are elevated and will rise during exacerbations and fall during remissions. IgE levels are also elevated in atopic asthma, but their overlap with normal levels reduces their value in distinguishing this form from other types of asthma.

Treatment

Avoidance: When possible, eliminating the allergen is the treatment of choice. This may require a change of diet, occupation, or residence; withdrawal of a drug; or removal of a household pet. Some locales, free of allergens such as ragweed, are havens for afflicted persons. When complete avoidance is impossible, as in the case of house dust, exposure may be reduced by removing dust-collecting furniture, carpets, and draperies, frequent wet-mopping and dusting, and installing a high-efficiency air-filtering system.

Symptomatic therapy: Relief of symptoms with drugs should not be neglected while the patient is being evaluated and specific control or treatment is being developed. The proper use of antihistamines, sympathomimetics, and corticosteroids is outlined for each disease category in the discussions which follow. In general, corticosteroids are appropriate for treatment of potentially disabling conditions which are self-limited and of relatively short duration (seasonal asthma due to pollens; serum sickness; infiltrative lung disease; severe contact dermatitis). In such cases there is little risk of the adverse effects of long-term corticosteroid treatment.

Desensitization (hyposensitization, immunotherapy): When it is not feasible to avoid an allergen or to control it sufficiently to relieve symptoms of atopic disease, desensitization can be attempted by injecting an extract of the allergen subcutaneously in gradually increasing doses. Several specific effects can be demonstrated although there is no test that correlates absolutely with clinical improvement. The titer of blocking (neutralizing) antibody increases proportionably to the dose administered. Sometimes, particularly when high doses of pollen extract can be tolerated, the serum IgE level falls significantly. In addition, peripheral blood leukocyte histamine release is reduced from pretreatment levels on incubation with antigen (or an increased amount of antigen is required to release 50% of the histamine in peripheral leukocytes). This effect is not specific—the reduced leukocyte hypersensitivity applies to antigens not used in desensitization as well.

Clinical results are most satisfactory when injections are continued year-round. Depending on the degree of sensitivity, the first dose is 0.1 ml of a dilution ranging from 1:100,000 to 1:100,000,000. The dose is increased weekly or biweekly by 75% (or less) until a maximum tolerated concentration has been reached; e.g., 0.3 ml of a 1:50 dilution. For crude pollen extracts, this amounts to about 30 μg of protein nitrogen (3000 protein nitrogen u.). Once the maximum dose has been reached, it can be maintained at monthly intervals year-round. Even in seasonal allergies this **perennial method** is superior to preseasonal or coseasonal treatment methods.

The major allergens used for desensitization are the inhalants which usually cannot be effectively avoided: pollens, house dust, and molds. Stinging insect extracts are used similarly to induce protection in patients who have experienced generalized reactions. There is rarely any indication for animal dander or food desensitization, and no good evidence that bacterial vaccines have any specific effect.

Patients are often extremely sensitive, particularly to pollen allergens, and if an overdose is given, can experience **constitutional reactions** varying from a mild cough or sneezing to generalized urticaria, severe asthma, and anaphylactic shock. To prevent such reactions, one must (1) check that the proper dilution is used, (2) increase the dose by small increments, (3) repeat the same dose (or even decrease it) if the local reaction from the previous injection is large (2.5 cm in diameter or greater), and (4) reduce the dose when a fresh vial is used. Reducing the dose of pollen extract during the pollen season is often wise also. Intramuscular and intravascular injection must be *avoided.*

Despite the best precautions, reactions will occur occasionally. The severe, life-threatening ones develop within 20 min; therefore, no patient should be allowed to leave earlier. The first signs of an impending reaction may be sneezing, coughing, and chest tightness, or a generalized flush, tingling sensations, and pruritus. A tourniquet should be applied above the injection site at once, and the site infiltrated with 0.2 ml of epinephrine 1:1000. If the reaction is mild, a double dose of an antihistamine can then be given orally (e.g., diphenhydramine 100 mg or chlorpheniramine 8 mg) and 0.3 ml of epinephrine 1:1000 can be given s.c. in the opposite arm. (The tourniquet should be released in 15 min.) However, if symptoms and signs of shock have developed, IV fluids should be started and epinephrine 1:1000, 0.3 to 0.5 ml IM, or 1:10,000, 1 to 2 ml IV, should be given, and other measures instituted for treatment of anaphylaxis (see below).

Occasionally, a generalized reaction such as urticaria may appear 30 min to several hours after an allergen injection. This can be treated with an antihistamine alone. Following any generalized reaction, the next dose of allergen should be reduced by one third or one fourth, and later increments kept as small as is practicable (usually 0.03 to 0.05 ml).

ALLERGIC RHINITIS

A symptom complex including hay fever and perennial allergic rhinitis, character-ized by seasonal or perennial sneezing, rhinorrhea, nasal congestion, pruritus, and often conjunctivitis and pharyngitis.

Hay Fever
(Pollinosis)

Hay fever, the acute seasonal form of allergic rhinitis, is generally induced by wind-borne pollens. The **spring** type is due to tree pollens (e.g., oak, elm, maple, alder, birch, cottonwood); the **summer** type, to grass pollens (e.g., Bermuda, timothy, sweet vernal, orchard, Johnson) and to weed pollens (e.g., sheep sorrel, English plantain); the **fall** type, to weed pollens (e.g., ragweed). Occasionally, seasonal hay fever is due primarily to airborne fungus spores.

Symptoms and Signs

The nose, roof of the mouth, pharynx, and eyes begin to itch gradually or abruptly after onset of the pollen season. Lacrimation, sneezing, and clear, watery nasal discharge accompany or soon follow the pruritus. Frontal headaches, irritability, anorexia, depression, and insomnia may appear. The conjunctiva is injected, and the nasal mucous membranes are swollen and bluish red. Coughing and asthmatic wheezing may develop as the season progresses. Many eosinophils are present in the nasal mucus during the season.

Diagnosis

The nature of the allergic process and even the responsible allergen is often suspected from the history. Diagnosis is confirmed by the above physical findings, skin tests, and the accompanying eosinophilia in blood or secretions.

Treatment

Symptoms may be diminished by avoidance of the allergen (see above). Most patients obtain adequate relief with oral antihistamines (e.g., chlorpheniramine, in sustained-release form, 12 mg q 8 h; triprolidine 2.5 mg q 8 h). If these drugs are too sedating, a different drug should be used (e.g., slow-release brompheniramine 12 mg orally q 8 h or phenindamine 25 mg orally q 4 h). Sympathomimetics are often used in combination with antihistamines. Phenylpropanolamine, phenyl-ephrine, or pseudoephedrine are available in many antihistamine-decongestant preparations. Ephedrine 25 mg orally q 4 h is more effective, but its central-stimulating effects limit its use.

When nasal symptoms are not relieved adequately by antihistaminic treatment, intranasal dexamethasone spray is usually effective. Two metered doses t.i.d. are used initially; each dose is freon-propelled from a container that delivers dexamethasone 0.084 mg/dose. When symptoms have been relieved, dosage is reduced to 1 dose b.i.d. for the remainder of the season. Severe intractable extranasal symptoms may require a short course of systemic corticosteroid treatment (prednisone 10 mg orally b.i.d., with gradual reduction in dose).

Desensitization treatment (see above) is advisable if drug treatment is poorly tolerated, if corticosteroids are needed during the season, or if asthma develops. It should be started soon after the pollen season has ended.

PERENNIAL ALLERGIC RHINITIS

In contrast to hay fever, symptoms of perennial rhinitis vary in severity (often unpredictably) throughout the year. Extranasal symptoms such as conjunctivitis are uncommon, but chronic nasal obstruction is often prominent and may extend to eustachian tube obstruction. The resultant hearing difficulty is particularly common in children. The **diagnosis** of allergic rhinitis is supported by a positive history of atopic disease, the characteristic bluish-red mucosa, numerous eosinophils in the nasal secretions, and positive skin tests (particularly to house dust, feathers, animal danders, or fungi, and occasionally to foods). Some patients have complicating sinus infections and nasal polyps.

Certain patients suffer from chronic rhinitis, sinusitis, and polyps and often have negative skin tests. These patients are not allergic but often have aspirin and indomethacin sensitivity and should be evaluated also for sensitivity to sodium benzoate (a food preservative) and tartrazine yellow (a food coloring) by a trial elimination of these food additives from the diet. Some patients with mild but annoying chronic continuous nasal obstruction or rhinorrhea have no demonstrable allergy, polyps, infection, or drug sensitivity, a condition identified as **vasomotor rhinitis** (see §17, Ch. 5).

Treatment

Management is similar to that for hay fever if specific allergens are identified, except that systemic corticosteroids, even though effective, should be avoided because of the need for prolonged use. Surgery (antrotomy and irrigation of sinuses, polypectomy, submucous resection) may be necessary after allergic factors have been controlled or ruled out. For many patients the only treatment is reassurance, antihistamine and vasoconstrictor drugs, and advice to avoid topical decongestants, which produce after-congestion and, when used continuously, may aggravate or perpetuate chronic rhinitis **(rhinitis medicamentosa).**

ALLERGIC PULMONARY DISEASE

The lungs can be involved in known or suspected allergic reactions in several ways, depending on the nature of the allergen and its route of entry. Specific disorders are discussed in §5, Ch. 12, and under BRONCHIAL ASTHMA in §5, Ch. 5.

ANAPHYLAXIS

An acute, often explosive, systemic reaction characterized by urticaria, respiratory distress, vascular collapse, and occasionally by vomiting, abdominal cramps, and diarrhea, that occurs in a previously sensitized person when he again receives the sensitizing antigen. This Type I reaction occurs when antigen reaches the circulation. The histamine and slow-reactive substances (SRS-A) released when the antigen reacts with IgE on basophils and mast cells cause the smooth muscle contraction and vascular dilation which characterize anaphylaxis. The most common causative antigens are foreign serum, certain drugs or diagnostic agents, desensitizing injections, or insect stings. **Anaphylactoid reactions** are clinically similar to anaphylaxis, but occur after the *first* injection of certain drugs (histamine, polymyxin, pentamidine, morphine, contrast media), and have a dose-related toxic-idiosyncratic mechanism rather than an immunologically mediated one.

Pathogenesis

The wheezing and gastrointestinal symptoms are caused by smooth muscle contraction. Vasodilation and escape of plasma into the tissues causes the urticaria and results in a decrease in effective plasma volume which is the major cause of shock. Fluid escapes into the lung alveoli and may produce pulmonary edema. Obstructive angioedema of the upper airway may also occur. Rarely, myocarditis develops if the reaction is prolonged.

Symptoms and Signs

Typically, in 1 to 15 min, the patient complains of a sense of uneasiness and becomes agitated and flushed. Palpitation, paresthesias, pruritus, throbbing in the ears, coughing, sneezing, and difficulty in breathing are other typical complaints. Nausea and vomiting are less common. The symptoms and signs of shock may develop within another 1 or 2 min, and the patient may become incontinent, convulse, become unresponsive, and die.

Prophylaxis

Patients with the greatest risk of anaphylactic reactions to a drug are those who have reacted previously to that drug. Yet anaphylactic deaths still occur in patients who do not give such a history. The risk of a reaction to horse serum is sufficiently high that routine skin testing before giving the serum is *mandatory* (see Horse Serum Sensitivity, below). Routine skin testing before other drug treatment is neither practicable nor reliable, except for penicillin. Tests for penicillin hypersensitivity are discussed under Drug Hypersensitivity, below.

Prophylaxis for the patient who needs antiserum (e.g., for botulism, diphtheria, gas gangrene, or snake bite) is described below, under Horse Serum Sensitivity.

Long-term desensitization is effective and appropriate for prevention of insect-sting anaphylaxis but has rarely been attempted in patients with a history of drug or serum anaphylaxis.

Treatment

Immediate treatment with epinephrine is imperative. It is a pharmacologic antagonist to the effects of the chemical mediators on smooth muscle, blood vessels, and other tissues.

For mild reactions such as generalized pruritus, urticaria, angioedema, mild wheezing, nausea, and vomiting, 0.3 to 0.5 ml of aqueous epinephrine 1:1000 should be given s.c. If an injected antigen has caused the anaphylaxis, a tourniquet should be applied above the injection site and 0.1 to 0.2 ml of epinephrine 1:1000 also injected into the site, in order to reduce systemic absorption of the antigen. This may suffice for a mild reaction, although a second injection of epinephrine s.c. may be required. Once symptoms have resolved, an oral antihistamine-ephedrine combination should be given for 24 h.

For more severe reactions, with massive angioedema but without evidence of cardiovascular involvement, patients should be given diphenhydramine 50 to 100 mg IM (for an adult) in addition to the above treatment, to forestall laryngeal edema and to block the effect of further histamine release. When the edema is responding, 0.3 ml of an aqueous suspension of epinephrine 1:200 s.c. can be given for its 6- to 8-h effect, and an oral antihistamine-ephedrine combination should be given for the next 18 h.

For severe respiratory reactions that do not respond to epinephrine, IV fluids should be started and aminophylline 6 mg/kg IV should be given over 10 to 20 min, followed by 1 mg/kg/h. Endotracheal intubation or tracheostomy may be necessary, with O_2 administration at 4 to 6 L/min.

The most severe reactions usually involve the cardiovascular system, causing immediate severe hypotension and vasomotor collapse. Epinephrine 1:1000, 0.3 to 0.5 ml IM should be given immediately. IV fluids should be started and the patient should be recumbent with legs elevated. The severe hypotension may be a result of vasodilation, hypovolemia from loss of fluid, or, rarely, myocardial insufficiency or a combination of these causes. Each has a specific treatment and often the treatment of one exacerbates the others. The appropriate therapy may be clarified if central venous pressure (**CVP**) and left atrial pressure can be obtained with a Swan-Ganz catheter. A low CVP and normal left atrial pressure indicate peripheral vasodilation and/or hypovolemia. Vasodilation should respond to the epinephrine (which will also retard the loss of intravascular fluid). In severe shock, however, 1 ml of epinephrine 1:1000 can be added to 10 ml of saline and given slowly IV, with a close watch for side effects such as headache, tremulousness, nausea, vomiting, or cardiac arrhythmias.

In most cases, hypovolemia is the major cause of the hypotension. The CVP and left atrial pressure are both low, and large volumes of saline must be given, with monitoring of the blood pressure, until the CVP rises to normal. Colloid plasma expanders such as dextran are rarely necessary. Only if fluid replacement does not restore normal blood pressure should one initiate treatment cautiously with adrenergic drugs such as metaraminol.

In the rare instance of myocardial insufficiency, both CVP and left atrial pressure will be elevated. Isoproterenol 1 mg is diluted in 500 ml of 5% dextrose and infused at a rate of 0.5 to 1 ml/min. The patient should be monitored carefully, for the isoproterenol may cause cardiac arrhythmias and hypotension due to peripheral vasodilation.

Cardiac arrest may occur, requiring immediate resuscitation and sodium bicarbonate IV (see CARDIAC ARREST AND CARDIOPULMONARY RESUSCITATION in §4, Ch. 4). Further therapy depends on ECG findings.

When all the above measures have been instituted, diphenhydramine (50 to 75 mg IV slowly over 3 min) and corticosteroids may then be given as a precaution against late-onset asthma, laryngeal edema, or hypotension. If the patient is still hypotensive, hydrocortisone sodium succinate 100 mg (or equivalent) should be given q 1 to 2 h until symptoms are controlled, then q 2 to 4 h for 24 h, and then discontinued. Diphenhydramine 50 to 75 mg IV can be given q 6 h if edema develops. Complications such as myocardial infarction and cerebral edema should be looked for and treated specifically.

Patients with severe reactions should remain in a hospital under observation for 24 h following recovery to ensure adequate treatment in case of relapse.

URTICARIA; ANGIOEDEMA
(Hives; Giant Urticaria; Angioneurotic Edema)

Urticaria: *Local wheals and erythema in the dermis.* **Angioedema:** *A similar eruption, but with larger edematous areas that involve subcutaneous structures as well as the dermis.*

Etiology

Acute urticaria and angioedema can be due to drug allergy, insect stings or bites, desensitization injections, or ingestion of certain foods (particularly eggs, shellfish, nuts, or fruits). Some food reactions occur explosively following ingestion of only minute amounts. Others (such as reactions to strawberries) may occur only after overindulgence, and possibly result from direct (toxic) histamine liberation. Urticaria may accompany or follow streptococcal and several viral infections, such as hepatitis. Some acute reactions are unexplained, even when recurrent. If acute angioedema is recurrent, and progressively more severe, a hereditary enzyme deficiency should be suspected (see HEREDITARY ANGIOEDEMA, below).

Chronic urticaria and angioedema lasting more than 3 wk are more difficult to explain and only in exceptional cases can a specific cause be found. They occur as commonly in nonatopic as in atopic subjects. Occasionally, unsuspected chronic drug or chemical ingestion is responsible; e.g., from penicillin in milk, from the use of nonprescription drugs, or from preservatives, dyes, or other food additives. Chronic underlying disease (SLE, polycythemia vera, chronic infection, lymphoma) should be ruled out. Though suspected frequently, controllable psychogenic factors are not often identified. Urticaria caused by physical agents is discussed in PHYSICAL ALLERGY, below.

Symptoms and Signs

In urticaria, pruritus, generally the first symptom, is followed shortly by the appearance of wheals which may remain small (1 to 5 mm) or may enlarge. The larger ones tend to clear in the center, and may be noticed first as large (more than 20 cm across) rings of erythema and edema. Ordinarily, crops of hives come and go, a lesion remaining in one site for several hours, then disappearing, only to reappear elsewhere. **Angioedema** is a more diffuse swelling of loose subcutaneous tissue: dorsum of hands or feet, eyelids, lips, genitalia, mucous membranes. Edema of the upper airway may produce respiratory distress and the stridor may be mistaken for asthma.

Diagnosis

This is usually obvious, though insect bites and scabies may closely simulate some eruptions. Identifying the responsible agent may be difficult because of the wide variety of possible causes. Skin tests are usually not helpful.

Treatment

Acute urticaria is a self-limited condition that generally subsides in 1 to 7 days; hence, treatment is chiefly palliative. If the cause is not obvious, all nonessential medication should be stopped until the reaction has subsided. Symptoms can usually be relieved with an oral antihistamine (e.g., diphenhydramine 50 to 100 mg q 4 h or cyproheptadine 4 to 8 mg q 4 h). Corticosteroids (e.g., prednisone 30 to 40 mg/day orally) may be necessary for the more severe reactions, particularly when associated with angioedema. Topical corticosteroids, however, are of no value. Epinephrine 1:1000, 0.3 ml s.c., should be the first treatment for **acute pharyngeal or laryngeal angioedema.** This may be supplemented with topical treatment; e.g., nebulized epinephrine 1:100. This will usually prevent airway obstruction, but one must be prepared to perform a tracheostomy and give O_2.

Although the specific cause of **chronic urticaria** can seldom be identified and removed, spontaneous remissions occur eventually in most cases. Control of stressful life situations often helps, and may even effect a permanent remission. Certain drugs (e.g., aspirin) may aggravate symptoms, as will alcoholic beverages, coffee, and tobacco smoking; if so, they should be avoided. When urticaria is produced by aspirin, sensitivity to related compounds (e.g., indomethacin) and to the food additives tartrazine yellow and sodium benzoate should be investigated (see PERENNIAL ALLERGIC RHINITIS, above). Oral antihistamines with a sedative effect are beneficial in most cases (e.g., cyproheptadine 4 to 8 mg q 4 h or hydroxyzine 25 to 50 mg t.i.d.). All reasonable measures should be used before resorting to corticosteroids, which are frequently effective but, once started, may have to be continued indefinitely.

HEREDITARY ANGIOEDEMA

A form of angioedema transmitted as an autosomal dominant trait and associated with a deficiency of serum inhibitor of the activated first component of complement. A positive family history is the rule, but there are exceptions. The edema is characteristically unifocal, indurated, painful rather than pruritic, and not accompanied by urticaria. Attacks are often precipitated by trauma or viral illness, and are aggravated by emotional stress. The gastrointestinal tract is often involved, with nausea, vomiting, colic, and even signs of intestinal obstruction. The condition may cause fatal upper airway obstruction. **Diagnosis** may be made by measuring C4, which is low, even between attacks, or more specifically by demonstrating deficiency of the C1 esterase inhibitor **(C1 Inh)** by immunodiffusion or bioassay technics.

Treatment

The usual symptomatic treatment used in angioedema is unsuccessful; the edema progresses until complement components have been consumed. Acute attacks which threaten to produce airway obstruction should therefore be treated promptly by establishing an airway. ε-Aminocaproic acid 10 to 16 Gm/day orally is effective in reducing the frequency and severity of attacks, but, partly because of side effects, such treatment is still experimental. Fresh-frozen plasma is used prophylactically prior to dental procedures or surgery to prevent an attack. It has also been used therapeutically during an attack. Although there is a theoretic concern that a complement substrate in the plasma might provoke an attack, in practice this has not been observed. Androgen treatment may help. A new anterior pituitary suppressant, danazol, not only seems effective, but in some patients increases the C4 and C1 Inh levels.

PHYSICAL ALLERGY

A condition in which allergic symptoms and signs are produced by exposure to cold, sunlight, heat, or mild trauma.

Etiology

The underlying cause is unknown in most cases. Photosensitivity (see in §20, Ch. 1, and CONTACT DERMATITIS in §16, Ch. 3) may sometimes be induced by drugs or topical agents, including certain cosmetics. Cold and light sensitivity, in many but not all cases, can be passively transferred with serum that contains a specific IgE antibody, suggesting an immunologic mechanism involving a physically altered skin protein as antigen. The serum of a few patients with cold-induced symptoms shows cryoglobulins or cryofibrinogen; these abnormal proteins may be associated with a serious underlying disorder such as a malignancy, a collagen vascular disease, or chronic infection. Cold may aggravate asthma or vasomotor rhinitis, but cold urticaria is independent of any other known allergic tendencies. Heat sensitivity usually produces cholinergic urticaria, which is also induced in the same patients by exercise and emotional stress. **Dermographism (dermatographia),** a wheal-and-flare reaction seen after scratching or firmly stroking the skin, is usually idiopathic but occasionally is the first sign of an urticarial drug reaction. In **pressure urticaria,** angioedema or wheals appear promptly or 8 to 12 h after the release of persistent pressure on the skin.

Clinical Features

Pruritus and unsightly appearance are the most common complaints. Cold sensitivity is usually manifested by urticaria and angioedema, which develop most typically after exposure to cold and during or after swimming or bathing. Sunlight may produce urticaria or a more chronic polymorphous skin eruption.

The skin lesions in cholinergic urticaria are small, highly pruritic, discrete wheals surrounded by a large zone of erythema. Cholinergic urticaria appears to be caused by an unusual sensitivity to acetylcholine, and administration of acetylcholine or methacholine should reproduce the lesions. The diagnosis is confirmed if methacholine 1:5000, 0.05 ml intradermally, causes satellite urticarial lesions; normal persons will develop a wheal.

Prophylaxis and Treatment

The use of drugs or cosmetics should be reviewed with the patient, particularly if photosensitivity is suspected. Protection from the physical stimulus is necessary, but most patients want more help than this when seeking medical attention. Management of photosensitivity is discussed in §20, Ch. 1, and under CONTACT DERMATITIS in §16, Ch. 3.

For relief of itching, an antihistamine with sedative effects should be given orally (diphenhydramine 50 mg orally q.i.d.; cyproheptadine 4 to 8 mg orally q.i.d.). Cyproheptadine has been noted to be the most effective in cold urticaria. Hydroxyzine 25 to 50 mg orally q.i.d. is more effective in cholinergic urticaria. Prednisone 30 to 40 mg/day orally should be given in severe light eruptions other than urticaria to shorten the clinical course; the dose is gradually reduced as treatment becomes effective.

ALLERGIC CONJUNCTIVITIS
(See also VERNAL CONJUNCTIVITIS in §19, Ch. 8)

Atopic conjunctivitis of an acute or chronic catarrhal form is usually part of a larger allergic syndrome such as hay fever, but may occur alone through direct contact with airborne substances such as pollen, fungus spores, various dusts, or animal danders.

Symptoms, Signs, and Diagnosis

Itching is prominent and may be accompanied by excessive lacrimation. The conjunctiva is edematous and hyperemic. The cause is often suggested by the history and may be confirmed by skin testing. If *atopic* conjunctivitis is suspected but skin tests are equivocal, an ophthalmic challenge (see TYPE I HYPERSENSITIVITY REACTIONS in §2, Ch. 4) occasionally will be positive. Since so few antigens can be tested in a reasonable period, ophthalmic challenge has limited application. *It should not be used for diagnosis of contact hypersensitivity.*

Treatment

An identified or suspected causative allergen should be avoided. Frequent use of a bland eyewash (e.g., buffered 0.65% saline) may reduce the irritation. Contact lenses should not be worn. In atopic conjunctivitis antihistamines given orally (see ALLERGIC RHINITIS, above) are helpful and may also be when used topically (e.g., 0.5% antazoline phosphate ophthalmic solution). The frequency of contact dermatitis is less than with topical dermatologic antihistamines. In severe cases and in most cases of contact hypersensitivity, more effective relief is provided by a corticosteroid ophthalmic ointment (e.g., hydrocortisone 2.5% or dexamethasone 0.05%) applied t.i.d. or q.i.d. Indications for desensitization are similar to those for hay fever; patients with contact hypersensitivity cannot be desensitized.

OTHER ALLERGIC EYE DISEASES

The **lids** may be involved by angioedema or urticaria, contact dermatitis, or atopic dermatitis. Contact dermatitis of the eyelids, a Type IV hypersensitivity reaction, may be caused by various ophthalmic medications or drugs conveyed by the fingers to the eyes (e.g., antibiotics by drug handlers) or by face powder, nail polish, or hair dye. The **cornea** may become involved by extension of allergic conjunctivitis or by a variant of superficial punctate keratitis.

Pain, photophobia, and circumcorneal inflammation indicate probable **uveitis,** which is due, rarely, to a specific environmental allergen. In most cases the cause is unknown, though bacterial hypersensitivity of the cell-mediated type (Type IV hypersensitivity) may be suspected. **Sympathetic ophthalmia** (see in §19, Ch. 11) is felt to be a hypersensitivity reaction to uveal pigment. **Endophthalmitis phacoanaphylactica** is caused by allergy to native lens protein. The reaction, which is severe, occurs typically in the remaining lens after one lens has been removed uneventfully, though it may follow trauma or inflammation involving the lens capsule. Prompt treatment by an ophthalmologist is required in these serious ophthalmic conditions.

GASTROINTESTINAL ALLERGY

An uncommon symptom complex due to ingestion of specific food or drug allergens, manifested by nausea, vomiting, crampy abdominal pain, and diarrhea. Gastrointestinal symptoms from food or drugs more commonly represent nonspecific intolerance or are secondary to digestive enzyme defects (as in celiac disease and disaccharidase deficiency), and hypersensitivity to food allergens is more commonly manifested as urticaria or angioedema.

Symptoms and Signs

The severe (but rare) acute reaction to food is characterized by nausea, vomiting, diarrhea, and violent abdominal pains associated with the other symptoms of anaphylaxis (see above). Less severe reactions—chronic crampy pain, diarrhea, and, often, urticaria—are more common. Most patients prone to severe reactions can detect traces of the offending food in their mouths by the rapid onset of mucosal burning or itching.

Occasionally, cheilitis, aphthae, pylorospasm, spastic constipation, irritable colon, pruritus ani, and perianal eczema have been attributed to food allergy, but the association is difficult to prove. **Eosinophilic enteropathy,** which may be related to specific food allergy, is an unusual form of protein-losing enteropathy that is associated with blood eosinophilia, eosinophilic infiltrates in the gut, and other signs of atopic disease.

Diagnosis

Severe food allergy is usually obvious to the patient. When it is not, diagnosis is difficult and the condition must be differentiated from functional gastrointestinal problems. Skin tests are of limited value. A detailed history, physical examination, and elimination diets will assist in establishing a diagnosis. The regular occurrence of symptoms after ingestion of a particular food (see discussion of provocative food testing under TYPE I HYPERSENSITIVITY REACTIONS in §2, Ch. 4) is usually the only practical diagnostic clue, but the association is not specific for allergy.

Treatment

Except for elimination of the offending foods, there is no specific treatment. When only a few foods are involved, abstinence is preferred. Sensitivity to one or more foods may disappear spontaneously. Oral desensitization (by first eliminating the offending food for a time and then giving small, daily increased amounts) has not been proved effective. Heating certain foods (e.g., milk) may reduce their antigenicity by protein denaturation. Antihistamines are of little value except in acute general reactions with urticaria and angioedema. Prolonged corticosteroid treatment is not indicated except in eosinophilic enteropathy.

For treatment of the severe, potentially fatal acute attack, see URTICARIA; ANGIOEDEMA, and ANAPHYLAXIS, above.

DRUG HYPERSENSITIVITY

Drug eruptions are discussed in §16, Ch. 10. Discussed here are other hypersensitivity reactions that can follow oral or parenteral drug administration. Contact dermatitis, which is a Type IV hypersensitivity reaction that follows topical use, is discussed in §16, Ch. 3; and drug reactions that result from other than immunologic mechanisms are also discussed in §22, Ch. 7.

Before attributing a given reaction to a drug, one should appreciate that placebos also may cause unwanted effects. Nausea, tachycardia, excessive sweating, epigastric disturbance with diarrhea, dry mouth, headache, easy fatigue, somnolence, even skin rashes have been reported by persons taking inert substances in double-blind studies. Nevertheless, true reactions due to drugs are important and constitute a major medical problem. The literature on specific drugs should be consulted for the most likely adverse reactions.

With **overdosage of a drug,** toxic effects occur in direct relation to the total amount of drug in the body, and can occur in any patient if the dose is large enough. *Absolute* overdosage results from an error in the amount or frequency of administration of individual doses. *Relative* overdosage may be seen in patients who, because of liver or kidney disease, do not metabolize or excrete the drug normally.

In **drug idiosyncrasy,** the adverse reaction develops on the first use of the drug. It may be the same toxic reaction ordinarily expected at higher doses, or it may be an exaggeration of a common mild side effect, such as antihistaminic sedation, or it may be unique. Reactions due to genetically determined enzyme deficiencies are being identified in steadily increasing numbers. Hemolytic anemia, for example, develops in patients with G6PD deficiency during treatment with any of several drugs. Succinylcholine apnea and isoniazid (INH) peripheral neuropathy are other examples from the field of pharmacogenetics.

Most toxic and idiosyncratic reactions (e.g., hyperergic reactions from anesthetic agents) differ sufficiently from allergic reactions to cause no confusion. There are a few exceptions. Toxic or idiosyncratic reactions from drugs with a direct histamine-releasing action (e.g., morphine, codeine, pentamidine, polymyxin) may present as urticaria or even as anaphylactoid reactions. Hemolytic anemia may be allergic (e.g., penicillin, stibophen) or due to enzyme deficiency. Drug fever may be allergic or may be toxic (e.g., amphetamine, tranylcypromine) or even pharmacologic (e.g., etiocholanolone).

Hypersensitivity reactions have the following characteristics: (1) The reaction occurs only after the patient has been exposed to the drug (not necessarily for therapy) one or more times without incident. (2) Once hypersensitivity has developed, the reaction can be produced by doses which are far below therapeutic amounts, and usually below those levels which give idiosyncratic reactions. (3) The clinical features of drug hypersensitivity reactions are restricted in their manifestations. Skin rashes (particularly urticaria), serum sickness, unexpected fever, anaphylaxis, and eosinophilic pulmonary infiltrates appearing during drug therapy are almost always due to hypersensitivity; some cases of anemia, thrombocytopenia, or agranulocytosis may be. Rarely, vasculitis develops after repeated exposure to a drug (e.g., sulfonamides, iodides, penicillin), and nephropathy (e.g., penicillin) and liver damage (e.g., halothane) have been reported in circumstances consistent with development of specific hypersensitivity.

Mechanisms of Drug Hypersensitivity

Protein and large polypeptide drugs can stimulate specific antibody production by straightforward immunologic mechanisms. Perhaps the smallest molecule which is potentially antigenic is **glucagon**, with a mol wt of about 3500. Most drug molecules are much smaller than this. By themselves the drugs cannot act as antigens, but as **haptens** some can covalently bind to proteins, and the resulting conjugates will stimulate antibody production specific for each chemical. It is likely that most drug hypersensitivity requires the prior formation of hapten-protein conjugates. The drug, or one of its metabolites, must be chemically reactive with protein, and must form a stable covalent bond. The usual serum-protein binding common to many drugs is much weaker and is of insufficient strength for antigenicity.

The specific immunologic reaction has been determined only for benzylpenicillin. This does not bind firmly enough with tissue or serum proteins to form an antigenic complex, but its major degradation product, benzylpenicillenic acid, can combine with tissue proteins to form benzylpenicilloyl **(BPO)**, the **major antigenic determinant** of penicillin. Several **minor antigenic determinants** are formed in relatively small amounts, by mechanisms that are not as well defined. IgE antibodies to the BPO determinant cause the urticaria that follows penicillin administration, while IgE antibodies to minor determinants are responsible for the anaphylaxis. In addition, IgG antibodies have been demonstrated to the major but not to the minor determinants. It is felt that these act as "blocking antibodies" to BPO, modifying or even preventing a reaction to BPO, while the lack of blocking IgG antibodies to the *minor* determinants would seem to explain the ability of these determinants to induce anaphylaxis.

A BPO-polylysine conjugate (benzylpenicilloyl-polylysine), which lacks antigenicity, is commercially available for skin testing. Since the minor determinants are not available, penicillin G in dilutions of 1000 u./ml and 10,000 u./ml may be used. Skin testing is first performed by the scratch technic with the more dilute, then with the more concentrated, dilution. Negative scratch tests may be followed by intradermal testing. If skin tests are positive, the patient risks an anaphylactic reaction if treated with penicillin. Negative skin tests minimize but do not exclude the risk of a serious reaction. Moreover, skin tests with penicillin are themselves sensitizing—they stimulate IgE production—so that in most instances a patient should be tested to rule out penicillin allergy only immediately before essential penicillin therapy is begun. Since they detect only Type I (IgE-mediated) reactions, skin tests will not predict the occurrence of morbilliform eruptions or hemolytic anemia.

The semisynthetic penicillins (ampicillin, oxacillin, nafcillin) and the cephalosporins all cross-react with penicillin, so that penicillin-sensitive patients often (though not always) react to them as well.

Hematologic Type II drug reactions may develop by any of three mechanisms, examples of which are as follows: (1) In penicillin-induced anemia, the antibody reacts with the hapten which is firmly bound to the RBC membrane, producing agglutination and increased destruction of RBCs. (2) In stibophen- and quinidine-induced thrombocytopenia, the drug forms a soluble complex with its specific antibody. The complex then reacts with nearby platelets (the "innocent bystander" target cells) and activates complement, which alone remains on the platelet membrane and induces cell lysis. (3) In other hemolytic anemias, the drug (e.g., methyldopa) appears to alter the RBC surface chemically, thereby uncovering an antigen which induces and then reacts with an autoantibody, usually of Rh specificity.

Diagnosis

Toxic-idiosyncratic and anaphylactic reactions are sufficiently unique in kind or in time that the offending drug is usually easily identified. Serum-sickness–type reactions are most often due to the penicillins or cephalosporins, but occasionally sulfonamides, phenylbutazone, sulfonylureas, or thiazides are responsible. Photosensitization is characteristic of sulfonamides, thiazides, tetracyclines, and griseofulvin. All drugs except those deemed absolutely essential should be stopped. When drug fever is suspected, the most likely drug is stopped (e.g., penicillin, aminosalicylic acid, phenytoin [diphenylhydantoin], barbiturates, quinidine). Reduction in fever within 48 h implicates that drug.

Diagnosis can be confirmed by challenge; i.e., by readministering the drug; but reproducing most allergic reactions to confirm the relationship may be risky, and is seldom warranted.

Laboratory tests for specific drug hypersensitivity (e.g., histamine release, basophil or mast cell degranulation, lymphocyte transformation) are either unreliable or remain experimental. Tests for hematologic drug reactions are an exception (see Diagnostic Tests under TYPE II HYPERSENSITIVITY REACTIONS in §2, Ch. 4).

Skin tests for immediate-type (Type I) hypersensitivity help in diagnosis of reactions to serum, protein hormones, and penicillin, but for most drugs they are unreliable.

Treatment

It is usually necessary to stop treatment with the offending drug if the reaction appears to be allergic, in contrast to toxic and some idiosyncratic reactions, where the dose can often be reduced and still be effective without causing a reaction. Sometimes a drug which may be life-saving must be continued despite allergic manifestations. Treatment of bacterial endocarditis with penicillin, for example, may be continued despite the appearance of a morbilliform eruption, urticaria, or drug fever. Urticaria is treated in the usual manner, including corticosteroids if necessary.

Most reactions will clear within a few days after a drug is stopped. Treatment can usually be limited to symptom control. For example, drug fever or a nonpruritic skin rash usually requires no treatment. However, if a patient is acutely ill, with signs of multiple system involvement, or with exfoliative dermatitis, intensive corticosteroid treatment is required (e.g., prednisone 40 to 80 mg/day orally). More information on treatment of specific clinical reactions will be found in the pertinent chapters throughout THE MANUAL.

HORSE SERUM SENSITIVITY

Anaphylaxis and serum sickness were frequent medical problems when antiserums, usually obtained from horses, were used extensively for passive immunization. Serum reactions have become infrequent with current active-immunization programs, antibiotics, and human immune serums for tetanus and for several viral diseases. However, horse antiserum is still used in the management of diphtheria, gas gangrene, botulism, and venomous snake bites; and antilymphocyte serum from horses and other species is being used increasingly to suppress immune reactions to transplanted organs.

Before giving any animal serum or animal serum product, it is imperative to ascertain whether the patient has ever received serum before and whether he has a history of asthma, hay fever, urticaria, or other allergic symptoms. A positive history calls for additional caution in giving serum; allergy to the animal species involved calls for *extreme caution* or, better, alternative treatment.

Regardless of history, any person about to receive a foreign serum *must be tested first.* Some written instructions still call for an intracutaneous test using 0.1 ml of a 1:10 dilution, but this procedure is unsatisfactory and may be dangerous: it produces many false-positive reactions and is likely to produce a generalized reaction in an allergic patient. A patient who is not atopic and who has not received horse serum previously should first be given a scratch test with a 1:10 dilution; if this is negative, 0.02 ml of a 1:10 dilution is injected intracutaneously. A wheal more than 0.5 cm in diameter will develop within 15 min if the patient is sensitive. All patients who have received serum previously *(whether or not they reacted)* and those with a suspected allergic history should be tested with more dilute serum (1:100 to 1:10,000, depending on the sensitivity suspected).

If the skin test is positive and serum must be used, serial dilutions should be used for skin testing to determine that dilution to which the patient is skin-test-negative. Desensitization is then carried out using 0.1 ml of the first skin-test-negative dilution injected s.c. If no reaction occurs in 15 min, the dose is doubled every 15 min until a dose approximating 1 ml of undiluted serum is reached. This amount of undiluted serum is then injected IM and if no reaction occurs in 15 to 20 min, the full dose can then be given. A syringe of 1:1000 epinephrine should always be on hand during sensitivity testing to initiate prompt treatment should a reaction occur (see ANAPHYLAXIS, above). If a patient does react, it may still be possible to proceed cautiously by reducing the amount injected after pretreatment with antihistamines and corticosteroids, given as for acute urticaria, and then increasing at small intervals. The treatment dose of antiserum for sensitive patients should be *twice* the usual dose to allow for some inactivation by the patient's antibodies.

SERUM SICKNESS

An allergic reaction usually appearing 7 to 12 days after administration of a foreign serum or certain drugs, characterized by fever, arthralgias, skin rash, and lymphadenopathy.

Etiology

The most common cause of serum sickness is not serum, but penicillin and related drugs (see DRUG HYPERSENSITIVITY, above). Reactions from horse serum antitoxins occur in at least 5% of persons given the serum for the first time. The injected serum or drug is slowly excreted, so that it remains in the circulation long enough to stimulate the production of specific IgG antibodies which form soluble complexes with the antigen to cause a Type III reaction; IgE antibodies and consequently a Type I reaction are also produced. (See §2, Ch. 4 for a discussion of the immunologic mechanisms.) Both types of reaction probably contribute to symptoms.

Symptoms and Signs

Onset is usually several days after injection of the serum or drug but may be much sooner than the usual 7 days if the patient has been exposed previously **(accelerated serum sickness).** Urticaria is the usual skin manifestation. Less frequently, the rash may be multiform or morbilliform; rarely, it is scarlatiniform or purpuric. Most patients have polyarthritis or periarticular edema. Temporomandibular arthritis may be severe, and has been confused with tetanus. When fever occurs, it is mild and lasts for only 1 or 2 days. Adenopathy develops in the region draining the injection site and may become generalized. Splenomegaly is sometimes present. Myocarditis may develop, but is rare. Peripheral neuritis is the only complication which may cause irreversible injury. Surprisingly, glomerulonephritis, so prominent in experimental serum sickness in animals, is rarely a problem.

Diagnosis

A history of serum or drug administration, plus the characteristic symptoms and signs, usually makes the diagnosis obvious. A positive immediate (IgE-mediated) skin test confirms the diagnosis but is of little help in predicting the development of serum sickness since the patient need not be sensitive at the time of testing. Theoretically, a positive skin test should predict accelerated serum sickness but this has not been established.

Treatment

Since the disease is self-limited, treatment is usually restricted to relief of symptoms. Pruritus is treated with an antihistamine as for acute urticaria; and arthralgias with salicylates (aspirin 0.6 to 1.5 Gm orally q 4 h). If these are not adequate, prednisone 30 mg/day orally is almost always effective. The corticosteroid dose is gradually reduced to zero after symptoms have been relieved. Early, intensive corticosteroid treatment is necessary if the rare complications of peripheral neuritis or myocarditis develop. Large doses of cyproheptadine (0.7 mg/kg/day) or hydroxyzine (5 mg/kg/day) given concomitantly with the serum have been effective in reducing symptoms, but this therapy is still experimental.

AUTOIMMUNE DISORDERS

Disorders in which the immune system produces autoantibodies to an endogenous antigen, with consequent injury to tissues.

Considered here are the pathogenetic immunologic mechanisms underlying autoimmune diseases. The specific disorders and their clinical aspects may be found elsewhere in The Manual.

Development of the Autoimmune Response

Although precise details of the autoimmune response are incompletely understood, there is no need to postulate a special mechanism by which organisms recognize their own antigens as "self" and thereby do not respond to them immunologically. The outcome of antigenic stimulation, whether antibody formation or activated T cells or tolerance, seems to depend on the same factors with autoantigen as with exogenous antigen.

Four possible mechanisms for developing an immune response to autoantigens are recognized:

1. Hidden or sequestered antigens (e.g., intracellular substances) may not be recognized as "self;" if released into the circulation they may induce an immune response. This occurs in sympathetic ophthalmia with the traumatic release of an antigen normally sequestered within the eye. Autoantibody alone may not produce disease because it cannot combine with the sequestered antigen. For example, antibody to sperm and heart muscle antigens are blocked by the basement membrane of the seminiferous tubules and myocardial cell membrane, respectively. Immunologically active T cells, however, may not have such restrictions and would be more effective in producing injury.

2. The "self" antigens may become immunogenic because of chemical, physical, or biologic alteration. Certain chemicals couple with body proteins and render them immunogenic, as seen in contact dermatitis. Photosensitivity exemplifies physically induced autoallergy: ultraviolet light alters skin protein, to which the patient becomes allergic. Biologically altered antigens are seen in New Zealand mice which develop autoallergic disease resembling SLE when persistently infected with an RNA virus known to combine with host tissues, altering them sufficiently to induce antibody.

3. Foreign antigen may induce an immune response that cross-reacts with normal "self"-antigen. Examples are the cross-reaction that occurs between streptococcal M protein and human heart muscle or the encephalitis that can follow rabies vaccination in which an autoimmune cross-reaction probably is initiated by animal brain tissue in the vaccine.

4. Autoantibody production may be a result of mutational change in immunocompetent cells. This may explain the monoclonal autoantibodies seen occasionally in patients with lymphoma.

The role of other complex mechanisms demonstrable experimentally still needs clarification. For example, adjuvants such as alum or bacterial endotoxin, while not antigenic themselves, enhance the antigenicity of other substances. Freund's adjuvant, an emulsion of antigen in mineral oil with heat-killed mycobacteria, is usually required in order to produce autoimmunity in experimental animals.

Genetic factors play a role in autoimmune disorders. Relatives of patients with autoimmune disorders often show a high incidence of the same type of autoantibodies, and the incidence of autoimmune disease is higher in identical than in fraternal twins. Women are more often affected than men are. The genetic contribution appears to be one of predisposition. In a predisposed population a number of environmental factors could provoke disease; in SLE, for example, these might be latent virus infection, drugs, or tissue injury such as occurs with ultraviolet light exposure. This situation would be analogous to the development of hemolytic anemia as a consequence of environmental factors in persons with G6PD deficiency, a predisposing genetically determined biochemical abnormality.

Pathogenetic Mechanisms

The pathogenetic mechanisms of autoimmune reactions are, in many cases, better understood than the way in which autoimmune antibodies develop. In some autoimmune hemolytic anemias, the RBCs become coated with Type II autoantibody; the complement system responds to these antibody-coated cells just as it does to similarly coated foreign particles, and the interaction of complement with the antibody complexed to the cell surface antigen leads to RBC phagocytosis or cytolysis.

The glomerulonephritis that follows "nephritogenic" β-hemolytic streptococcal infections may be the result of autoantibodies (cross-reacting with streptococcal antigens) formed against soluble components from the kidney, causing complement-activating antigen-antibody (IgG) complexes which aggregate in the glomeruli. The same kind of Type III autoimmune hypersensitivity reaction occurs in patients with SLE, who form complexes of DNA and other nuclear antigens with autoantibody and complement which are deposited in the glomeruli in similar fashion.

A variety of autoantibodies are produced in SLE and other systemic (as opposed to organ-specific) autoimmune diseases. Antibodies to formed elements in the blood account for hemolytic anemia, and probably leukopenia and thrombocytopenia; antibodies to nuclear material result in the Type III deposition of antigen-antibody complexes, not only in glomeruli, but also in vascular tissues and synovial linings of joints. A similar synovial deposition of aggregated IgG-RF-complement complexes occurs in rheumatoid arthritis. Rheumatoid factor (RF) is usually an IgM globulin (occasionally IgG) with specificity for a receptor on the constant region of the heavy chain of autologous IgG. Although the deposition occurs chiefly within the joints, the IgG-RF-complement aggregates can also be found within neutrophils, where they cause the release of lysosomal enzymes that contribute to the inflammatory joint reaction. Plasma cells are also present in large numbers within the joint, synthesizing IgG at a rapid rate. Although the antigen inducing the IgG synthesis is unknown, it is presumed also to be intrasynovial, perhaps a normal joint constituent or a microorganism. In SLE the low serum complement level reflects the widespread immunologic reactions taking place; in rheumatoid arthritis, by contrast, serum complement is normal, but intrasynovial complement levels are low.

In pernicious anemia, autoantibodies capable of neutralizing intrinsic factor can be found in the gastrointestinal lumen. Autoantibodies against the microsomal fraction of gastric mucosal cells are even more common. It is postulated that a cell-mediated autoimmune attack against the parietal cells results in the atrophic gastritis which, in turn, reduces the production of intrinsic factor but still allows absorption of sufficient vitamin B_{12} to prevent the megaloblastic anemia. If autoantibodies to intrinsic factor should also develop in the gastrointestinal lumen, however, B_{12} absorption will cease and pernicious anemia will develop.

Hashimoto's thyroiditis is associated with autoantibodies to thyroglobulin, the microsomes of thyroid epithelial cells, a thyroid cell-surface antigen, and a second colloid antigen. Tissue injury and eventual myxedema may be mediated both by the cytotoxicity of the microsomal antibody and by the activity of specifically committed T cells.

An unusual situation obtains in some cases of thyrotoxicosis (Graves' disease), since here an IgG autoantibody to a purported cell surface antigen stimulates rather than destroys cells. The antibody, long-acting thyroid stimulator (LATS), may induce such an effect by binding to the same thyroid cell receptors that TSH normally binds to, thereby having the same effect on thyroid cell function that TSH normally has.

---

6. TRANSPLANTATION

The transfer of living tissues or cells from one individual to another, with the objective of maintaining the functional integrity of the transplanted tissue in the recipient.

GENERAL CONSIDERATIONS

The clinical use of transplantation as a remedy for disease is still limited for most organ systems despite surgical technics that make transplantation of almost any tissue feasible. The greatest obstacle is the **rejection reaction** which generally destroys the tissue shortly after transplantation (except in special circumstances, such as corneal grafts or transplants between identical twins). Nevertheless, with new understanding of the mechanisms of immunologically mediated tissue destruction and use of improved methods of preventing rejection, organ transplantation has saved many patients with otherwise fatal disease. In fact, kidney transplantation is preferred for most patients with terminal renal failure.

Transplants are categorized by the genetic relationship between donor and recipient and by the site of transplantation. An **autograft** is a transfer of tissue from one location to another in the same individual (e.g., bone grafting for fracture stabilization). **Isografts** are grafts between identical twins. An **allograft (homograft)** is a transplant between members of the same species, and a **xenograft (heterograft)** is one between members of different species. A tissue or organ graft is **orthotopic** if it is transferred to an anatomically normal recipient site—as in a heart transplant. If the transplant is to an anatomically abnormal site, it is **heterotopic**—as in the transplantation of a kidney into the iliac fossa of the recipient

IMMUNOBIOLOGIC PRINCIPLES

Allografts or xenografts may be rejected through either a cell-mediated or a humoral immune reaction of the recipient against antigenic components that are present on the donor's cell membranes. These **transplantation, or histocompatibility, antigens** are found on all nucleated cells of the body. The strongest antigens are governed by a complex of genetic loci termed **HLA** (see below); together with the major blood group (ABO) antigens, they are the chief transplantation antigens in man, although others may eventually be detectable. Because transplantation antigens can be identified by their effects in vitro, tissue typing (described below) is possible.

The role of humoral antibody in graft rejection is obvious when the recipient has been presensitized (by pregnancy, blood transfusion, or previous transplantation) to HLA antigens present in the graft. Transplantation in these circumstances almost invariably leads to **hyperacute rejection,** causing destruction of the graft within hours or even minutes after revascularization. This **antibody-mediated rejection reaction** is characterized by small vessel thrombosis and graft infarction and cannot be reversed by any known immunosuppressive technics. A similar result usually occurs if a graft is transplanted in defiance of the blood group barriers normally observed in blood transfusions. Therefore pre-transplant evaluation must include verifying the ABO compatibility between donor and recipient and a negative cross-match for tissue antibodies (lack of reactivity between donor leukocytes and recipient serum in vitro), as well as tissue typing for HLA compatibility. The role of humoral antibody in more delayed graft destruction is probably also important but is still unclear.

Acute **lymphocyte-mediated immune reaction** against transplantation antigens (the usual **host-vs.-graft reaction**) is the principal mechanism of rejection. A delayed hypersensitivity response similar to the tuberculin reaction, it causes graft destruction days to months after transplantation and is characterized histologically by a mononuclear cellular infiltration of the allograft with varying degrees of hemorrhage and edema. Usually vascular integrity is maintained, in contrast to antibody-mediated rejection, and thus cell-mediated rejection may be reversed in many cases by intensifying immunosuppressive therapy. After successful reversal of an acute lymphocyte-mediated rejection episode, histologic examination shows that severely damaged elements of the graft have healed by fibrosis, and the remainder of the graft appears to be normal.

Occasionally **late graft deterioration** occurs in immunosuppressed patients. This chronic type of rejection is often insidious but relentless in progression despite increased immunosuppressive measures. The pathologic picture differs from that of acute rejection. The vascular endothelium is primarily involved, with extensive proliferation that gradually occludes the vessel lumen, resulting in ischemia and fibrosis of the graft.

THE HLA SYSTEM

A group of tissue antigens governed by a chromosomal region bearing a number of genetic loci, each with multiple alleles, that have relevance to transplantation rejection reactions and other immune phenomena.

It has been established that a group of genetically linked antigens are the major cause of most graft rejection episodes in organ transplantation. In recent years, there has also been a growing awareness of the statistical association of certain of these antigens with a variety of diseases. Although some of these disorders may have immunologic features, the pathogenetic meaning of such associations is unknown.

The antigens (see TABLE 2-6), termed **HLA** (for human leukocyte group **A**), are controlled by a complex of genes at several closely linked loci located on the 6th chromosome. Four genetic loci (designated Locus A, B, C, and D) for these genes have been identified to date. The genes are allelic—that is, a number of different forms of each gene are found in the population. To date, 19 alleles have been identified for Locus A, 20 for Locus B, 5 for Locus C, and 6 for Locus D. By mendelian laws, each person has 2 alleles from each locus (or, of course, a pair of identical alleles).

Because the alleles were numbered before their loci were identified, those on Loci A and B are not numbered consecutively. Those alleles which are still provisional are designated with a "w." The difficulties encountered in identifying and sorting out this complex allelic system led to much confusion in original nomenclature. This problem has been resolved by a simple revised designation for the HLA system, which is listed in TABLE 2-6 together with the most common previous designations.

The antigens associated with Loci A, B, and C are identified serologically, and are therefore often referred to as **SD** (**s**erologically **d**etermined) antigens. The antigens governed by Locus D are best identified by a mixed lymphocyte culture reaction, and are often termed **MLR** or **LD** (lymphocyte **d**etermined); these antigens show significant functional differences from the A-, B-, and C-locus antigens, and are probably different structurally.

While any of the HLA antigens may participate in transplantation reactions, there has been a suggestion, as yet incompletely confirmed, that those located on Locus D are of special importance. The antigens having a statistical association with various presumably autoimmune disorders and with lymphoid-cell neoplasms are primarily B- and D-locus antigens. Evidence is now accumulating to suggest that other immunologic disorders, such as atopic allergy, are also associated with a particular HLA genotype. In addition, complement components C2, C4, C8, and properdin Factor B have been found to be governed by genes closely linked to the D locus.

Statistical associations between the following **disorders and HLA antigens** are considered to be established: B27 and ankylosing spondylitis, Reiter's syndrome, and psoriatic spondylitis; B13 and Bw17 with psoriasis. Probable associations include A2 with chronic glomerulonephritis; and B5, Bw35, Bw15, and B18 with Hodgkin's disease. A possible association with B27 has also been reported in enteropathic spondylitis, *Yersinia* arthritis, juvenile rheumatoid arthritis, anterior uveitis, and asthma (which also was associated with A1). A great many other associations have been reported, some of them negative. For example, persons with Hodgkin's disease or malignant lymphomas were reported to have a decreased incidence of A11; those with psoriasis, a decreased incidence of B12; and those with rheumatic fever, a decreased incidence of A3. However, because of the difficulties of testing for individual HLA antigens, the reliability of such associations, both negative and positive, depends on accumulating more data.

TISSUE TYPING

Prior to transplantation, histocompatibility (or tissue) typing of peripheral blood or lymph node lymphocytes is usually performed. The problem is to identify the HLA antigens serologically and, by appropriate donor selection, to minimize the antigenic differences between donor and recipient.

A good primary source for HLA tissue-typing antibodies is the serum of multiparous women, who have formed antibodies to fetal transplantation antigens that were inherited from the father but are absent on the mother's cells. Another

TABLE 2-6. HISTOCOMPATIBILITY ANTIGENS: NOMENCLATURE*

New Designation	Previous Designation	New Designation	Previous Designation
Locus A	First, LA locus	**Locus C**	Third, AJ locus
HLA-A1	HL-A1	HLA-Cw1	T1
HLA-A2	HL-A2	HLA-Cw2	T2
HLA-A3	HL-A3	HLA-Cw3	T3
HLA-A9	HL-A9	HLA-Cw4	T4
HLA-A10	HL-A10	HLA-Cw5	T5
HLA-A11	HL-A11		
HLA-A28	W28		
HLA-A29	W29		
HLA-Aw23	W23	**Locus D**	LD, MLC-1, MLR-S
HLA-Aw24	W24	HLA-Dw1	LD 101, LD-W5a
HLA-Aw25	W25	HLA-Dw2	LD 102, LD-7a
HLA-Aw26	W26	HLA-Dw3	LD 103, LD-8a & b
HLA-Aw30	W30	HLA-Dw4	LD 104
HLA-Aw31	W31	HLA-Dw5	LD 105
HLA-Aw32	W32	HLA-Dw6	LD 106
HLA-Aw33	W19.6,Fe55		
HLA-Aw34	Malay 2		
HLA-Aw36	Mo		
HLA-Aw43	Bk		

New Designation	Previous Designation
Locus B	Second locus, "four" series
HLA-B5	HL-A5, 4c
HLA-B7	HL-A7
HLA-B8	HL-A8
HLA-B12	HL-A12
HLA-B13	HL-A13
HLA-B14	W14
HLA-B18	W18
HLA-B27	W27
HLA-Bw15	W15
HLA-Bw16	W16
HLA-Bw17	W17
HLA-Bw21	W21
HLA-Bw22	W22
HLA-Bw35	W5
HLA-Bw37	TY
HLA-Bw38	W16.1
HLA-Bw39	W16.2
HLA-Bw40	W10
HLA-Bw41	Sabell
HLA-Bw42	MWA

* New nomenclature for factors of the HLA system was adopted in 1975 by the WHO–International Union of Immunologic Societies Committee on Leukocyte Nomenclature. The entire complex of loci is now called "HLA." Genetic loci belonging to the system are designated by one or more letters following HLA. Individual alleles of each locus, and the corresponding specificities, are designated by numbers following the locus symbols. Provisionally identified specificities continue to carry the letter "w" (for "Workshop"), now inserted between the locus letter and the allele and specificity number.

source is serum from patients who have previously rejected an allograft. In each case, the antiserums are multispecific; i.e., they contain antibodies against many or all of the transplantation antigens that were present in the fetus or allograft but absent in the mother or graft recipient. As a result, tissue typing requires large test-cell panels in which the antiserums can be grouped to represent a specific antigen identified in common by each group. Newer technics for isolating single transplantation antigens from cell membranes have been developed, and monospecific antiserums have been produced by immunization of volunteer donors and suitable serum absorption reactions to remove unwanted antibodies. The use of histocompatibility typing has significantly improved functional survival of transplants between related individuals, but because the complex histocompatibility differences in an outbred population introduce many more variables, this technic has only slightly improved the results of transplants between unrelated individuals.

IMMUNOSUPPRESSION

Immunosuppressive agents are used to control the rejection reaction caused by antigenic differences that remain after tissue typing and donor-recipient matching. Since these drugs suppress *all* immunologic reactions and also the metabolism of rapidly dividing cells, overwhelming infection is the leading cause of death in transplant recipients. Nevertheless, carefully selected and administered immunosuppressive treatment has been primarily responsible for the present success of clinical transplantation.

Except after isografts, immunosuppressive therapy can rarely be stopped completely after transplantation. However, intensive immunosuppression is usually required only during the first few weeks after transplantation or during rejection crises. Subsequently, the graft often seems to become accommodated and can be maintained with relatively small doses of immunosuppressives and fewer adverse effects.

The antimetabolite **azathioprine** is one of the most important immunosuppressive drugs. It is given orally or IV, usually beginning at the time of transplantation; doses of 1.5 to 3 mg/kg are usually tolerated indefinitely by the transplant recipient. Its primary toxic effects are bone marrow depression and hepatitis (although here a reactivation of viral hepatitis may be the underlying factor).

Cyclophosphamide has been substituted in patients who do not tolerate azathioprine; equivalent doses are apparently equal in immunosuppressive activity. This alkylating agent is also used as one of the primary immunosuppressive drugs in bone marrow transplantation, but much larger doses are required (see below) and severe toxicity (hemorrhagic cystitis, alopecia, and infertility) is not unusual.

Prednisone or **methylprednisolone** is usually given in high doses (2 to 30 mg/kg) at the time of transplantation and then reduced gradually to a maintenance dose of 10 to 20 mg/day given indefinitely. Should allograft rejection occur, the dose is sharply increased again, risking serious side effects (see in §22, Ch. 15), especially an increased susceptibility to a variety of infections.

Because prednisone causes persistent adrenal suppression, supplemental corticosteroids are needed during periods of increased stress such as major trauma or surgery—for example, hydrocortisone sodium succinate 300 mg IV on the day of surgery, 200 mg on the first postoperative day, and 100 mg on the second postoperative day, after which the previous prednisone doses are resumed. Corticosteroid therapy need not be increased for a minor stress such as a viral URI.

Irradiation, one of the first immunosuppressive treatments, is now of limited clinical use in transplantation. The graft and local recipient tissues are sometimes irradiated, either as an adjunctive prophylactic immunosuppressive measure or during treatment for established rejection. The total dose is usually 400 to 600 rads, which is below the threshold that might cause serious radiation injury of the graft itself. Extracorporeal irradiation of the recipient's blood or lymph as it traverses a surgically created fistula has been successful but is too cumbersome for use on a large clinical scale. In the treatment of refractory leukemia, whole-body irradiation in 1000-rad doses has been used in combination with chemotherapy, which is sufficient to destroy the host's immunologic capability (and residual leukemic cells as well). The irradiation is followed by a bone-marrow allograft.

Attempts have been made to specifically suppress *cellular* immunity with equine or rabbit antiserum against human lymphocytes or thymus cells. This method leaves the recipient's *humoral* immunologic response intact, preserving his defenses against many bacterial infections. **Antilymphocyte serum (ALS)** or its **globulin fraction (ALG)** may be useful adjuncts, allowing other immunosuppressive measures to be used in lower, less toxic, doses. However, preparations and regimens for their use have not been standardized, and thus the clinical role of ALS and ALG is still investigational. Possible adverse reactions to these heterologous serums include anaphylactic reactions, serum sickness, or antigen-antibody-induced glomerulonephritis, but using highly purified serum fractions and giving them IV as well as combining them with other immunosupressive agents seems to reduce the incidence of these reactions.

KIDNEY TRANSPLANTATION

Since long-term success can be expected in over two thirds of renal allografts, all patients with terminal renal failure should be considered for transplantation except those who are extremely old or are suffering from a malignancy or other life-threatening condition. Pretransplant preparation includes hemodialysis to ensure a relatively normal metabolic state, and provision of a functional, infection-free lower urinary tract, by surgery if needed. Bladder reconstruction, nephrectomy of infected kidneys, or construction of an ileal conduit for draining the allograft may be required. Prolonged hemodialysis is avoided in pretransplant patients if possible, since the repeated transfusions that are often required may sensitize the patient to transplantation antigens.

Donor Selection

Kidney allografts may be obtained from living relatives or cadaver donors. Donors with malignant disease, except possibly neoplasms originating in the CNS, are excluded. Living donors are also carefully evaluated for emotional stability, normal bilateral renal function, freedom from other systemic disease, and histocompatibility. HLA antigens, because of their mode of inheritance, are identical in 25% of siblings. Transplantation between HLA-compatible siblings is successful in over 90% of cases and less immunosuppression may be needed. Transplants from other siblings and from parents tend to be less successful, depending upon the degree of histoincompatibility between donor and recipient.

A living donor gives up reserve renal capacity, may have complex psychologic conflicts, and faces some morbidity in the nephrectomy. Today more than half of kidney transplants are from cadavers, in many instances from previously healthy subjects who have sustained fatal brain damage but maintain stable cardiovascular and renal function. (The concept of brain death is gaining widespread acceptance, and the Uniform Anatomical Gift Act of 1973 allows adults to assign their organs for later use as transplants under such circumstances.) After determination of brain death or after circulatory arrest, the kidneys are removed as quickly as possible and cooled by perfusion with a heparinized electrolyte solution. With this technic, a kidney can be kept viable for 6 to 8 h before transplantation. If necessary, kidneys can be preserved for up to 48 h by means of continuous perfusion with an oxygenated plasma-based perfusate.

Transplant Procedure and Immunosuppression

The transplanted kidney is usually placed retroperitoneally in the iliac fossa. Vascular anastomoses are performed to the iliac vessels, and ureteral continuity is established. Although prophylactic immunosuppressive therapy is begun just before or at the time of transplantation, most recipients undergo one or more acute rejection episodes in the early post-transplant period. Rejection is suggested by deterioration of renal function, hypertension, weight gain, tenderness and swelling of the graft, fever, and appearance of protein, lymphocytes, and renal tubular cells in the urine sediment. Rejection may be reversed if immunosuppressive therapy is intensified, or it may progress until the transplant is no longer functioning. If the rejection cannot be easily reversed, immunosuppression is stopped, the patient is supported on hemodialysis, and the graft is removed.

Most rejection episodes and other complications occur within 3 to 4 mo after transplantation. After that time most patients return to more normal health and activity, but immunosuppressive medication (usually azathioprine and prednisone) must be maintained and infections must be avoided. Immunosuppression is not interrupted unless toxicity or severe infection occurs, since even brief cessation may precipitate rejection.

Late Complications

Some patients suffer chronic graft rejection with progressive hypertension and gradual deterioration of renal function which is difficult to reverse and may necessitate nephrectomy and retransplantation. Other possible late complications include azathioprine toxicity, increasing side effects of prednisone administration, recurrent glomerulonephritis, chronic infections, and the sudden development of pneumonia, septicemia, or other infections.

BONE MARROW TRANSPLANTATION

The primary indications for bone marrow transplantation have been restoration of immunologic competence in patients with congenital immunodeficiency syndromes and reestablishment of functional marrow in aplastic anemia. It is now also being used to replace neoplastic marrow in leukemia.

Although the procedure involves simple aspiration of marrow from the donor and its IV infusion into the recipient, several factors contribute to its complexity. First, prospective bone marrow recipients are usually more susceptible to infection and hemorrhage than are other immunosuppressed patients. Second, since immunologically competent cells are being transferred to an immunosuppressed patient, these cells may attack the cells of the host to cause a **graft-vs.-host (GVH) reaction.** The resulting syndrome of fever, exfoliative dermatitis, hepatitis, diarrhea, and weight loss has been responsible for many deaths after marrow transplants, thus limiting possible donors almost exclusively to HLA-identical siblings of the recipients.

For pretransplant immunosuppression, high doses of cyclophosphamide (30 to 50 mg/kg) are given daily for several days, or large doses of ALG are given for 7 to 10 days, or total-body irradiation may be used. Methotrexate is administered weekly for the first 4 mo after the transplantation to prevent a GVH reaction. An established GVH reaction has sometimes been successfully reversed by giving ALG.

The major causes of failure of marrow transplantation are failure of engraftment, with continuing aplasia, immunoincompetence, and sepsis; GVH reaction;

or recurrence of leukemia. With long-term success of the graft (> 5 yr) a stable population of host and donor marrow cells existing compatibly (**chimerism**) develops. It is often possible to stop the immunosuppressive therapy after several months of stable chimerism without resultant graft rejection or recurrent GVH reaction. Thus, many long-term survivors are on no therapy, in contrast to patients with long-surviving allografts of other tissues.

SKIN TRANSPLANTATION

Skin allografts are of great value in patients with extensive burns or other massive skin loss. Covering the denuded area reduces fluid and protein losses and discourages invasive infection. By alternating strips of autografts and allografts the entire denuded area can be covered in a patient with insufficient donor sites to permit the use of autografts alone. The allografts are rejected, but these secondarily denuded areas can then be re-covered with autografts, taken from healed original donor sites. Allografts have also been used as dressings for infected burns or wounds; the wounds rapidly become sterile and develop well-vascularized granulations on which autografts will take readily.

Recently, patients (especially children) with extensive (usually lethal) burns have been treated early with immunosuppression, followed by excision of the burns and wound closure with allografts. The allografts can be maintained for several months with immunosuppression, usually with ALG. During this time, the patient's own skin is repeatedly harvested and used to replace the allografts. Once the burns are completely autografted, immunosuppression is stopped. The risk of fatal infections in these immunosuppressed patients is acceptable since patients with burns covering as much as 85% of their body surface have been saved.

TRANSPLANTATION OF OTHER ORGANS

Thymus implants have proved to be of definite benefit in restoring immunologic responsiveness to children with thymic aplasia and consequent lack of normal development of the lymphoid system.

Transplantation of liver, heart, lung, and endocrine organs is still experimental, but some recipients have survived several years with allografts. Because only cadaver donors can be used and because no artificial organs are available to sustain terminal patients awaiting transplantation, the logistic problems are more formidable than with kidney transplantation.

The technical feasibility of **liver transplantation,** using an accessory heterotopic organ or an orthotopic replacement, has been demonstrated. Heterotopic transplantation is less traumatic, but auxiliary livers tend to atrophy if excluded from the portal circulation and have not had significant clinical success. The occurrence of large septic infarcts of the allograft, possibly due to an immunologic reaction, is another major problem. ALG and prednisone are usually given for immunosuppression since large doses of azathioprine are not well tolerated in liver transplantation patients.

Cardiac transplantation has become progressively restricted to a few centers because of the massive clinical and laboratory effort involved. Most recipients have had severe coronary disease with advanced secondary changes due to congestive failure. Immunosuppressive regimens used are similar to those for kidney transplantation. Rejection is diagnosed by ECG changes, serum enzyme elevations, and transvenous cardiac biopsies. Because no artificial organ is available to sustain them during periods of depressed cardiac function, recipients often die during severe rejection. Since some recipients have survived in good condition for as long as 5 yr, considerable interest is maintained in the potential of this technic.

Lungs are particularly difficult to transplant, primarily because infection has a devastating effect in a transplanted organ that is continually exposed to nonsterile ambient air and depends on the cough mechanism, which is disrupted by transplantation. In addition, doubts concerning the functional capacity of a lung immediately after transplantation have discouraged widespread attempts at lung transplantation.

Endocrine transplants have limited clinical application since satisfactory exogenous replacement therapy is available for most deficiencies. Pancreatic transplants have been performed in severe juvenile diabetes mellitus, but with only short-term success.

---

7.   TUMOR IMMUNOLOGY

Evidence for the occurrence of immune responses to a variety of human tumors is increasing. Tumor-specific (or tumor-associated) transplantation antigens have been demonstrated in most experimental animal tumors and in several human neoplasms. It seems likely that the presence of these surface markers on neoplastic cells would allow their recognition by immunocompetent host cells as well as their reaction with antibodies directed against immunogenic surface configurations. The significance of such recognitions and reactions in the pathogenesis and control of tumors is currently the object of intensive laboratory and clinical investigations.

Spontaneous regressions of human neoplasms have encouraged interest in the possibility of immunologic therapy for neoplastic diseases. Present immunotherapy in human neoplasia is based on recent advances in knowledge of humoral and cellular immunity, immunosuppression, human transplantation antigens, and immunologic tolerance (a state in which a substance normally capable of inducing an immune response fails to do so).

TUMOR-SPECIFIC TRANSPLANTATION ANTIGENS (TSTA)

Most induced or transplanted experimental animal tumors have been shown to immunize syngeneic recipients against subsequent challenge with the same tumor but not against transplantation of normal tissues or other tumors. Such findings indicate the presence of antigens which are associated with the tumor cells but are not apparent on normal cells. These antigens are known as **tumor-specific** or **tumor-associated transplantation antigens (TSTA).** (The term "tumor-associated" may be more accurate, since such markers may be normally inapparent cell components which become manifest during the neoplastic process, as explained below.)

The findings are particularly well demonstrated by chemical-carcinogen–induced tumors, which tend to have individual antigenic specificity that varies from tumor to tumor, even with tumors induced by the same carcinogen; and by virus-induced tumors, which tend to show cross-reactivity between tumors induced by a given virus.

Suggested **mechanisms for the origin of such antigens** include: (1) new genetic information introduced by a virus; (2) alteration of genetic function by carcinogens, possibly through derepression, by which genetic material that is normally inactive, except perhaps during embryonic development, is activated and becomes expressed in the cell phenotype; (3) uncovering of antigens that are normally "buried" in the cell membrane, through the inability of neoplastic cells to synthesize membrane constituents such as sialic acid; (4) release of antigens that are normally sequestered in the cell or its organelles, through the death of neoplastic cells.

Numerous **technics to demonstrate TSTA** in animal tumors have been used. These include standard tissue transplantation methods, immunofluorescence, cytotoxicity tests using dye uptake or radioisotope release, prevention of tumor growth in vitro or in vivo by exposing the tumor to lymphoid cells or serum from immunized donors, delayed hypersensitivity skin tests, and lymphocyte transformation in vitro.

Evidence for TSTA in human neoplasms has been demonstrated with several neoplasms, including Burkitt's lymphoma, neuroblastoma, malignant melanoma, osteosarcoma, and some gastrointestinal carcinomas. Choriocarcinomas in women possess paternally derived histocompatibility antigens which may serve as "tumor-specific" antigens in eliciting an immune response. The complete cure of choriocarcinomas by chemotherapy may be attributable, at least in part, to such an immune response.

HOST RESPONSES TO TUMORS

CELLULAR IMMUNITY

The importance of lymphoid cells in tumor immunity has been repeatedly demonstrated in experimental animal tumor systems. In humans, the growth of tumor nodules has been inhibited in vivo by mixing suspensions of a patient's lymphocytes and tumor cells, suggesting a cell-mediated reaction to the tumor. In vitro studies have demonstrated that lymphoid cells from patients with certain neoplasms show cytotoxicity against corresponding human tumor cells in culture. This has been found with neuroblastoma, malignant melanoma, sarcomas, and carcinomas of the colon, breast, cervix, endometrium, ovary, testis, nasopharynx, and kidney. Similar antitumor cytolytic properties have been demonstrated with lymphocytes from members of the families of neuroblastoma and osteosarcoma patients, suggesting common exposure to a suspected environmental agent.

HUMORAL IMMUNITY

Humoral antibodies that react with tumor cells in vitro are produced in response to a variety of animal tumors induced by chemical carcinogens or viruses. However, antibody-mediated protection against tumor growth in vivo has only been demonstrable in certain animal leukemias and lymphomas. By contrast, lymphoid-cell-mediated protection in vivo occurs in a broad variety of animal tumor systems.

Anti-tumor antibodies may include the following types. (1) **Cytotoxic antibodies:** These are generally complement-fixing antibodies directed against surface antigens of relatively high density. In general, IgM antibodies are more cytotoxic in transplantation systems than are IgG antibodies. (2) **Enhancing** or **blocking antibodies:** Generally IgG antibodies, possibly complexed with soluble antigen, these *favor* the growth of a tumor rather than inhibit it. The mechanism for such immunologic enhancement is not understood but may involve (a) binding with TSTA and blocking their immunogenicity (afferent enhancement); (b) reacting with and inhibiting immunologically competent cells (central enhancement); (c) coating of tumor cells and thus preventing their interaction with lymphoid cells (efferent enhancement). The enhancement of human tumors seems likely since blocking antibodies have been demonstrated in vitro. (3) **Unblocking factors:** These factors are not yet characterized completely but may be antibodies. They decrease the blocking activity of enhancing antibodies or antigen-antibody complexes. They have been detected in the serum of patients following surgical removal of all clinically apparent tumor tissue. (4) **"Arming" factors:** Possibly antibodies or antibody-antigen complexes, these have been found in serum from tumor-bearing animals. They can confer specific "synergistic cytotoxicity" on lymph node cells from nonsensitized donor animals. (5) **Cytophilic antibodies:** The role of these antibodies in tumor immunology has not been established, but they are thought to react with macrophages, conferring on them the ability to bind to surface antigens of other cells. The exact relationship of cytotoxic, blocking, unblocking, and arming factors is not yet clear; i.e., whether or not the presumed antibodies involved are distinct from each other is not known.

Humoral antibodies directed against *human* tumor cells or tumor cell constituents have been demonstrated in vitro in the serum of patients with Burkitt's lymphoma, malignant melanoma, osteosarcoma, neuroblastoma, and digestive system carcinomas. Antibodies to melanoma cells and to carcinoembryonic antigen (see below) are usually found in patients *without* disseminated disease. Why this is so is still unknown. It may be that a failure to produce such antibodies permits metastasis; or perhaps antibodies are formed but are promptly absorbed by the large tumor mass.

Increasing interest is being directed toward "anti-antibodies" in human malignancy. Antibodies have been demonstrated in melanoma patients which appear to interact with the $F(ab')_2$ fragment of anti-melanoma cytoplasm IgG antibodies. This complicated and possibly delicate balance between potentially beneficial and potentially detrimental immune responses requires clarification to assist in planning immunotherapeutic maneuvers.

ALTERATIONS OF HOST IMMUNE REACTIVITY

Tumors that possess TSTA are able to grow in vivo, which suggests a deficient host response to the TSTA. Possible mechanisms include the following: (1) Specific immunologic tolerance to TSTA (e.g., because of prenatal exposure to the antigen, possibly viral in origin). (2) Suppression of the immune response by chemical or viral carcinogens. (3) Suppression of the immune response by treatment, especially cytotoxic chemotherapy and radiation therapy. The occurrence of more than 100 times the expected incidence of tumors in patients undergoing immunosuppressive therapy for renal transplantation suggests an impairment of postulated "immune-surveillance" mechanisms, which are theorized to inhibit growth of newly transformed neoplastic cells, or an impairment of immunity to oncogenic viruses, among possible explanations. Also, tumors have been inadvertently transplanted to immunosuppressed human kidney recipients, and these may regress when immunosuppression is discontinued. (4) Suppression of the immune response by the tumor itself. Deficient cellular immunity can be associated with recurrence and dissemination of tumors. This has been repeatedly demonstrated with a variety of human tumors, most dramatically in Hodgkin's disease, which appears to involve a variable defect in T cell function. However, whether this association precedes and contributes to the dissemination or results from it is not established. Deficient humoral immunity occurs in association with neoplasms involving abnormal B cell derivatives, such as multiple myeloma and chronic lymphocytic leukemia. Some apparent humoral "deficiencies" may be the result of anti-tumor antibody removal by "anti-antibodies" as noted above.

NONIMMUNE HOST RESPONSES

Certain host responses are not considered "immune" in the classic sense, although they involve potentially immunocompetent cells. A variety of animal tumors will grow in syngeneic hosts but are inhibited when transplanted to nonimmunized F_1 hybrids **(allogeneic inhibition)**. This has raised the speculation that interactions of lymphoid cells with cells possessing different surface antigens may serve as a surveillance mechanism that is capable of rapidly eliminating neoplastic cells in the absence of specific immunity.

IMMUNOTHERAPY OF HUMAN TUMORS

The observation of complete regression with chemotherapy in at least three types of disseminated human tumors—choriocarcinoma, Burkitt's lymphoma, and neuroblastoma—concurrent with the demonstration of immunologic reactions to these tumors, supports an optimistic expectation of increasing application of immunologic approaches to human tumor therapy. Recent attempts at immunotherapy have often involved preterminal patients with very large tumor cell burdens whose already impaired immune mechanisms had little chance of being effectively augmented. However, the possibility exists of *enhancing* tumor growth through immune manipulation in patients who might otherwise have favorable prognoses—for example, through stimulation of blocking antibodies or anti-antibodies. Cautious investigation of immunotherapy with patients who have relatively poor prognoses, but at a time when their disease is limited, seems justifiable at present; e.g., in a patient whose recurrent malignant melanoma in lymph nodes has been surgically resected.

Experimental Therapeutic Methods

Large tumor masses are, if possible, reduced by prior surgery, radiotherapy, or chemotherapy to permit immune mechanisms to be effective.

1. Active immunization with tumor cells. (a) **Autochthonous tumors** (tumors arising in the same host) have been used as vaccines after irradiation or neuraminidase treatment in malignant melanoma patients. Clinical improvement has been rare in the presence of metastases, but prolonged remissions have occurred in series of patients with minimal residual tumor. (b) **Allogeneic tumor cells** (cells from other patients) have been used after their irradiation in acute lymphoblastic leukemia and acute myeloblastic leukemia in conjunction with BCG or other adjuvants, after remission has been induced by intensive chemotherapy and radiotherapy. Prolongation of remissions has been reported in some series but not in others. It is estimated that the patient's body burden of leukemic cells must be reduced by chemotherapy and radiotherapy from an initial 10^{12} down to 10^5 cells before immunologic defenses can be effective. (c) **Tumor cell extracts** have not been extensively used as antigens in human immunotherapy, although they are used for delayed hypersensitivity skin testing. They are also used to characterize TSTA in animal studies. (d) **Activation of autologous lymphocytes in vitro:** Lymphoid cells from the thoracic duct have been incubated with tumor cells in vitro and then reinfused. Autologous blood lymphocytes have also been activated in vitro with phytohemagglutinin (a hemagglutinin from plants, capable of inducing blast transformation and mitosis in lymphocytes) and then reinfused. Increased numbers of blood lymphoid cells can be obtained by large-scale culture or with centrifugal blood cell separators.

2. Passive immunization. (a) **Antiserum:** Antilymphocyte serum has been used in chronic lymphocytic leukemia, resulting in a temporary decrease in lymphocyte counts. However, the possibility cannot be ignored that such humoral antibodies might induce immunologic enhancement in certain tumor systems. (b) **Lymphoid cells:** Allogeneic blood leukocytes, from donors previously grafted with the recipient's tumor, have been transfused ("adoptive" immunotherapy) in studies with malignant melanoma and other tumors. Some remissions have occurred. Concomitant immunosuppressive therapy may permit survival of the donor lymphoid cells and graft-vs.-host reactions may result, as with bone marrow transplantation. (c) **Transfer factor:** This dialyzable leukocyte extract, capable of transferring delayed hypersensitivity reactivity from one individual to another, has been studied as a means of transferring antitumor immunity in malignant melanoma, breast carcinoma, sarcomas, and Hodgkin's disease, among others, with some results suggesting an anti-tumor effect.

3. Nonspecific immunotherapy. (a) Skin malignancies have regressed after induction of delayed hypersensitivity to dinitrochlorobenzene and subsequent direct application of dinitrochlorobenzene to the tumor. (b) Immunologic adjuvants, such as BCG, extracts of BCG such as MER (methanol extraction residue), or killed suspensions of *Propionibacterium acnes (Corynebacterium parvum, C. acnes)* have been used in controlled trials, with or without added tumor antigen, in malignant melanoma, acute leukemia, lymphomas, and breast and colon carcinoma. Direct injection of BCG into melanoma nodules almost always leads to regression of the injected nodules, and occasionally of distant, noninjected nodules as well. Intensive BCG administration in recurrent melanoma (Stage III) after surgical resection appears to have improved survival. Some patients with Stage III and Stage IV Hodgkin's disease who achieve a complete remission with chemotherapy are receiving BCG as "maintenance" immunotherapy in a randomized chemotherapy–immunotherapy study, without conclusive results to date. That BCG may shift the delicate balance of antitumor factors and enhancing factors toward either the host's or the tumor's advantage must be kept in mind.

TUMOR IMMUNODIAGNOSIS

Many tumors release antigenic substances into the circulation. These antigenic macromolecules may eventually provide sensitive indicators of the presence of a variety of malignancies, yielding a valuable immunologic approach to the early diagnosis of neoplastic disease, particularly if detectable by technics appropriate for mass screening programs. They can also aid in monitoring patients for tumor recurrence after therapy.

Carcinoembryonic antigen (CEA) is a protein-polysaccharide complex found in colon carcinomas and in normal fetal gut, pancreas, and liver. Use of a sensitive radioimmunoassay has led to the detection of increased levels in the blood of patients with colon carcinoma. However, the specificity of this technic is currently under investigation since positive tests have also occurred in cirrhosis, in ulcerative colitis, and with other cancers. α-**Fetoprotein** is an antigen migrating with the α-globulins in electrophoresis, and is found in serum from patients or animals with primary hepatoma and from patients with ovarian or testicular embryonal carcinoma. γ-**Fetoprotein** is found in a variety of human tumors and in fetal serum.

4. HEMORRHAGIC DISORDERS *(Cont'd)*

1. ANEMIAS

Conditions in which RBC (or Hb) production is impaired, RBC destruction is premature, or blood loss has been excessive, usually resulting in one or more of the quantitative RBC measurements (Hb, Hct, RBC count) being below normal.

Classification and Terminology

This etiologic classification will be followed in the subsequent presentation:

  I. Anemias Due to Excessive Blood Loss
      A. Acute posthemorrhagic anemia
      B. Chronic posthemorrhagic anemia
 II. Anemias Due to Deficient Red Cell Production
      A. Deficiency of factors related to erythropoiesis
          1. Iron deficiency
          2. Copper and (experimentally) cobalt deficiencies
          3. Vitamin B_{12} and folic acid deficiencies (pernicious anemia and related megaloblastic anemias)
          4. Experimentally: pyridoxine, riboflavin, and pantothenic acid. In man: protein deficiency, rarely other specific vitamin deficiencies

General Symptoms and Signs

The clinical manifestations of anemia *are directly related to its severity and acuteness* because they are caused by tissue hypoxia and represent the cardiovascular-pulmonary compensatory responses. Subjective symptoms which may be associated with severe anemia are weakness, vertigo, headache, tinnitus, spots before the eyes, easy fatigability, drowsiness, irritability, and psychotic behavior. Amenorrhea, loss of libido, or low-grade fever occasionally develops. Gastrointestinal complaints and congestive heart failure may develop. Jaundice and splenomegaly occur in some anemias.

Laboratory Evaluation

The basic diagnostic evaluation of an anemic patient mandates a CBC including RBC indices, platelet count, reticulocyte count, and review of a well-prepared peripheral blood smear.

The normal range of RBCs at sea level is 5.4 million/cu mm $\pm$ 0.8 for males, and 4.8 million $\pm$ 0.6 for females. At birth, the blood count is slightly higher; by the third month it falls to levels of about 4.5 million $\pm$ 0.7, at which it remains for several years, and then gradually rises from age 4 yr until puberty. An adult male is considered anemic if the RBC count is < 4.5 million/cu mm or the Hb is < 14 Gm/100 ml of blood, and an adult female if the RBC count is < 4 million/cu mm or the Hb is < 12 Gm/100 ml of blood.

For the RBC count to remain constant, dying cells must be replaced by new cells (reticulocytes) released from the bone marrow. Since the normal life span of an erythrocyte is about 120 days, 1/120th of the total RBC mass must be replaced daily, or about 40,000 to 50,000 new cells/cu mm. This is 0.8 to 1% of the total RBC count and is the normal reticulocyte count, an important gauge of marrow activity.

Normally, the Hb level is 16 $\pm$ 2 Gm/100 ml of blood for males, and 14 $\pm$ 2 Gm for females. The normal volume of packed RBCs (hematocrit—**Hct**) is 47 $\pm$ 5 ml/100 ml of blood for men, and 42 $\pm$ 5 ml for women.

RBC indices (the mean corpuscular volume **[MCV]**, mean corpuscular Hb **[MCH]**, and mean corpuscular Hb concentration **[MCHC]**) can be derived from the

RBC count, Hb, and Hct. Anemias with an MCV < 80 are termed **microcytic;** with an MCV > 94, **macrocytic.** MCH and MCHC values of < 27 and 32, respectively, are indicative of Hb deficiency, or **hypochromia.** Anemias with an MCH > 32 are **macrocytic;** because of the greater cell size, the MCHC remains normal. Examination of RBCs on a well-stained peripheral smear gives similar information regarding RBC morphology and, together with the indices, permits a classification of anemias which correlates well with etiologic classification (see TABLE 3-1, p. 262) and greatly aids diagnostic evaluation.

Patients with anemias due to defective nucleoprotein synthesis have macrocytic cells with a high MCH (but a normal MCHC), in contrast to the hypochromic, microcytic anemias of iron deficiency. Anemias due to bone marrow inhibition, replacement, or failure are normocytic and normochromic. When replacement of the bone marrow has occurred, the smear usually shows some immature WBCs and nucleated RBCs; in marrow failure, pancytopenia is present.

In addition to variations in size (anisocytosis) and Hb content, abnormalities in the shape of RBCs **(poikilocytosis)** and nucleated erythrocytes may be seen in the smear. **Polychromasia** refers to cells that stain various shades of blue and red with Wright's stain due to variations in ribonucleic acid (RNA) content. **Stippled cells** contain blue-staining granules, remnants of nucleoprotein. **Spherocytes** are relatively small, round corpuscles which stain bright red and show no central pallor. **Schistocytes** are fragments of red corpuscles which are tiny elliptical, triangular, or otherwise diminished and irregular shapes ("burr" cells, pyknocytes, spiculed cells). **"Target" cells** are thin cells with a peripheral rim and a central dot of Hb. The presence of immature leukocytes and plasma cells is also abnormal.

Reticulocyte levels are increased in anemias due to excessive blood loss or destruction and decreased in those caused by inadequate blood formation. It is important to think in terms of absolute reticulocyte levels. For example, 1% of 5 million RBCs is 50,000 cells, a normal number, but 1% of 2 million would fall far below normal.

Bone marrow biopsy and evaluation should be done whenever the nature of the anemia is not readily evident. These procedures are well tolerated, rarely contraindicated, and specimens are usually available for review within 1 h, though clot and biopsy sections may require more time. The nature of the anemia (e.g., iron deficiency, hypoplasia, megaloblastosis, ineffective erythropoiesis, etc.) should be definable by combining evaluation of the peripheral counts, RBC indices, smear, and bone marrow.

General Therapeutic Considerations

Treatment of anemia should always be specific. Response to specific therapy is part of the diagnostic evaluation. Therefore, a clinical trial with broad-spectrum hematinics ("shotgun therapy") is never appropriate. In deficiency states, treatment should not be discontinued prematurely. After normal laboratory values have been achieved and the underlying cause has been corrected, it may be prudent to continue therapy for weeks (folic acid deficiency) or months (iron deficiency) in order to replenish the stores. In some instances, the cause of the deficiency is not reversible (pernicious anemia, hereditary hemorrhagic telangiectasia) and replacement therapy is lifelong.

Blood transfusion is reserved for patients with active bleeding, with recent bleeding when more is expected, or when the patient has hypoxemic symptoms or signs. Transfusion procedures and blood components are discussed in detail in

Ch. 2, below. Physicians should feel gratified when a patient with an acquired anemia is managed successfully without transfusion.

ANEMIAS DUE TO EXCESSIVE BLOOD LOSS

ACUTE POSTHEMORRHAGIC ANEMIA

Anemia caused by the rapid loss of a large amount of blood.

Etiology and Pathogenesis

Massive hemorrhage may be due to traumatic rupture or incision of a large blood vessel, erosion of an artery by lesions such as peptic ulcer or a neoplastic process, spontaneous rupture of aneurysms or varices, or the hemorrhagic diatheses. The immediate effects depend on the rapidity and amount of blood loss. Sudden loss of one third of the blood volume may be fatal, but as much as two thirds may be lost over a 24-h period without fatality. Symptoms are due both to the sudden decrease in blood volume and to subsequent hemodilution, with decrease in O_2-carrying capacity of the blood.

Symptoms and Signs

Faintness, dizziness, thirst, sweating, weak and rapid pulse, and rapid respiration (at first deep, then shallow) may occur. Orthostatic hypotension is common. Blood pressure may at first rise slightly because of reflex arteriolar constriction, then gradually fall. If bleeding continues, blood pressure may fall to shock levels and death may ensue.

Laboratory Findings

During and immediately after hemorrhage, the RBC count, Hb, and Hct are deceptively high because of vasoconstriction. Within a few hours, fluid begins to enter the circulation from the tissues, resulting in hemodilution and a drop in the RBC count and Hb proportional to the severity of bleeding. The resultant anemia is normocytic. Polymorphonuclear leukocytosis as high as 35,000, and a rise in platelet count to as high as 1 million/cu mm may take place within the first few hours. Evidence of blood regeneration appears several days after bleeding has ceased. Blood smears at this time may disclose polychromatophilia, reticulocytosis, slight macrocytosis, and occasional normoblasts and immature WBCs.

Treatment

Immediate therapy consists of measures to stop the bleeding, restore blood volume, and combat shock. Blood transfusion is the only reliable means of rapidly restoring blood volume and is indicated for severe bleeding with threatening vascular collapse. Plasma is the most satisfactory temporary substitute for blood. Saline or dextrose infusions have only a transient beneficial effect. Absolute rest, fluids by mouth as tolerated, and other standard measures for treatment of shock are indicated.

Subsequent treatment includes a high-protein diet supplemented with vitamins, and iron therapy.

CHRONIC POSTHEMORRHAGIC ANEMIA

A hypochromic microcytic anemia caused by prolonged moderate blood loss, as from a chronically bleeding peptic ulcer, menometrorrhagia, or bleeding hemorrhoids. The clinical features and treatment of this condition are discussed below, under IRON-DEFICIENCY ANEMIA.

TABLE 3-1. CHARACTERISTICS OF COMMON ANEMIAS

Etiology or Type	Morphologic Changes	Special Features
Acute blood loss	Normochromic, normocytic; marrow hyperplastic	In severe hemorrhage may be nucleated RBCs & left shift of WBCs; also leukocytosis
Chronic blood loss	See ANEMIA DUE TO IRON DEFICIENCY; may show features of Acute Blood Loss if recent severe hemorrhage has supervened	
Iron deficiency	Hypochromic, microcytic, aniso- & poikilocytosis; marrow hyperplastic, with delayed hemoglobinization	Achlorhydria, smooth tongue, & spoon nails may be present; stainable marrow iron absent; serum iron low; total iron-binding capacity increased
Vitamin B_{12} deficiency	Oval macrocytes; megaloblastic marrow; granular leukocytes hypersegmented	Serum B_{12} level < 150 pg/ml; frequent GI & CNS involvement; stainable marrow iron plentiful; indirect serum bilirubin elevated; cholesterol decreased
Folic acid deficiency	Same as vitamin B_{12} deficiency	Serum folate < 5 ng/ml; nutritional deficiency & malabsorption (sprue, pregnancy, infancy, alcoholism)
Marrow failure	Normochromic, normocytic; marrow aspiration often fails or may show hypoplasia of erythroid series or of all elements	Occasionally idiopathic, but usually a history of exposure to toxic drugs or chemicals (e.g., chloramphenicol, atabrine, hydantoins, insecticides)
Pyridoxine-responsive anemia	Usually hypochromic; rarely normocytic or macrocytic; marrow hyperplastic, with delayed hemoglobinization; siderocytes may be present	Inborn or acquired metabolic defect; stainable marrow iron plentiful; response to pyridoxine partial, rarely complete
Acute hemolysis	Normochromic, normocytic; marrow, normoblastic hyperplasia	Increased serum bilirubin (indirect) & increased stool & urine urobilinogen; hemoglobinuria in fulminating cases

Condition	Blood findings	Other findings
Chronic hemolysis	Normochromic, normocytic; marrow, normoblastic hyperplasia; basophilic stippling (especially in lead poisoning)	Survival studies show shortened RBC life span; radio-iron turnover increased
Hereditary spherocytosis (congenital hemolytic jaundice)	Spheroidal microcytes in smear	Erythrocytes show increased osmotic fragility; shortened survival of labeled RBCs; radioactivity buildup over spleen
Paroxysmal nocturnal hemoglobinuria	Normocytic (may be hypochromic due to iron deficiency)	Dark morning urine; hemosiderin present; positive acid hemolysis & sugar-water tests; reticulocytes may be decreased
Paroxysmal cold hemoglobinuria	Normocytic, normochromic	Follows exposure to cold; due to a cold agglutinin. Usually associated with congenital or acquired syphilis
Sickle cell anemia	Aniso- & poikilocytosis; some sickle cells in smear; all sickle in wet preparation	Limited to Negroes; electrophoresis shows S Hb; painful crises & leg ulcers may occur; bony changes shown by x-ray
Thalassemia	Hypochromic, microcytic; thin cells; target cells; basophilic stippling; aniso- & poikilocytosis; nucleated RBCs in homozygotes	Decreased osmotic fragility; elevated A_2 & F Hb; Mediterranean ancestry; homozygotes anemic from infancy; splenomegaly; bony changes on x-ray
Infection or chronic inflammation	Normochromic, normocytic; marrow normoblastic; iron plentiful	Serum iron decreased; total iron-binding capacity decreased
Marrow replacement (myelophthisis)	Aniso- & poikilocytosis; nucleated RBCs; early granulocyte precursors; marrow aspiration may fail, or show leukemia, myeloma, or metastatic cells	Liver and spleen may be enlarged; bone changes may be demonstrable; radio-iron uptake greater over spleen and liver than sacrum; reticulocytes may be slightly increased if many normoblasts in blood

ANEMIAS DUE TO DEFICIENT RED CELL PRODUCTION

ANEMIAS DUE TO DEFICIENCY OF FACTORS RELATED TO ERYTHROPOIESIS
(See also discussions of vitamin and element deficiencies in §11, Chs. 3 and 4)

IRON-DEFICIENCY ANEMIA
(Anemia of Chronic Blood Loss; Hypochromic Microcytic Anemia; Chlorosis; Hypochromic Anemia of Pregnancy, Infancy, and Childhood)

Chronic anemia characterized by small, pale RBCs and depletion of iron stores.

Etiology

Iron deficiency is the most common cause of anemia, and may be due to increased iron requirement, diminished iron absorption, or both. Iron deficiency is especially likely to develop during the first 2 yr of life because of the demands of rapid growth and the inadequate iron content of milk. Adolescent girls with marginal iron stores may become iron-deficient from menstruation. In adult males, the most frequent cause of iron-deficiency anemia is chronic occult blood loss, usually from the gastrointestinal tract. In adult females, pregnancy is a common cause of iron-deficiency anemia unless supplemental iron is given. Decreased absorption of dietary iron may occur after gastrectomy, with disorders of the small bowel mucosa, and with the eating of clay or laundry starch that is habitual in some cultures.

Pathophysiology

The **first stage** of iron-deficiency anemia is iron depletion, in which the loss of iron exceeds the gain and in which storage iron is progressively depleted but Hb and plasma iron remain normal. As storage iron decreases, there is a compensatory increase in absorption of dietary iron and in the level of transferrin. In the **second stage,** the stores are exhausted and the available iron is insufficient to meet the needs of the erythroid marrow. The plasma iron level drops progressively and the plasma transferrin level continues to increase. The decreasing plasma iron level leads to a progressive decrease in marrow sideroblasts. When the plasma iron falls to $< 50 \mu g/100$ ml and the transferrin saturation to $< 16\%$, erythropoiesis is impaired. In the **third stage,** anemia begins to develop because of an insufficient supply of iron to the marrow, but there is no discernible change in the peripheral smear or RBC indices despite mild anemia. In the **fourth stage,** hypochromic-microcytic changes appear. Microcytosis precedes hypochromia. Finally, in the **fifth stage,** symptoms and signs of tissue iron deficiency develop.

Symptoms and Signs

The symptoms of chronic severe iron-deficiency anemia may include a craving for dirt or paint **(pica)** or ice **(pagophagia),** and, in rare advanced cases, dysphagia associated with a postcricoid esophageal web **(Plummer-Vinson syndrome).** The signs of far-advanced iron-deficiency anemia may include a smooth tongue **(glossitis),** cracking of the skin at the corners of the mouth **(cheilosis),** and brittle, longitudinally ridged fingernails with progressive concavity or "spooning" **(koilonychia).** Glossitis and cheilosis are not specific for iron-deficiency anemia and will not develop until the anemia is severe.

Diagnosis

Iron-deficiency anemia is the only anemia with absent marrow iron stores. Diagnosis depends upon an understanding of the progressive stages of the anemia. There are no specific symptoms or signs, and differential diagnosis mainly involves the hypochromic-microcytic anemias associated with the thalassemias, chronic diseases, and the sideroblastic anemias (see TABLE 3-2).

Iron-deficiency anemia **in the adult** is almost always due to chronic blood loss. When the clinical picture does not indicate a site (e.g., menorrhagia), occult gastrointestinal bleeding should be investigated even in the absence of demonstrable blood in random stool samples. Chronic intravascular hemolysis with hemoglobinuria and hemosiderinuria, a rare cause of iron deficiency, should be sought in patients with fragmented RBCs on smear or with pancytopenia.

Treatment

Iron is provided by ferrous sulfate or ferrous gluconate 300 mg orally t.i.d. Oral iron is safer than parenteral iron; the rate of response is the same with either route. Parenteral iron should be reserved for patients who do not tolerate or will not take oral iron, or for patients who lose large amounts of blood steadily due to disorders such as hereditary hemorrhagic telangiectasia. Iron in enteric-coated capsules is not well absorbed.

A maximal reticulocyte response usually occurs 7 to 12 days after iron replacement is begun. There is little rise in Hb for 2 wk, but thereafter the rise should be 0.7 to 1 Gm/100 ml/wk in cases of severe anemia. A subnormal response may result from continued blood loss, underlying infection or malignancy, insufficient intake of iron by the patient, or, rarely, malabsorption of oral iron. As Hb rises, the rate of rise decreases, but the anemia should be fully corrected within 2 mo. Therapy should be continued for another 3 to 4 mo to replenish stores.

COPPER AND COBALT DEFICIENCIES

Deficiencies of these two minerals can be produced experimentally, but in man cobalt deficiency has never been described and copper deficiency is rare. A syndrome has been observed in infants in which the anemia, like experimental copper-deficiency anemia, is microcytic and hypochromic. The condition is associated with hypocupremia and hypoferremia, as well as hypoproteinemia, and a protein-losing enteropathy can often be demonstrated. True copper deficiency has also been reported in severely undernourished infants being rehabilitated on high-caloric, low-copper diets. Copper supplementation produced a dramatic response in some of these infants.

TABLE 3-2. DIFFERENTIAL DIAGNOSIS OF THE HYPOCHROMIC-MICROCYTIC ANEMIAS

	Iron Deficiency Anemia	Anemia of Chronic Diseases	Sideroblastic Anemia
Plasma iron	Low	Low	Normal to high
Total iron-binding capacity	High	Low	Normal
% Saturation	< 16	> 16	Normal to high
Iron stores	Absent	Normal to high	Normal to high
Sideroblasts	Decreased	Decreased	Ringed forms

VITAMIN B₁₂ AND FOLIC ACID DEFICIENCIES

Deficiency of either vitamin B_{12} or folic acid may result in defective nucleoprotein synthesis. In order for cells to divide, there must be a doubling of deoxyribonucleic acid (**DNA**), the nucleoprotein of the chromosomes. The coenzymes of B_{12} and folic acid are necessary for DNA synthesis. If either of these substances is deficient, nucleoprotein synthesis is impaired, resulting in an anemia characterized by megaloblastic hemopoiesis with the production of enlarged, oval macrocytes with an abnormally short life span. Iron turnover studies indicate increased activity in the marrow, evidence of dyspoiesis in which many cells are destroyed before they can circulate (ineffective erythropoiesis).

Anemia Due to Vitamin B₁₂ Deficiency

Vitamin B_{12} is present in meat and other animal protein foods. Absorption occurs in the terminal ileum and requires the intact presence of "**intrinsic factor**," a specific substance secreted by the gastric parietal cells in the fundus and body of the stomach, to transport the vitamin across the intestinal mucosa. B_{12} is stored in the liver in sufficient quantities to sustain physiologic needs for 3 to 5 yr.

Etiology and Pathophysiology

Decreased B_{12} absorption is the major pathophysiologic mechanism and may be due to one of several factors. In **pernicious anemia,** the most common cause of B_{12} deficiency, the atrophic gastric mucosa fails to secrete intrinsic factor. Gastrectomy, chronic atrophic gastritis, and myxedema may also cause deficient intrinsic factor secretion. Deficiency of intrinsic factor is rarely congenital. Competition for available B_{12} and cleavage of the intrinsic factor may occur in the blind loop syndrome (bacterial B_{12} utilization) and in fish tapeworm infestation. Ileal absorptive sites may be congenitally absent or destroyed by inflammatory regional enteritis or surgical resection. Less common causes of decreased B_{12} absorption include chronic pancreatitis, malabsorption syndromes, and administration of certain drugs (e.g., oral calcium chelating agents, aminosalicylic acid, biguanides). Inadequate B_{12} intake in vegetarians, or increased B_{12} utilization in hyperthyroidism and pregnancy may also be causative.

Symptoms and Signs

Anemia is present in most patients, developing insidiously and progressively as the large hepatic stores of B_{12} are depleted. It is often more profound than would be expected from the symptoms since physiologic adaptation can occur with its slow evolution. Splenomegaly and hepatomegaly may occasionally be seen. Various gastrointestinal manifestations may be present, including anorexia, intermittent constipation and diarrhea, and poorly localized abdominal pain. Glossitis, usually described as "burning of the tongue," is an early symptom. Considerable weight loss is common.

Neurologic involvement may be present even in the absence of anemia. Transient paresthesias of the upper extremities, peripheral neuropathy, irritability, mild depression, delirium, and paranoia may occur early. Spinal cord involvement begins in the dorsal column with loss of vibratory sensation in the lower extremities, loss of position sense, and ataxia; lateral column involvement follows, with spasticity, hyperactive reflexes, and a Babinski's sign. Yellow-blue color blindness occurs rarely.

FUO may occur and responds promptly to B_{12} therapy. Endocrine deficiencies, especially hypothyroidism and adrenal insufficiency, may occur in association with pernicious anemia and suggest an autoimmune basis for the gastric mucosal atrophy. Hypogammaglobulinemia may be associated with pernicious anemia.

Laboratory Findings

The anemia is macrocytic, with an MCV > 100. The smear shows macroovalocytosis, aniso- and poikilocytosis, and basophilic stippling of the RBCs. Howell-Jolly bodies are common; Cabot's rings and nucleated RBCs may be seen in severe cases. Usually, polychromatophilia is not present and reticulocytes are reduced sharply unless the patient has been treated or is undergoing a spontaneous remission. Hypersegmentation of the granular leukocytes is one of the earliest findings; leukopenia develops later. Thrombocytopenia is observed in about half the severe cases, and the platelets are often bizarre in size and shape. The bone marrow demonstrates erythroid hyperplastic and megaloblastic changes in proportion to the severity of the anemia. Giant metamyelocytes and nuclear twinning are seen in the granulocytic series.

Serum vitamin B_{12} is below 150 pg/ml. Propionic and methylmalonic aciduria are present. Serum bilirubin is elevated due to ineffective erythropoiesis. Autoantibodies to gastric parietal cells can be identified in 80 to 90% of patients with pernicious anemia and in 40 to 50% of those with intrinsic factor deficiency.

Achlorhydria is present in patients with pernicious anemia. Fasting gastric analysis demonstrates a small volume of gastric secretions (achylia gastrica) with a pH > 6.5; achlorhydria is confirmed if the pH rises to between 6.8 and 7.2 following histamine administration. Absent gastric intrinsic factor secretion is seen in patients with pernicious anemia.

An excellent diagnostic test is the absorption of radioactive B_{12} with and without intrinsic factor (Schilling test). It is particularly useful in establishing the diagnosis in patients who have been treated and are in remission. As done by Schilling, it consists of giving 0.5 μg of ^{57}Co-labeled B_{12} orally, followed in 2 h by an injection of 1000 μg of unlabeled B_{12}. The urine for the next 24 h should contain > 8% of the labeled material. Pernicious anemia patients characteristically excrete < 2%, unless the labeled dose is given with intrinsic factor, in which case absorption and excretion are restored to the normal range. Subnormal absorption of B_{12}, uncorrected by intrinsic factor, is seen in sprue and other malabsorption syndromes. The test need not be performed before the completion of therapeutic trials.

Because of the increased incidence of gastric cancer in patients with pernicious anemia, gastrointestinal x-rays should be taken in every patient with this diagnosis. These may disclose other causes of megaloblastic anemia (e.g., intestinal diverticula or blind loops, or abnormal small bowel patterns characteristic of sprue). Careful inquiry into the dietary and drinking habits of such patients is essential. Hypothyroidism may be accompanied by a macrocytic anemia; a common cause of refractory macrocytic anemia is occult leukemia.

Treatment

The amount of B_{12} retained by the body is in proportion to the amount given. Calculation of the specific amount of therapeutic B_{12} required is difficult since repletion must include restoration of the hepatic stores, normally 3000 to 10,000 μg, and B_{12} retention declines as restoration of stores is achieved. Vitamin B_{12} 1000 μg is given IM 2 to 4 times/wk until the hematologic abnormalities are corrected. Although hematologic correction usually occurs within 6 wk, stable neural improvement may take up to 18 mo. Folic acid administration in the B_{12}-deprived state is associated with fulminant neurologic deficit and is **contraindicated.** Oral iron therapy is given if iron deficiency is diagnosed by an absence of stainable iron in the bone marrow prior to B_{12} treatment.

B_{12} maintenance therapy must be given for life unless the pathophysiologic mechanism for the deficiency is corrected. At least 100 μg/mo IM is given, but larger doses (1000 μg/mo) may be required to prevent neurologic recrudescences.

Anemia Due to Folic Acid Deficiency

Etiology and Pathophysiology

The metabolism, several pathophysiologic mechanisms, and causes of folate deprivation are also discussed in §11, Ch. 3.

Folic acid is most plentiful in green leafy vegetables, yeast, liver, and mushrooms. It is absorbed in the duodenum and upper jejunum. Hepatic storage of folate is limited, providing only a 2- to 4-mo supply in the absence of intake. Dietary deficiency of folic acid is not uncommon. In addition, vitamin C is essential in the initial stages of the reduction of folic acid to its metabolically active form, tetrahydrofolic acid. Alcohol interferes with the intermediate metabolism of folic acid. Therefore, persons living on a marginal subsistence diet ("tea-and-toasters") and chronic alcoholics are prone to develop macrocytic anemia from folic acid deficiency, as are those with chronic liver disease. Infants deficient in vitamin C may have **"megaloblastic anemia of infancy."** Since the fetus obtains its folic acid from maternal supplies, pregnant women are susceptible to developing a megaloblastic anemia.

Intestinal malabsorption is another common cause of folic acid deficiency. In **tropical sprue,** the malabsorption itself is secondary to the atrophy of intestinal mucosa resulting from lack of folic acid. Even minute doses will correct both the anemia and the steatorrhea in most of these patients.

Folic acid deficiency may develop in some epileptics receiving sodium phenytoin because of a biochemical antagonism between drug and vitamin. Folate deficiency also develops in patients treated with antagonists to folate (e.g., methotrexate) or purine (6-mercaptopurine).

Diagnosis

Other than anemia, pallor, fatigue, and glossitis, there are few physical symptoms and signs. There are no neurologic abnormalities. The peripheral blood and bone marrow examinations show the characteristic megaloblastic dyspoiesis described above for B_{12} deficiency. Serum folic acid levels below 3 ng/ml are suggestive of deficiency. Erythrocyte folate levels are low (normal, 90 to 450 ng/ml) and are diagnostic of deficiency.

Treatment

Folic acid 1 mg/day is given orally. The patient's awareness of the importance of adequate folic acid intake is critical; approximately 50 μg of folate is required daily, with 2 to 3 times that amount required in pregnancy and childhood.

OTHER B VITAMIN DEFICIENCIES

Animal studies show that various B vitamins other than B_{12} and folic acid play a role in blood formation, but clinical deficiencies are rare or not well defined. Kwashiorkor, which is characterized by signs of malnutrition (e.g., weight loss, a characteristic "pavement" dermatitis, a reddish alteration in hair color), is due mainly to protein deficiency but is frequently associated with deficiencies of iron and of various B vitamins, including riboflavin. The term **"pyridoxine deficiency"** refers to a pyridoxine-responsive anemia (see SIDEROBLASTIC ANEMIAS, below) which rarely, if ever, is due to actual deficiency of this vitamin. However, experimentally produced pyridoxine deficiency does cause severe microcytic, hypochromic anemia. This differs from that seen in iron deficiency in that the serum iron is elevated and the tissues are heavily loaded with iron. Experimental **riboflavin deficiency** is normocytic. **Pantothenic acid** is necessary for heme synthesis, but the associated anemia is moderate in degree and normocytic.

ASCORBIC ACID DEFICIENCY

Deficiency of ascorbic acid is often associated with anemia. This is hypochromic and may be normocytic, microcytic (if there has been long-standing blood loss), or, occasionally, macrocytic. The last is probably the consequence of associated folic acid deficiency.

ANEMIAS OF BONE MARROW FAILURE

HYPOPLASTIC AND APLASTIC ANEMIAS

Normochromic, normocytic anemias with associated leukopenia and thrombocytopenia, a hypoplastic or aplastic bone marrow, and a prolonged plasma iron clearance. Rarely, the bone marrow is normocellular or even hypercellular, even though pancytopenia is present.

Etiology and Pathogenesis

About half of cases of aplastic anemia are "**idiopathic**"; they are most common in adolescents and young adults. The **Fanconi syndrome** (familial aplastic anemia, bone abnormalities, microcephaly, hypogenitalism, and olive-brown skin pigmentation) appears in young children and is associated with chromosomal aberrations.

Exposure to certain **chemical agents** (e.g., benzene, inorganic arsenic, acetylsalicylic acid, phenytoin), **antineoplastic agents** (e.g., nitrogen mustard and congeners, methotrexate, 6-mercaptopurine and other antimetabolites), and **ionizing radiation** can result in aplastic anemia. The reaction is only occasionally associated with some substances (e.g., chloramphenicol, quinacrine, phenylbutazone, mephenytoin, gold compounds, potassium chlorate, possibly certain sulfonamides and insecticides) and is then presumably idiosyncratic. A possible relationship has been proposed with hepatitis, miliary tuberculosis, and SLE.

Pure RBC aplasia refers to cases in which only the red corpuscles and their precursors are affected; the WBCs, platelets, and their marrow precursors are normal. Pure RBC aplasia is usually idiopathic, but drugs such as chloramphenicol and phenytoin may be causative. A congenital form (**Blackfan-Diamond syndrome**) has been described. Erythroid aplasia may occur transiently during various infections and hemolytic disorders (aregenerative crisis, acute erythroblastopenia), and in association with tumors of the thymus.

Symptoms and Signs

Onset is usually insidious, often occurring over weeks or months after exposure to a toxic agent. However, it is occasionally explosive. Clinical manifestations vary with the severity of the pancytopenia. General symptoms of anemia are usually severe. Waxy pallor of skin and mucous membranes is characteristic. Chronic cases may show considerable brown skin pigmentation. If severe thrombocytopenia is present, blood may extravasate into the mucous membranes and skin. Hemorrhages into the ocular fundi are frequent. Agranulocytic angina (severe sore throat associated with a sharp reduction in the number of granulocytes) may occur. Splenomegaly is absent, unless induced by transfusion hemosiderosis.

Laboratory Findings

The anemia is severe and is normochromic and normocytic (rarely, macrocytic). A WBC count of 1500 or lower is common, the reduction occurring chiefly in the granulocytes. Platelets are reduced severely. Reticulocytes are rare. The aspirated bone marrow is usually acellular but occasionally is normal or even hyperplastic. In the latter case, the majority of the cells may be histiocytes and plasma cells. There is no evidence of hemolysis and no alteration of gastric acidity. The serum iron is elevated.

Diagnosis

This is readily apparent in the presence of normochromic anemia, agranulocytosis, thrombocytopenia, and aplastic bone marrow, especially if a history of exposure to a toxic substance is obtained. An "aleukemic" leukemia may produce a similar peripheral blood picture, but the bone marrow is hyperplastic with young cells predominating, and splenomegaly and lymphadenopathy are frequently present. Rarely, a pancytopenia secondary to the replacement of bone marrow hemopoietic tissue by neoplastic tissue may simulate an aplastic anemia.

Prognosis

In cases caused by a toxic agent, removal of the offending substance may be followed by spontaneous recovery. In idiopathic cases, recovery is less frequent despite repeated blood transfusions. Survival after the development of anemia may be less than 6 mo, but 30 to 50% of patients live 1 yr or more.

Treatment

The essential therapy is whole blood transfusion in order to prolong life until the marrow resumes its function. Transfusions must be used sparingly to avoid hemosiderosis. Drugs that might be injurious to the marrow should be avoided, and substances that might stimulate the marrow (e.g., androgens, corticosteroids) should be tried. Infection is controlled with antibiotics, but "prophylactic" antibiotic therapy is unnecessary and unwise and may permit the growth of resistant organisms. With rare exceptions, bone marrow transplants have been successful only in identical twins.

SIDEROBLASTIC ANEMIAS

A group of anemias of unknown etiology, largely refractory to therapy, which differ from the aplastic anemias in that the erythroid bone marrow is hyperplastic and contains numerous iron-laden developing normoblasts ("sideroblasts"). In some of the cells, the iron granules tend to form a ring around the nucleus ("ringed" sideroblasts). The anemia is often hypochromic and microcytic, sometimes dimorphic, or, more rarely, normocytic or macrocytic. In contrast to the hypochromic, microcytic anemia of iron deficiency, the serum iron concentration is increased and the iron-binding protein is nearly completely saturated.

Etiology and Pathophysiology

Sideroblastic anemia may be hereditary or acquired. **The most common hereditary type** is the pyridoxine-responsive, X-linked anemia of young males. Pyridoxine in its active form, pyridoxal phosphate, is required in the condensation of glycine and succinyl coenzyme A to form δ-aminolevulinic acid. Patients with pyridoxine-responsive sideroblastic anemia have a block in the synthesis of heme, so that incoming iron is not incorporated normally but is deposited in the mitochondria to form the ringed sideroblast. This block is partly overcome by pharmacologic doses of pyridoxine.

Acquired sideroblastic anemia is usually seen in middle-aged or elderly patients. It may be associated with certain diseases (e.g., rheumatoid arthritis, polyarteritis nodosa, myelofibrosis, and myeloma, Hodgkin's disease, or other malignancies), toxins, or drugs, or may be idiopathic. Lead, ethanol, isoniazid, and, to a lesser extent, cycloserine and pyrazinamide are most commonly implicated. Chronic alcoholism can produce a sideroblastic anemia associated with folate deficiency, but discontinuation of alcohol rapidly corrects both abnormalities.

Symptoms, Signs, and Diagnosis

Sideroblastic anemia is characterized by either hypochromic-microcytic or dimorphic red cells, erythroid hyperplasia, increased iron stores, and ringed sideroblasts on marrow iron stain. Since iron is not being incorporated into heme, serum iron levels and saturation of transferrin are often increased, and ferrokinetic studies reveal a pattern of "ineffective erythropoiesis" that results from early death in the marrow of the abnormal red cells. This ineffective erythropoiesis is suggested clinically by extensive poikilocytosis on the peripheral smear and by a low reticulocyte count despite a striking marrow erythroid hyperplasia. Thus, sideroblastic anemia can be diagnosed readily from signs of ineffective erythropoiesis, elevated serum iron values, and the presence of ringed sideroblasts. Differentiation from iron-deficiency anemia and the hypochromic-microcytic anemia associated with chronic disease is shown in TABLE 3-2 on p. 265.

Prognosis

Although some patients with idiopathic acquired sideroblastic anemia are preleukemic and later develop acute myeloblastic leukemia, most patients follow a relatively benign course with a median survival of 10 yr. A complete hematologic response rarely occurs with treatment regimens, but occasionally there is a partial response. Many of the deaths result from nonhematologic causes. The prognosis in hereditary forms varies greatly. Often the anemia in the X-linked form responds in part to pyridoxine therapy; these patients can lead relatively normal lives.

Treatment

Therapy for **X-linked sideroblastic anemia** consists of pyridoxine 50 mg orally t.i.d. Therapy for **acquired sideroblastic anemia** involves a trial of pyridoxine 50 mg orally t.i.d., often in combination with folic acid 1 mg orally t.i.d. Possible causative drugs should be eliminated, although the sideroblastic anemia associated with isoniazid can be corrected by giving pyridoxine with isoniazid.

Periodic transfusions of packed RBCs may be necessary but should be used cautiously because of the dangers of viral hepatitis and iron overload. A 3- to 6-mo trial of oral androgen therapy (such as oxymetholone 2 mg/kg/day) should be considered for refractory cases needing frequent transfusions.

ANEMIAS DUE TO EXCESSIVE RED CELL DESTRUCTION (HEMOLYTIC ANEMIAS)

The normal life span of the RBC is about 120 days. As they age, RBCs are removed by components of the reticuloendothelial system, principally in the spleen, where Hb catabolism takes place. The essential feature of hemolytic anemia is a shortened red cell "life span" no longer compensated by accelerated RBC production. General aspects of hemolytic anemias will be described below first, followed by a description of specific hemolytic disorders.

Pathogenesis

Most hemolysis occurs extravascularly; i.e., in the phagocytic cells of the spleen, liver, and bone marrow. Hemolysis is usually due to (1) abnormalities within the RBC (Hb or metabolism); (2) abnormalities of the RBC membrane (permeability, structure, or lipid content); or (3) abnormalities extrinsic to the RBC (serum antibodies, trauma in the circulation, or infectious agents). The spleen is involved in all cases, and the resulting splenomegaly jeopardizes the survival of normal red cells. The spleen detects and destroys mildly abnormal RBCs. More severely abnormal RBCs are destroyed in the liver, which (because of its large blood flow) is more efficient in removing damaged cells from the circulation.

Although intravascular hemolysis is uncommon, it leads to hemoglobinuria when the Hb released into plasma exceeds the Hb-binding capacity of plasma haptoglobin. Hb is reabsorbed into renal tubular cells where the iron is converted to hemosiderin, part of which is assimilated for reutilization and part of which reaches the urine when the tubular cells slough.

Clinical Manifestations

The systemic manifestations of hemolytic anemias resemble those of other anemias. Hemolysis may be acute, chronic, or episodic. Acute severe hemolysis **(hemolytic crisis)** is uncommon and may be accompanied by chills, fever, pain in the back and abdomen, prostration, and shock. Severe hemolysis is also accompanied by manifestations of increased red cell destruction (jaundice, splenomegaly, and, in certain types of hemolysis, hemoglobinuria and hemosiderinuria) and increased red cell production (reticulocytosis and hyperactive bone marrow). Anemia of chronic hemolysis may be exacerbated by a temporary failure of red cell production **(aplastic crisis)**; this is usually related to an infection.

Jaundice occurs when the conversion of Hb to bilirubin exceeds the liver's capacity to form bilirubin glucuronide and to excrete it into bile. Thus, unconjugated ("indirect") bilirubin accumulates. Increased pigment catabolism is manifested by increased stercobilin in the stool and urobilinogen in the urine. Pigment gallstones frequently complicate chronic hemolysis.

The only definitive estimate of the hemolytic process is a measure of red cell survival, preferably with ^{51}Cr. Tests indicative of increased destruction and production of RBCs are also helpful in defining a hemolytic state. Red cell morphology should also be assessed; morphology is specific to each hemolytic disease. Other tests include hemoglobin electrophoresis, assay of glucose-6-phosphate dehydrogenase, autohemolysis, osmotic fragility, Coombs test, cold agglutinins, and acid hemolysis or sucrose lysis tests. Specific enzyme assays may be indicated.

Treatment

Treatment is individualized to specific hemolytic disorders. For massive acute hemolysis, urine flow should be maintained with mannitol and IV fluids; alkalinization of the urine with sodium bicarbonate is recommended. Hemoglobinuria may necessitate iron replacement therapy. Splenectomy is beneficial when the red cell defect is not severe enough to be detected by the liver or to cause intravascular RBC destruction.

HEMOLYSIS DUE TO INTRINSIC RED CELL DEFECTS

ABNORMALITIES OF RED CELL METABOLISM—HEREDITARY ENZYME DEFICIENCIES

Glucose is the prime energy source for the RBC. Following its entry into the RBC, glucose is converted to lactate either by anaerobic glycolysis **(the Embden-Meyerhof pathway)** or via the **hexosemonophosphate** shunt. Hemolytic anemias may result from hereditary deficiencies in the enzyme systems involved in these pathways of glucose metabolism.

These diseases are all relatively rare and share the following characteristics: The trait is an autosomal recessive, and hemolytic anemia is seen only in homozygotes; spherocytes are absent, but small numbers of crenated spheres are present; and hemolysis and anemia persist after splenectomy, though there may be some improvement. The disorders are characterized by deficiency of **pyruvate kinase, triosephosphate isomerase, hexokinase, glucose phosphate isomerase,** or other enzymes that participate in this metabolic pathway.

Glucose-6-Phosphate Dehydrogenase (G6PD) Deficiency, Drug-Sensitive Variety (Intrinsic Red Cell Defect Plus Extrinsic Factor)

This X-linked disorder (see also in §22, Ch. 6) is fully expressed in males and homozygous females and variably expressed in heterozygous females. It occurs in about 10% of American Negro males and a smaller percentage of Negro females. There is a very low frequency among peoples from the Mediterranean basin; e.g., Italians, Greeks, Arabs, and Sephardic Jews.

In affected Negroes and most affected Caucasians, hemolysis occurs in older RBCs after exposure to drugs or other substances that permit the oxidation of Hb and RBC membranes by O_2. These include primaquine, aspirin, sulfonamides, nitrofurans, phenacetin, naphthalene, some vitamin K derivatives, and, in some Caucasians, fava beans. Acute viral and bacterial infections and diabetic acidosis also may precipitate hemolysis. Anemia, jaundice, and reticulocytosis develop. Heinz bodies may be seen early during the hemolytic episode, but they do not persist in patients with spleens. Often the best diagnostic clue is the presence of "bite cells" in the peripheral blood. These are RBCs which appear to have had one or more bites (1 μ in size) taken from the cell periphery, possibly as a result of Heinz body removal by the spleen. Since only the older cells are destroyed, hemolysis is self-limited, usually affecting at most 25% of the RBC mass in Negroes. However, in Caucasians, hemolysis may be profound, with a sufficient intramuscular component to lead to hemoglobinuria and acute renal failure. If the offending drug is not stopped, RBCs continue to undergo destruction as their level of G6PD declines during cell aging, but the acute destruction of the large number of older cells that were present during the initial drug exposure ends. Chronic congenital hemolysis in the absence of drugs occurs in some Caucasians.

A large number of screening tests for G6PD are available. Following hemolysis, false negative results may be obtained due to the absence of older, more deficient RBCs and the presence of reticulocytes which are rich in G6PD. Specific enzyme assays are the best diagnostic test. Affected patients should be advised so that they can avoid offending agents.

Congenital Erythropoietic Porphyria
(See in PORPHYRIAS in §11, Ch. 7)

ABNORMALITIES OF THE RED CELL—DEFECTS OF MEMBRANE STRUCTURE AND PERMEABILITY

Hereditary Spherocytosis
(Chronic Familial Icterus; Congenital Hemolytic Jaundice; Chronic Acholuric Jaundice; Familial Spherocytosis; Spherocytic Anemia)

An inherited chronic disease characterized by hemolysis of spheroidal RBCs, anemia, jaundice, and splenomegaly.

Etiology and Pathogenesis
Hereditary spherocytosis results from an inherited abnormality of the red cell membrane, the precise nature of which is unknown. Cell membrane lipids are decreased, and the cell membrane surface area is decreased out of proportion to the lipid lack. Structural instability of the membrane to sodium requires the ex-

penditure of excess energy (in the form of adenosine triphosphate) to extrude sodium. The decreased surface area impairs the cell's ability to change shape as needed to traverse the microcirculation of the spleen. Therefore, RBCs are trapped in the spleen and destroyed. The condition is inherited as a simple mendelian dominant trait. There is usually a history of one or more family members with jaundice, anemia, or splenomegaly. However, one or more generations may be skipped due to variations in the degree of penetrance of the gene.

Symptoms and Signs

Symptoms and signs are usually mild. Moderate jaundice and symptoms of anemia are present in severe cases. Aplastic crises (fever, abdominal pain, rapidly increasing jaundice) due to intercurrent infection may exacerbate the anemia. Splenomegaly is almost invariable and, rarely, may cause abdominal discomfort. Hepatomegaly may be present, and cholelithiasis is common. Leg ulcers and bone changes as seen in sickle cell anemia may be present. Congenital skeletal abnormalities, such as tower-shaped skull and polydactylism, are seen occasionally.

Laboratory Findings

The anemia varies greatly in degree. The RBC count is usually between 3 and 4 million, but during an aplastic crisis it may fall to less than 1 million. The Hb level drops proportionately with the cell count. Since RBCs are spheroidal and the MCV is normal, the mean corpuscular diameter is somewhat below normal, giving the appearance of microspherocytosis. Reticulocytosis of 15 to 30% and leukocytosis are common.

The osmotic fragility of RBCs is characteristically increased, but in mild cases it may be normal unless the sterile defibrinated blood is first incubated at 37 C (98.6 F) for 24 h. The Coombs test is negative. Autohemolysis is increased but can be corrected with glucose.

Prognosis and Treatment

Splenectomy is the only treatment. At surgery the gallbladder should be palpated for the presence of stones and should be removed if diseased. Splenectomy is usually followed by abatement of symptoms and a rise in the RBC count. Since spherocytosis persists following splenectomy, the osmotic fragility of the blood is still increased.

Hereditary Elliptocytosis
(Ovalocytosis)

This rare disorder is inherited as an autosomal dominant trait. The RBCs are oval or elliptical in shape. Hemolysis is usually absent or only slight, and there is no anemia. Splenomegaly is often present. Splenectomy frequently relieves the hemolysis.

Membrane Lipid Defects

A few patients with severe alcoholic cirrhosis or other severe liver dysfunction acquire RBCs that are spiculated in shape and rigid due to excess cholesterol in the cell membrane **("spur cells")**. They morphologically resemble acanthocytes in abetalipoproteinemia. Hemolysis may be marked with Hb values less than 7.0 Gm; however, values of 8 or 9 Gm are more common. Hemolysis is alleviated by splenectomy, but the morbidity and mortality of this procedure are high.

HEMOLYSIS DUE TO ABNORMALITIES EXTRINSIC TO THE RED CELL

IMMUNOLOGIC ABNORMALITIES

Reactions to Incompatible Blood
(See §3, Ch. 2)

Idiopathic Immune Hemolytic Anemia
(Autoimmune Hemolytic Anemia)

In this condition, RBCs become coated with IgG antibodies that arise spontaneously or after stimulation by a drug (α-methyldopa, L-dopa, mefenamic acid). The antibodies may be specific for common blood groups, most frequently a portion of the Rh locus. Hemolysis is mild to severe and is accompanied by spherocytosis. The Coombs test is positive. A thrombotic tendency often accompanies the hemolysis. Dopa drugs may cause only a positive Coombs test without hemolysis, in which case the drug can be continued. Penicillin and the cephalosporins in high doses may cause hemolytic anemia. The antibody in these circumstances is against an antibiotic-RBC membrane complex; the RBCs are involved passively. A positive Coombs test without hemolysis may also occur with the cephalosporins, due to nonspecific protein-coating of the RBCs rather than to an immunohemolytic process.

Immune hemolysis may complicate chronic lymphocytic leukemia, lymphosarcoma, and SLE. Transfusion reactions are discussed in Ch. 2, below, and erythroblastosis fetalis in §9, Ch. 12.

Treatment

In idiopathic cases, the anemia responds to corticosteroids, but splenectomy is frequently required to control the hemolytic process. Immunosuppressive agents have been used in patients refractory to steroids and splenectomy.

In all drug-induced hemolytic anemias, withdrawal of the drug decreases the hemolytic rate. With α-methyldopa and related drugs hemolysis ceases, usually within 3 wk; however, the positive Coombs test may persist for a year or more. Corticosteroids occasionally are used if hemolysis is very severe. With penicillin-type drugs, hemolysis ceases as soon as the drug is cleared from the plasma.

Cold Agglutinin Disease

Patients with lymphoproliferative diseases, infectious mononucleosis, or mycoplasma pneumonia may develop IgM antibodies frequently directed against the I or i antigen of red cells. Reactivity is high at low temperatures but minimal above 30 C (86 F). No cause is found in some patients. Agglutination and complement fixation result, but intravascular lysis does not occur. Hemolysis is usually mild or absent but may transiently be severe. Avoidance of cold is usually sufficient therapy. Chemotherapy is sometimes necessary.

Paroxysmal Nocturnal Hemoglobinuria
(PNH; Marchiafava-Micheli Syndrome)

This rare disorder of the hemopoietic system is characterized by episodes of hemolysis and hemoglobinemia, the latter accentuated during sleep. The cause is unknown, but it seems to be due to defective RBCs that are unusually susceptible to normal complement in plasma. Thus, PNH is an acquired membrane defect with sensitivity to a serum component. PNH is most common in males in their 20s, but it occurs at any age. Crises may be precipitated by infection, administration of iron or vaccines, or, in females, menstruation.

Abdominal and lumbar pain may occur, along with splenomegaly, hemoglobinemia, hemoglobinuria, and symptoms of severe anemia. The anemia is normocytic and normochromic. Protracted urinary Hb loss may result in iron deficiency even though some organs, particularly the kidneys, may be saturated with hemosiderin. Leukopenia and thrombocytopenia are common. Gross hemoglobinuria is common during crises, and the urine may contain hemosiderin. Affected patients are strongly predisposed to both venous and arterial thrombi, and this is a common cause of death.

Diagnostic tests include the acid hemolysis test in which hemolysis usually occurs if blood is acidified with CO_2, incubated for 1 h, and centrifuged. The "sugar-water" test of Hartman, which depends on the enhanced hemolysis of complement-dependent systems in isotonic solutions of low ionic strength, is also useful.

Treatment is symptomatic. Blood transfusions containing plasma (complement) should be **avoided**. Saline-washed RBCs may be given during crises. Heparin should be used cautiously since it may accelerate hemolysis in some patients, but its use in thrombotic disease appears warranted. Oral iron supplements are useful.

Paroxysmal Cold Hemoglobinuria
(PCH; Donath-Landsteiner Syndrome)

In this rare disease, hemolysis occurs minutes to hours after exposure to cold; exposure may be localized (e.g., drinking cold water, handwashing in cold water). Intravascular hemolysis is caused by an autohemolysin that unites with RBCs at low temperatures and hemolyzes them only after warming. The cold hemolysin is a 7S-immunoglobulin. PCH due to such a cold-activated autohemolysin occurs in some patients with congenital or acquired syphilis, and antisyphilitic therapy may cure the PCH. Other cases may represent an autoimmune hemolytic process.

Symptoms include severe pain in the back and legs, headache, vomiting, diarrhea, and passage of dark brown urine. Findings include hemoglobinuria, mild anemia, and moderate reticulocytosis. There may be temporary hepatosplenomegaly. Mild hyperbilirubinemia may follow the attack.

TRAUMATIC HEMOLYTIC ANEMIAS
(Microangiopathic Hemolytic Anemias)

RBCs fragment when exposed to excessive shear or turbulence in the circulation. The persistence of fragments in the circulation aids diagnosis. The fragments appear as triangles, helmet shapes, etc. Trauma may be (1) external to the vessel, as occurs in march hemoglobinuria or during karate or bongo playing; (2) within the heart, as in aortic stenosis and with faulty aortic valve prostheses; (3) in arterioles, as in malignant hypertension and some malignant tumors; or (4) in end arterioles in thrombotic thrombocytopenic purpura and disseminated intravascular coagulation **(DIC)**. Coagulation factor deficits occur only in DIC (see §3, Ch. 4). Treatment is directed toward the underlying process. Iron-deficiency anemia occasionally is superimposed on hemolysis as a result of hemosiderinuria, and, when demonstrated, may respond to iron therapy.

HEMOLYSIS DUE TO INFECTIOUS AGENTS

Infectious agents may produce hemolytic anemia by the direct action of toxins (e.g., from *Clostridium perfringens*, α- or β-hemolytic streptococci, or meningococci), or by invasion and destruction of the RBC by the organism (e.g., plasmodia and bartonellae).

ANEMIAS DUE TO BOTH DECREASED PRODUCTION AND INCREASED DESTRUCTION (HEMOLYSIS) OF RED CELLS

DEFECTIVE HEMOGLOBIN SYNTHESIS

HEMOGLOBINOPATHIES

Genetically transmitted abnormalities of the Hb molecule manifested by alterations in its chemical characteristics, electrophoretic mobility, or physical properties.

The normal adult Hb molecule **(Hb A)** consists of two pairs of polypeptide chains designated α and β. Fetal Hb **(Hb F)** is present at birth, gradually decreases in the first months of life, and makes up less than 2% of total Hb in adults. In Hb F, γ chains are substituted for β chains. In certain disorders of Hb synthesis and in aplastic and myeloproliferative states, Hb F may be increased. Normal blood also contains up to 2.5% of Hb A_2, which is composed of α chains and δ chains.

The type of chains and the chemical structure of individual polypeptides in the chains are controlled genetically. Genetic defects may result in Hb molecules with abnormal physical or chemical properties, some of which may result in anemia. Such anemias are severe in homozygotes and mild in heterozygous carriers of the trait. Some individuals may be heterozygous for two such abnormalities and show an anemia with characteristics of both traits.

The abnormal hemoglobins are distinguished by their electrophoretic mobility and have been designated by letters. The first to be discovered was sickle cell Hb (Hb S). The designations since then have followed alphabetical sequence in order of discovery: thus, C, D, E, G, H, etc. Structurally different hemoglobins with the same electrophoretic mobility are named also by the city in which they were discovered (e.g., Hb C_{Harlem}, Hb $S_{Memphis}$). The important hemoglobinopathies in the USA are those due to Hb S and Hb C and the thalassemias.

Sickle Cell Anemia
(Hb S Disease; Drepanocytic Anemia; Meniscocytosis)

A chronic hemolytic anemia occurring almost exclusively in Negroes and characterized by sickle-shaped RBCs due to homozygous inheritance of Hb S.

Etiology, Incidence, and Pathogenesis

Homozygotes have sickle cell anemia (about 0.3% of Negroes in the USA); **heterozygotes** (8 to 13% of Negroes) are not anemic, but the sickling trait **(sicklemia)** can be demonstrated in vitro.

In Hb S, valine is substituted for glutamic acid in the sixth peptide of the β chain. This alters its electrical charge and makes it move more slowly than Hb A in zone or paper electrophoresis. Hb in the peripheral blood is in the deoxygenated form because of the low O_2 tension in the tissues. Deoxy- Hb S is much less soluble than deoxy- Hb A and forms a semisolid gel of rodlike tactoids, thus causing sickling of the RBCs. The distorted RBCs are unable to pass through small arterioles and capillaries, and plugs of RBCs lead to thrombosis and infarction. Because sickled RBCs are more fragile than normal RBCs and less able to withstand the mechanical trauma caused by circulation in blood, hemolysis occurs when they are released into the circulation. Repeated episodes lead ultimately to severe anemia.

Symptoms and Signs

In homozygotes, the clinical manifestations are due to anemia and to thrombosis and infarction. Anemia is usually severe, and many patients are moderately jaundiced. Anemia may be exacerbated in children by acute sequestration crisis. More common is the so-called "aplastic crisis" in both children and adults occurring when marrow RBC production slows during acute infections. Episodes of arthralgia with fever may occur, and aseptic necrosis of the femoral head is common. Chronic punched-out ulcers about the ankles are a recurrent problem. Episodes of severe abdominal pain with vomiting may simulate severe abdominal disorders, and such painful crises are usually associated with back and joint pain. Hemiplegia, cranial lobe palsies, and other neurologic disturbances may result from cerebral thromboses.

Patients usually are poorly developed and often have a relatively short trunk with long extremities and a tower-shaped skull. Chronic overactivity of the marrow causes bone changes that can be seen on x-ray; widening of the diploic spaces of the skull and the "sun-ray" appearance of the diploid trabeculations are characteristic. The long bones frequently show cortical thickening, irregular densities, and evidence of new bone formation within the medullary canal. Hepatosplenomegaly is common in children, but because of repeated infarctions and subsequent fibrosis, the spleen in adult patients is rarely palpable. The heart is usually enlarged, with a prominent pulmonary conus. Heart murmurs may simulate rheumatic or congenital heart disease. Cholelithiasis is common.

In the heterozygous state, affected individuals are normal and do not experience hemolysis, painful crises, or thrombotic complications. Hyposthenuria is common. Unilateral hematuria occurs occasionally but is self-limited and should never be treated by nephrectomy. Failure to recognize the heterozygous sickle cell state is an unfortunate cause of needless nephrectomy.

Laboratory Findings

The anemia is normocytic with the RBC count usually between 2 and 3 million and the Hb reduced proportionally. The pathognomonic laboratory finding is sickling (crescent-shaped RBCs, often with elongated or pointed ends) in an unstained drop of blood that has been prevented from drying or has been treated with a reducing agent (see under CLINICAL HEMATOLOGY in §24, Ch. 2). Dry stained smears may show only a few sickled cells.

Normoblasts are frequently seen in the peripheral blood, and a reticulocytosis of 10 to 40% or more is common. Leukocytosis may be as high as 25,000 with a shift to the left. The platelets may be increased. The bone marrow is hyperplastic, with normoblasts predominating; it may become aplastic during sickling crises or severe infections. Serum bilirubin is usually elevated, and fecal and urinary urobilinogen values are high. The ESR is low.

Prognosis and Treatment

Few homozygous patients live beyond age 40. Common causes of death are intercurrent infections (especially tuberculosis), multiple pulmonary emboli, or thrombosis of a vessel supplying a vital area.

Therapy is symptomatic. Splenectomy and hematinics are valueless. Transfusions should be given only for symptomatic anemia or during aplastic crises accompanying severe infections, and not for treatment of painful crisis alone. A partial exchange transfusion may break a cycle of closely spaced painful crises.

Urea orally or parenterally is of no value and may be harmful. Cyanate therapy is being evaluated.

Hemoglobin C Disease

A moderately severe anemia due to an inherited abnormality of Hb formation. From 2 to 3% of American Negroes show the trait. Heterozygotes are usually not anemic. Symptoms are similar to those of sickle cell anemia, but milder. The spleen is usually enlarged, and arthralgia is common. There may be abdominal pain but the abdominal crises of sickle cell anemia do not occur. The patient may be mildly jaundiced.

The anemia is normocytic and hypochromic, with 30 to 100% target cells in the smear. Reticulocytes are increased slightly, and nucleated RBCs may be present. The RBCs do not sickle. Electrophoresis shows that all the Hb is type C. Serum bilirubin is slightly elevated, and urobilinogen is increased in the stools and urine. There is no specific **treatment.** The anemia is usually not severe enough to require blood transfusion.

Hemoglobin S-C Disease

Since 10% of Negroes carry the Hb S trait, the incidence of the heterozygous S-C combination is much greater than that of the homozygous Hb C disease. Many cases of anemia in patients with sicklemia may represent undetected examples of the S-C combination.

The anemia in Hb S-C disease is similar to that of Hb C disease, but milder. However, gross hematuria, retinal hemorrhages, and aseptic necrosis of the femoral head are common in Hb S-C disease.

Stained blood smears show target cells and a few sickled cells. All the cells sickle in a sickling preparation.

THALASSEMIAS
(Mediterranean Anemia; Hereditary Leptocytosis; Thalassemia Major and Minor)

A group of chronic, familial, hemolytic anemias occurring in populations from countries bordering the Mediterranean and from Southeast Asia, and characterized by defective Hb synthesis and ineffective erythropoiesis.

Etiology and Pathogenesis

Thalassemia results from unbalanced Hb synthesis due to defective production rates of either β (and, in some cases, δ) or α polypeptide chain synthesis. β-Thalassemia, common in Italians and Greeks, results from a decreased synthesis of β polypeptide chains. It is inherited as an autosomal dominant trait; heterozygotes **(thalassemia minor)** are usually asymptomatic, but typical symptoms occur in homozygotes **(thalassemia major).** Since the genetic control of α chain synthesis involves more than one pair of genes, the inheritance pattern for α thalassemia, which results from a decreased α chain synthesis, is more complex. Silent carriers are free of demonstrable abnormality but carry the gene for a mild impairment of α chain synthesis. Heterozygotes show few characteristics of thalassemia and carry a defective major α chain synthetic gene. Double inheritance of the heterozygous state and the silent carrier state results in demonstrable impairment of α chain synthesis. The deficiency of α chains causes the formation of tetramers of β chains **(Hb H)**, or, in infancy, γ chains **(Bart's Hb).** The homozygous state is lethal since Hb lacking α chains does not transport O_2.

Symptoms and Signs

The clinical features of all thalassemias are similar but vary in severity. Symptoms of severe anemia occur in β-thalassemia major (Cooley's anemia). Patients are jaundiced, and leg ulcers and cholelithiasis occur as in sickle cell anemia. Splenomegaly is common, and the spleen may be huge. If splenic sequestration develops, the survival time of transfused, normal RBCs is shortened. Hyperactivity of the bone marrow causes thickening of the cranial bones and malar eminences, producing "hemolytic facies." The bone changes are similar to those in sickle cell anemia. Pathologic fractures are common. Iron deposits in cardiac muscle may cause cardiac dysfunction and ultimately cardiac failure.

Patients with Hb H disease are mildly to moderately anemic and have hypochromic RBCs of varied size and shape.

Laboratory Findings

In thalassemia major, anemia is severe, often with an RBC count of 2 million or less. The Hb is always proportionately lower than the RBC count, and the MCV and MCHC are below normal. The reticulocyte count is elevated. The smear is virtually diagnostic, with large numbers of nucleated erythroblasts, target cells, small pale RBCs, and punctate and diffuse basophilia.

The mechanical fragility of the RBCs is increased, but hemolysis in hypotonic saline does not begin at levels $> 0.40\%$, and complete hemolysis may never be achieved. The marrow is hyperplastic, with increased numbers of RBC precursors predominating. Serum bilirubin and fecal and urinary urobilinogen are increased. Hb F is usually increased, sometimes to as much as 90% in homozygotes; Hb A_2 is also elevated to $> 3\%$ in most cases.

Skeletal x-rays show findings characteristic of chronic overactivity of the marrow. The cortices of the skull and the long bones are thinned, and the marrow space is widened. The diploic spaces in the skull may be accentuated, with the trabeculae giving a "sun ray" appearance. Areas of osteoporosis in the long bones may occur. The vertebral bodies and the skull may have a somewhat granular or "ground glass" appearance. The phalanges may lose their normal shape and appear rectangular or even biconvex.

Prognosis

The outlook varies. Some patients with β-thalassemia major live to puberty or beyond. Life expectancy is not altered for individuals with minor forms of the disease.

Treatment

Children should receive as few transfusions as possible, since iron overload can ultimately result. Attempts to suppress hemopoiesis by chronic transfusion in severely affected patients are being studied, and this therapy is being coupled with attempts to remove the resulting iron overload. Splenectomy is not beneficial and may increase the peripheral erythroblastosis. Thalassemia minor requires no treatment.

ANEMIA ASSOCIATED WITH CHRONIC DISEASES

A chronic, predominantly hypoproliferative, normocytic or microcytic anemia commonly seen in patients with chronic inflammation or infection and sometimes neoplasms.

Etiology and Pathogenesis

Anemia is seen with a wide variety of chronic diseases (long-standing infections, noninfectious inflammatory diseases such as rheumatoid arthritis, malignancies, renal insufficiency, hepatic disease, and certain endocrine deficiency states). The anemias of infection, rheumatoid arthritis, and cancer appear to be related in that they are accompanied by hypoferremia and reticuloendothelial siderosis. They have been called **"anemias of chronic disorders."** The anemias accompanying the other diseases mentioned above are discussed separately, below.

In the anemia of chronic disorders, erythropoietin is decreased and the bone marrow appears to be unable to compensate for a mild to moderate decrease in erythrocyte life span. The cellularity of the marrow is normal. In addition, serum iron and iron-binding capacity are decreased, iron stores are increased, sideroblast iron is decreased and free erythrocyte protoporphyrin is increased. Thus, there appears to be a barrier to the normal flow of iron from the reticuloendothelial cells to plasma. The bone marrow remains capable of responding to erythropoietin or to measures which stimulate erythropoietin production, such as anoxia or hemorrhage, but, for reasons unknown, the production of erythropoietin is usually less than would normally be expected with the given degree of anemia. There is usually a mild reduction in RBC survival, insufficient to explain the anemia.

When anemia is found in association with **malignancy,** factors other than those discussed above may play a role or may even be more important; e.g., blood loss, impaired intake or malabsorption of necessary dietary factors.

Symptoms, Signs, and Laboratory Findings

Clinical findings are usually those of the underlying condition unless the anemia is severe. The anemia is usually normocytic or microcytic and normochromic, with subnormal reticulocyte counts. The anemia is usually mild to moderate; if the Hb is consistently < 9 Gm/100 ml other causes should be sought. The smear appears normal except in severe degrees of anemia, when some aniso- and poikilocytosis may be present. RBC indices are normal or slightly reduced. The WBC count reflects the associated pathologic state; i.e., it may be elevated in some infections like osteomyelitis, or low in conditions like rheumatoid arthritis. The serum iron and total iron-binding capacity are low; the transferrin saturation is not so depressed as in iron deficiency, and may be normal.

Treatment

Basic therapy is that of the associated disease. Supportive measures include adequate diet and vitamins. These chronic anemias are generally well tolerated, and blood transfusions are rarely indicated. Iron, liver extract, vitamin B_{12}, and folic acid have no value in treatment.

ANEMIA OF RENAL DISEASE

Pathogenesis

Anemia is seen with uremia, regardless of the nature of the underlying renal disease. A crude correlation exists between the degree of anemia and the degree of renal insufficiency. Unlike the anemia of other chronic disorders (see above), hypoferremia is not a consistent feature. The anemia is characterized by a shortened RBC survival and diminished erythropoietin production with a subnormal marrow response. The subnormal marrow response usually predominates. Less frequently, shortened RBC life span predominates and the anemia is more clearly hemolytic. There is a general relation between anemia and the products which are retained in renal insufficiency. Radioiron marrow transit time is prolonged and correlates with lack of marrow stimulation by erythropoietin.

In a very rare patient, renal arteriolar microvascular disease may be associated with hypertension, marked hemolysis, and increased reticulocyte production. This so-called **hemolytic-uremic syndrome** is generally associated with widespread platelet consumption and occlusion of the microvasculature, and convincingly demonstrates a dissociation between renal exocrine and endocrine functions (decreased glomerular filtration but with increased erythropoietin and renin production).

Laboratory Findings

The anemia may be severe (Hb < 8 Gm/100 ml). It is usually normocytic and normochromic and the reticulocyte count is normal or reduced. In the hemolytic form, however, macrocytosis, reticulocytosis, polychromatophilia, stippling, normoblasts, and aniso- and poikilocytosis are found. Particularly characteristic is the presence of "burr cells," distorted or fragmented RBCs with peripheral sharp projections. Serum iron and total iron-binding capacity levels are typically normal. The WBC count is usually normal. Platelets may be normal or somewhat reduced. The marrow is normal or shows erythroid hypoplasia.

Treatment

Therapy should be directed at the underlying renal disease. If adequate renal function is reestablished, the anemia is relieved. In patients treated with long-term dialysis, increased erythropoiesis has been observed as the patient's general condition has improved, but it rarely returns to normal. When anemia is severe, blood transfusions may help, but should be given sparingly. Routine transfusions may delay recovery of erythropoiesis and increase the risk of immunization against tissue antigens that might preclude eventual renal transplantation.

ANEMIA OF LIVER DISEASE

Multiple factors are implicated in the pathogenesis of the anemia seen with liver disease; e.g., blood loss from esophageal varices, and malnutrition. Nutritional folic acid deficiency not uncommonly accompanies cirrhosis in alcoholics. Alcohol itself can cause depression of RBC production. RBC survival is moderately shortened due to hypersplenism. In some patients, marked hemolysis associated with spur cells occurs.

The RBCs are normal or increased in size and tend to be targeted in appearance. Spherocytes reflect cells which have lost membrane in relation to surface volume.

ANEMIA OF MYXEDEMA

Pathogenesis of the anemia associated with myxedema is obscure. Lessened consumption of O_2 by the tissues may be a factor. An ill-defined metabolic disturbance may cause the anemia encountered in adrenocortical insufficiency and hypopituitarism.

The anemia is usually moderate in degree and normocytic but may be macrocytic. Iron and folic acid deficiency may be present.

Correction of the hormone deficiency relieves the anemia, but the response is usually slow. Other (vitamin and mineral) deficiencies may require specific replacement.

ANEMIAS DUE TO BONE MARROW REPLACEMENT OR INVASION
(Myelophthisic Anemias)

Anemia, usually normocytic, associated with space-occupying lesions of the bone marrow.

Etiology and Pathogenesis

Replacement of bone marrow with neoplastic tissue or fibrosing or sclerosing lesions has been assumed to cause myelophthisic anemia by decreasing the amount of functioning hemopoietic tissue. There is little foundation for this hypothesis. Measurements of RBC production rates have, in fact, yielded normal or increased values in some cases. RBC life span is often reduced. A metabolic fault related to the underlying disease and, in some cases, erythrophagocytosis have been considered pathogenetic factors.

The most common cause is carcinoma metastasizing to bone marrow from primary tumors, most often located in the breast, prostate, kidney, lung, or adrenal or thyroid gland. Another frequent cause is myelofibrosis, which may be of undetermined origin, or, in some instances, a late stage of polycythemia vera. Other causes include marble-bone disease of Albers-Schönberg, other congenital bone diseases, multiple myeloma, leukemia, and Hodgkin's disease.

Unfortunately, loose terminology is often used in referring to this condition, with resulting confusion. **Myeloid metaplasia** refers to the extramedullary hemopoiesis in the liver and spleen that accompanies myelophthisis from any cause, including myelofibrosis. **Myelofibrosis** is a replacement of marrow by fibroblastic cells. In one variant of this process, large numbers of megakaryocytes may be seen among the fibroblasts. This is a proliferative process and may occur concurrently with the extramedullary hemopoiesis in the liver, spleen, and other organs which are infiltrated in a manner similar to leukemia.

Symptoms and Signs

In severe cases, the usual symptoms of anemia may be present (see General Symptoms and Signs at the beginning of this chapter), as well as symptoms referable to the underlying disease. Splenomegaly, sometimes massive, occurs and associated hepatomegaly is common.

Laboratory Findings

The anemia, usually of moderate severity, is characteristically normocytic but may be slightly macrocytic. Morphologic alterations in the erythrocytes may be extreme, with wide variation in size and shape. Another outstanding feature is the presence in the blood of nucleated RBCs, mostly normoblasts, and immature WBCs. These may be only a few, or so numerous as to suggest leukemia (so-called **leuko-erythroblastic anemia**). Polychromatophilia and reticulocytosis are often present. Reticulocytosis is due to premature release of reticulocytes (**"shift reticulocytosis"**) and is not an index of blood regeneration. The WBC count may be normal, reduced, or increased. The platelet count is often low, and giant bizarre-shaped platelets may be seen.

Kinetic studies with labeled iron may be diagnostic if they indicate hemopoietic activity in the spleen and/or the liver. The marrow aspirate, if obtainable, is hypocellular. Diagnosis is confirmed by marrow trephine biopsy. Metastatic cancer cells in the marrow may establish the diagnosis.

X-rays of the skeletal system may disclose bony lesions characteristic of the underlying cause of the anemia.

Treatment

Therapy is that of the underlying disorder. Blood transfusions are indicated if the anemia is severe. In some instances, this type of anemia, particularly that due to myelofibrosis, has been treated successfully with androgens and/or corticosteroids to increase RBC production and, perhaps, to decrease their destruction.

---

2. BLOOD TRANSFUSION

The procedure of transferring human blood or a component of blood from a normal donor to a sick or injured recipient.

Blood is a living tissue; transfusion of blood or its cellular components is a form of transplantation. More than 7,400,000 transfusions of blood and components are given yearly, and the number is steadily increasing. The decision to transfuse is a *clinical* judgment that requires weighing the possible benefits and known hazards with alternative treatments. A transfusion that is not specifically indicated is contraindicated. Clinical use of blood and components is discussed below.

Collection and Storage of Blood

Blood is taken from normal healthy people and screened by interviewing the donor, performing an Hb test, and taking the donor's temperature, pulse, and blood pressure. Detailed criteria have been established by the FDA, American National Red Cross, and American Association of Blood Banks. **Causes for disqualification** are history of (1) hepatitis, (2) heart disease, (3) cancer, (4) severe asthma, (5) bleeding disorder or convulsions. **Temporary deferments** are: (1) malaria, (2) exposure to malaria, (3) exposure to hepatitis, (4) pregnancy, (5) major surgery, (6) hypertension, (7) hypotension, and (8) anemia. Some of these criteria protect would-be donors from possible ill effects of blood donation; others protect the recipient. Donation is limited to once every 2 mo.

Paid blood donation is being discouraged because of abuses inherent in the "skid row" blood banks in big cities, because blood from such banks has five to ten times the usual rate of hepatitis infectivity, and because of a desire to encourage voluntary blood donation and thus broaden the donor base.

The standard blood donation is 450 ml, taken into a plastic bag containing either Citrate Phosphate Dextrose **(CPD)** or Acid Citrate Dextrose **(ACD)** anticoagulant, preferably CPD. Heparin is a poor preservative but is occasionally used, mostly for pediatric heart surgery or exchange transfusion.

Stored whole blood differs considerably from circulating blood. Changes that occur in blood during refrigerated storage are collectively referred to as the "storage lesion." Some of these changes (see FIGS. 3-1 and 3-2) may affect certain recipients.

Before use, blood must be tested for classification and suitability. This includes ABO and Rh typing (see below), antibody screening, STS, and a test for hepatitis B surface antigen (HB$_s$Ag). The container label gives the results of these tests and other important information and cautions.

Blood Components

The various components of blood can be separated, concentrated, and stored individually; replacement should be restricted to those items definitely needed by the patient.

Anticoagulants used for whole blood storage are designed to protect RBCs and are not optimal for other components. Labile components are best stored after separation from whole blood. The demand for components such as platelets, antihemophilic factor **(AHF)**, and fresh plasma for fractionation is so high that blood banks must separate components from a majority of freshly collected bloods. To do this and continue to supply whole blood ad lib wastes donors' RBCs, which are a by-product of component separation. Whole blood is now considered more of a raw material than a transfusion medium.

For anything other than simple RBC transfusion, consulting the blood bank physician before writing orders provides optimal choices and service. TABLE 3-3 shows some characteristics of blood and components as ordinarily prepared by the blood bank, not including purified manufactured derivatives which are essentially pharmaceutical rather than blood bank items. Clinical indications for individual components are discussed below (amounts must always be individualized).

Red blood cells (RBCs) are transfused to replace Hb or O$_2$ carrying capacity, including blood lost at surgery and in priming extracorporeal circuits. When volume expansion is required, other fluids can be used concurrently or separately (see SHOCK, in §4, Ch. 3).

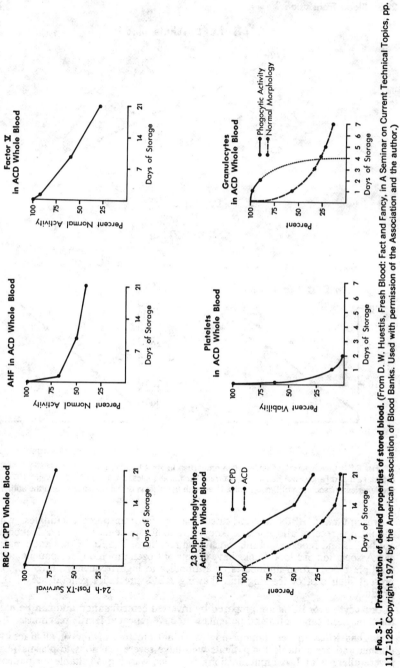

FIG. 3-1. Preservation of desired properties of stored blood. (From D. W. Huestis, Fresh Blood: Fact and Fancy, in A Seminar on Current Technical Topics, pp. 117–128. Copyright 1974 by the American Association of Blood Banks. Used with permission of the Association and the author.)

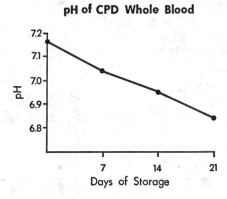

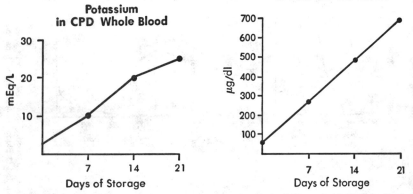

FIG. 3-2. **Development of undesirable properties in stored blood.** (From D. W. Huestis, Fresh Blood: Fact and Fancy, in A Seminar on Current Technical Topics, pp. 117–128. Copyright 1974 by the American Association of Blood Banks. Used with permission of the Association and the author.)

Frozen-thawed RBCs are indicated mainly for transplant candidates, who should not receive allogeneic leukocytes, and for patients who have leukocyte antibodies and repeated febrile transfusion reactions. The Red Cross and American Association of Blood Banks have depots of frozen rare blood for patients with multiple blood group antibodies or antibodies to high frequency antigens. The present high cost of freezing and thawing RBCs precludes general use of this product.

Leukocyte-poor RBCs are prepared by inverted centrifugation and can be used for transplant candidates and patients who have repeated febrile reactions.

Washed RBCs (by continuous-flow washing) are free of almost all traces of plasma and are suitable for patients who have severe reactions to plasma (e.g., severe allergies or IgA immunization). Modified washing is suitable for patients

TABLE 3-3. BLOOD COMPONENTS AS PREPARED FROM CPD* WHOLE BLOOD

Component	Storage Period	Storage Temperature (C)	Hct (%)**	Vol/unit (ml)**	Remarks
RBCs*	21 days	4 to 6	70	300	
Frozen glycerolized RBCs	2 or more yr	−85 (high glyc.) −190 (low glyc.)	n.a.* n.a.	n.a. n.a.	There are several different freeze-thaw protocols having somewhat different characteristics
Thawed deglycerolized RBCs	24 h	4 to 6	70 to 90	200 to 300	
Leukocyte-poor RBCs	21 days	4 to 6	85 to 90	200 to 230	
WB*	21 days	4 to 6	40	513	
WB, heparinized	48 h	4 to 6	40 to 45	477	Deteriorates during 2nd 24 h
Platelet concentrate	3 days 3 days	4 to 6 20 to 22	n.a. n.a.	25 to 30 30 to 50	Best given fresh Best given fresh. Must be agitated continuously during storage
Cryoprecipitated AHF*	1 yr	below −18	0	10	Contains (/unit) about 100 u. AHF and 300 mg fibrinogen
Fresh frozen plasma	1 yr	below −18	0	220	Contains all clotting factors except platelets, but unconcentrated
Granulocytes	48 h (?)	4 to 6	n.a.	Depends on technic	Several technics, all still experimental

* CPD = citrate phosphate dextrose solution; RBCs = red blood cells; WB = whole blood; AHF = antihemophilic factor; n.a. = not applicable.
** Approximate.

with congestive heart failure and hypervolemia, or for pediatric heart surgery to avoid citrate.

Whole blood is becoming less available because of the demand for plasma, components, and fractions. It is sometimes necessary when components are not available, and is also used for rapid massive blood loss and exchange transfusions. When whole blood is not available, RBCs and other fluids or components can be used.

Whole blood, heparinized, has nearly gone out of use but is still requested for some cases of pediatric heart surgery, primarily to eliminate citrate. Frozen-thawed RBCs or RBCs subjected to a single saline wash may be substituted. Heparinized blood is also sometimes used in exchange transfusions for adults with fulminant hepatitis and for babies with severe hemolytic disease.

Platelet concentrates are used for severe thrombocytopenia (platelet count < 10,000/cu mm) or for a bleeding tendency related to less severe thrombocytopenia (e.g., counts between 10,000 and 50,000/cu mm). They are also sometimes necessary for surgical patients who exhibit a bleeding tendency following massive transfusion or prolonged periods on extracorporeal circulation. Since a single fresh platelet concentrate in an adult usually causes a rise of about 12,000 in the platelet count, 6 to 8 concentrates are usually needed. A purpuric patient often shows no rise in count because the transfused platelets are immediately used.

Cryoprecipitated antihemophilic factor (AHF) is a concentrate prepared by rapid freezing and slow thawing of fresh plasma. It is used almost exclusively for hemophiliacs in a dosage depending on the patient's size and AHF deficiency. Each concentrate contains about 100 u. AHF plus about 300 mg fibrinogen, and can also be used as a source of the latter.

Fresh frozen plasma is an unconcentrated source of all clotting factors except platelets. It can be used to correct a bleeding tendency of unknown cause, or one associated with liver failure. It can also supplement RBCs when whole blood is not available for exchange transfusion.

Granulocyte or **"buffy coat"** transfusion is still experimental, used primarily in conjunction with chemotherapy for cancer or leukemia when normal marrow activity is temporarily abolished and sepsis occurs.

"Fresh" blood is required in few conditions and most of these are better handled with blood components. TABLE 3-4 gives definitions of "fresh" to fit certain clinical situations and also gives suitable component alternatives.

Infusion Technic

Before starting any blood transfusion, the label and the cross-match report should be checked to make sure that the blood is indeed for the patient concerned, that it is compatible, and that the component is correct.

An 18-gauge needle, or larger, is desirable. Smaller needles may have to be used in pediatric patients, but hemolysis may occur if excess pressure is necessary. A Y blood-administration set with a proper filter should be used, with the RBCs attached to one limb and isotonic saline to the other. Since most transfusions are RBCs, which are more viscous than whole blood, 50 to 100 ml of saline are allowed to run into the RBCs before starting. No IV solution other than isotonic saline should be allowed into the blood bag or in the same tubing with blood since many solutions exert deleterious effects. For example, D/W causes clumping and decreased survival of RBCs; Ringer's solution causes clotting. Infusion of a single unit of RBCs should not take more than 2 h.

Close observation is important during the first 15 min, since most severe reactions will be evident by then. The patient should be kept warm and well covered

TABLE 3-4. USE OF "FRESH" BLOOD, AND REASONABLE ALTERNATIVES

Clinical Indication	Realistic Definition of "Fresh" Blood (Assuming CPD RBCs or WB)*	Reasonable Substitutes
Bleeding due to massive blood replacement	< 12 h	Platelet concentrates plus RBCs**
Open-heart surgery, before and during extracorporeal circulation	Preferably < 1 wk	Bank or frozen-thawed RBCs plus volume expanders
Open-heart surgery, oozing after extracorporeal circulation	< 12 h	Platelet concentrates plus bank RBCs
Optimal RBC survival and function	< 1 wk	Frozen-thawed RBCs
Exchange transfusion	< 1 wk	Bank or frozen-thawed RBCs plus fresh plasma
Liver failure	< 1 wk	Bank or frozen-thawed RBCs plus fresh plasma
Chronic renal disease	< 1 wk	Frozen-thawed or leukocyte-poor RBCs

* CPD=citrate phosphate dextrose solution; RBCs=red blood cells; WB=whole blood.
** Some patients may also need fresh plasma and occasionally fibrinogen or cryoprecipitated antihemophilic factor (AHF).

From D. W. Huestis, Fresh Blood: Fact and Fancy, in A Seminar on Current Technical Topics. Copyright 1974 by the American Association of Blood Banks. Used with permission of the Association and the author.

to prevent chills which might otherwise be interpreted as a reaction. Transfusions should not be given at night if possible, because observation of the patient is more difficult and his sleep is disturbed.

If any untoward reaction appears to be related to transfusion (see COMPLICATIONS OF TRANSFUSIONS, below), the transfusion should be stopped and the blood bank notified so that an investigation can be started. **That unit should not be restarted.** It is best not to give further transfusions until the cause of the reaction is known.

Divided transfusions (one half one day, one half the next) should be avoided since this increases the hazard of bacterial growth. When incipient heart failure or hypervolemia is a concern, washed RBCs should be used and a whole unit given in the usual way. Otherwise, to prevent overload, some of the patient's own blood may have to be removed as RBCs are given. For small pediatric transfusions, the blood bank can provide blood or RBCs in multiple interconnected bags which can be subdivided with safety.

IMMUNOHEMATOLOGY

General Principles

Clotted blood is optimal for determining antigens on the RBCs and antibodies in the serum. Blood from a skin puncture may be added directly to isotonic saline for RBC typing. Packed RBCs from blood citrated, oxalated, or anticoagulated with EDTA may also be used when appropriately washed and resuspended. Cells are tested against antiserums and serum against test RBCs of known type, and the presence or absence of agglutination or hemolysis is recorded. Careful and meticulous attention to both technical and clerical details is important to avoid errors that may have catastrophic consequences. Reagent manufacturers' instructions should be followed.

ABO and Rh Typing

The four ABO blood groups are determined by testing for the presence or absence of A and B antigens on the RBCs using Anti-A and Anti-B reagents (forward or cell typing), and by testing for Anti-A and Anti-B in the serum using reagent A and B RBCs (serum or reverse typing). See TABLE 3-5 for the test results seen in each of the four blood groups. Both cell typing and serum typing are done routinely, because the serum and cell grouping occasionally do not agree. When this occurs, the true blood group must be identified by testing with additional reagents before proceeding with a transfusion. Cell typing may be done in test tubes or on slides. Reverse typing should be done by a tube technic because, with the less sensitive slide method, weakly agglutinating Anti-A and Anti-B in some individuals may give rise to misclassification.

Rh typing should be done routinely whenever ABO typing is done. The test determines whether the Rh factor, $Rh_o(D)$, is present (Rh-positive) or absent (Rh-negative) in the patient's or donor's RBCs.

Rh_o Variant (D^u) Test

Occasionally, RBCs that have a weakly reacting Rh factor, called Rh_o Variant (D^u), will react negatively in the Rh typing test but will be agglutinated by Anti-$Rh_o(D)$ if the more sensitive indirect antiglobulin method is used. If an apparently Rh-negative blood specimen is from a blood donor or a pregnant woman or her husband, the test for Rh_o Variant (D^u) should always be done. If the Rh-negative blood specimen is from a prospective recipient of a blood transfusion, the Rh_o Variant (D^u) test need not be done. Persons positive for D^u are considered Rh-positive.

Screening for Unexpected Antibodies

Modern blood-banking practice requires that screening for unexpected RBC antibodies be done routinely on each blood specimen submitted for blood grouping; i.e., blood from donors, recipients, and prenatal patients. Unexpected antibodies are specific for RBC blood group antigens other than A and B, such as $Rh_o(D)$, Kell (K), Duffy (Fy^a), and hr'(c). Early detection of such antibodies is important because they can cause hemolytic disease of the newborn and serious transfusion reactions, and they greatly complicate the cross-matching and procurement of compatible blood. Serum is screened for the presence of such an

TABLE 3-5. CHARACTERISTICS AND REACTIONS
OF THE FOUR ABO BLOOD TYPES

ABO type	Red Cells				Serum		
	Antigens present	Reactions with reagents			Antibody present	Reactions with reagents	
		Anti-A	Anti-B	Anti-A, B		A Cells	B Cells
O	Neither	−	−	−	Anti-A & -B	+	+
A	A	+	−	+	Anti-B	−	+
B	B	−	+	+	Anti-A	+	−
AB	A&B	+	+	+	Neither	−	−

antibody by multiple agglutination tests including the sensitive indirect antiglobulin technic, using Group O reagent human RBCs. This reagent is a pool of carefully selected Group O Rh-positive and Rh-negative RBCs that are jointly positive for most important RBC antigens.

Antibody Identification

Once an unexpected antibody is demonstrated by screening, its identity should be determined by testing the serum against a panel of Group O reagent RBCs of known antigenic composition. Further studies such as antibody elution and absorption and subtyping of the patient's RBCs may be required. Knowing the identity of an irregular RBC antibody is helpful for future transfusion therapy and for prognosis and management of hemolytic disease of the newborn when such an antibody is found in the serum of a pregnant woman.

Antibody Titration

When an irregular RBC antibody is identified in the serum of a pregnant woman, it should be titrated to estimate its strength, even though there is poor correlation between the maternal antibody titer and the severity of hemolytic disease in the incompatible fetus. A significant rise in antibody titer means that the fetus carries the antigen and may be affected. In such cases, repeated spectrophotometric examination of the amniotic fluid for bilirubin is essential in order to monitor the condition of the fetus.

Antiglobulin Testing

The **direct antiglobulin (Coombs) test** demonstrates whether the patient's RBCs are coated with antibody. It is performed by treating washed RBCs with antihuman Ig serum and observing for agglutination. The direct antiglobulin test is done on the cord blood of babies of Rh-negative mothers, or of any babies suspected of having hemolytic disease of the newborn caused by maternal antibody. The direct antiglobulin test is also done in the investigation of anemias. If positive, it suggests the presence of autoimmune hemolytic anemia which may be spontaneous but is more likely to indicate lymphoma or SLE.

The **indirect antiglobulin test** is done by in vitro incubation of RBCs with an unknown serum. The presence of antibody coating the cells will be detected by agglutination after washing the test RBCs and adding the antihuman Ig serum. This is part of the cross-match and antibody detection routines, and is sometimes positive in autoimmune hemolytic anemias.

Cross-Match Testing

After determining the ABO and Rh type and doing antibody screening on both prospective recipient and donor bloods, cross-matching tests must be done. The **cross-match** ensures that the recipient's serum does not contain antibodies that will react with the transfused RBCs.

Even if the antibody screening test on the patient's serum is negative, it is still possible to find an incompatibility on cross-match since the donor RBCs may have some antigen not present in the reagent red cells used for screening, or may have an antigen in a more reactive form. If the recipient has a positive screening test, his antibody should be identified and candidate donors should be pretested with the corresponding reagent antibody, if it is available and if there is time, to select blood donor units negative for the RBC antigen concerned. In an emergency, units compatible by cross-match may be transfused before such identification and donor testing have been completed.

As a rule, the cross-match must be compatible before a transfusion is given. The few exceptions to this rule are mostly in patients with autoantibodies.

Donor blood having an irregular antibody is not usually used for transfusion, although it is quite suitable for the preparation of frozen-thawed or washed

RBCs. A "minor" cross-match, testing donor serum against recipient's RBCs, can be done, but most authorities consider it superfluous if a proper antibody screening test is done.

Rh Immune Globulin

$Rh_o(D)$ immune globulin must be given to every Rh-negative mother immediately after every abortion or delivery (live or stillborn) unless it is proved to be unnecessary. $Rh_o(D)$ immune globulin can be omitted only if the baby is $Rh_o(D)$- or D^u-negative, or if the mother's serum already contains Anti-$Rh_o(D)$.

Preparatory testing is done on dual specimens: (1) **Cord blood** is analyzed for ABO and Rh type, including Rh_o Variant (D^u); and a direct antiglobulin test is done. (2) **Maternal blood** drawn immediately postpartum is analyzed for ABO group and Rh type, including Rh_o Variant (D^u); and antibody screening and identification are done. An apparent maternal D^u-positive result may indicate a feto-maternal bleed and should be interpreted with caution.

Genotyping of Husbands

The husband of every Rh-negative woman should be Rh-typed. If he is also Rh-negative, there need be no concern about Rh hemolytic disease in the newborn. If the husband is Rh-positive, his zygosity for the Rh factor (Rh genotype) should be determined for purposes of genetic counseling and for prognosis and management if maternal anti-Rh appears during a pregnancy. *If the husband of an Rh-sensitized woman is homozygous Rh-positive, every fetus will be affected with Rh hemolytic disease;* if he is heterozygous, there is a 50% chance that each fetus will be Rh-negative and, therefore, free from hemolytic disease. The most probable zygosity is determined by testing the father's RBCs with the common Rh reagents, anti-$Rh_o(D)$, anti-rh'(C), anti-rh''(E), anti-hr'(c), and anti-hr''(e), and evaluating the results statistically.

COMPLICATIONS OF TRANSFUSION

Reactions that accompany or follow IV administration of blood or blood components. The more important reactions occur during the transfusion.

HEMOLYTIC REACTIONS

Reactions accompanied by hemolysis of the recipient's or the donor's RBCs— usually the latter—during or following the administration of solutions, plasma, blood, or blood components. The most severe reaction occurs when donor RBCs are hemolyzed by antibody in the recipient's plasma.

Etiology

Hemolysis can result from blood group incompatibility, incompatible plasma or serum, hemolyzed or fragile RBCs (e.g., by overwarming stored blood or contact with inappropriate IV solutions), injections of distilled water or nonisotonic solutions, or instillation of water into the bladder following transurethral prostatic resection.

Incompatibility is the most frequent cause of hemolysis despite advances in blood grouping and cross-matching. Human error (e.g., mislabeling and confusion of samples and of blood containers) is usually responsible. Poor laboratory technic, including inadequate cross-matching or failure to identify correctly the ABO group or Rh type of both donor and recipient, is less common.

Except in an emergency, Rh-negative recipients should receive only Rh-negative blood. Routine typing for other factors (e.g., hr'[c]) is unnecessary. Recipients who have formed any blood group antibody must *always* receive blood negative for the antigen in question.

Cross-matching procedures are designed to detect IgG as well as IgM antibodies. A high-protein procedure or enzyme-modified RBCs may be used, but the indirect antiglobulin test is essential in all cases.

Antibodies against blood group antigens other than ABO or Rh may occur naturally or may be acquired as a result of transfusion or pregnancy. They can cause a hemolytic transfusion reaction or fetal erythroblastosis. The most important of these are anti-Kell (K) and anti-Duffy (Fy^a). Cross-matching will detect almost all such antibodies, though an occasional patient will have a hemolytic reaction despite negative pretransfusion tests.

The **use of "high-titer" Group O blood** refers to the use of any Group O blood, the plasma of which contains Anti-A and Anti-B of the hemolytic or IgG (incomplete) form. This kind of dangerous antibody presents a potential risk when Group O blood must be given in emergencies to a recipient with another blood group. Tests to determine hemolytic or incomplete Anti-A and Anti-B are unreliable. The plasma containing most of the antibody should be removed first. Adding specific A and B substances to Group O blood is not recommended since the dangerous IgG antibodies are not neutralized and the material itself may cause anaphylactic reactions.

Symptoms, Signs, and Diagnosis

Hemolytic reactions vary in severity depending on the degree of incompatibility, the amount of blood given, the rate of administration, and the integrity of the kidney, liver, and heart. Onset is usually acute and may occur during or immediately following a blood transfusion; rarely, later. The patient complains of discomfort and anxiety, or may have no symptoms. Difficulty in breathing, precordial oppression, a bursting sensation in the head, flushing of the face, and severe pain in the neck, the chest, and especially the lumbar area, may be present. Evidence of shock may appear, with a rapid feeble pulse, cold clammy skin, dyspnea, fall in blood pressure, nausea, and vomiting. This acute phase usually develops within 1 h. Free Hb may be found in the plasma and urine, followed by an elevated serum bilirubin and clinical jaundice.

After the acute phase, one of several courses may follow: (1) no further symptoms; (2) temporary oliguria with mild nitrogen retention, then complete recovery; (3) more persistent oliguria, then possibly anuria and uremia, with death in 5 to 14 days. Prolonged oliguria is a poor prognostic sign. When recovery occurs, it is usually marked by diuresis with elimination of retained nitrogenous wastes.

Hemolytic reactions may occur under general anesthesia, when most of the symptoms will be masked. The only evidence may be uncontrollable bleeding at the site of incision and bleeding from mucous membranes, caused by an associated disseminated intravascular coagulation syndrome.

An important quick aid to diagnosis is to take a blood sample from the patient immediately, centrifuge it, and examine it visually for serum Hb. Significant hemolysis will be clearly visible as a pink to dark red color.

For medicolegal reasons, pretransfusion specimens of both the donor's and the patient's blood should be retyped and again cross-matched. Post-transfusion samples from patient and donor blood should also be regrouped and cross-matched again to check on any possible technical or clerical errors or mislabeling of the initial samples.

Prognosis

This depends primarily on the amount of blood given, the degree of incompatibility, and the clinical condition of the patient. Shock at the time of the reaction is a grave prognostic sign. Diuresis is usually a good prognostic sign. Significant permanent kidney damage is unusual.

Prophylaxis

Hemolytic reactions may be avoided by meticulous identification and indelible labeling of patient blood samples intended for cross-matching, and by equally careful identification of donor blood and of the recipient at the time of transfusion. Also important are proper storage of blood; avoidance of warming of blood; allowing 15 min to give the first 50 ml, with close observation for untoward reactions; and careful and complete laboratory procedures to detect incompatibilities. Serious sequelae may be avoided by prompt interruption of the transfusion at the onset of symptoms and adequate treatment.

Treatment

The transfusion should be stopped. Immediate manifestations are treated symptomatically. Blankets may be used to alleviate chill. To establish osmotic diuresis, an infusion of 10% mannitol solution should be started at once and continued at a rate of 10 to 15 ml/min until 1000 ml have been given.

If diuresis ensues, the mannitol infusion should be continued until hemoglobinemia and hemoglobinuria have cleared. If no urine appears, acute renal failure should be suspected and the patient treated accordingly (see §6, Ch. 7).

FEBRILE REACTIONS

Reactions consisting of chills, fever with a rise of at least 1 C, and sometimes headache and back pain, rarely progressing to cyanosis and shock.

In some patients, after many transfusions or pregnancies, leukocyte antibodies appear in response to the antigens of transfused or fetal WBCs. These antibodies may react with the WBCs in succeeding transfusions to produce such a reaction. When these symptoms occur repeatedly with the use of otherwise compatible blood, succeeding transfusions should be attempted with leukocyte-poor or frozen-thawed RBCs. Rarely, febrile reactions can be caused by bacterial pyrogens in solutions or tubing, but these have been almost completely eliminated by the use of disposable infusion sets.

ALLERGIC REACTIONS

Reactions due to hypersensitivity of the patient to an unknown component in the donor's blood. These are common and are usually due to allergens in the donor plasma, or, less often, to the transmission of antibodies from an allergic donor. Immunized IgA-deficient patients may react violently (anaphylaxis) to IgA in donor plasma.

Symptoms and Signs

Allergic reactions are usually mild, with urticaria, edema, occasional dizziness, and headache during or immediately after the transfusion. Less frequently, dyspnea, wheezing, and incontinence may be present, indicating a generalized spasm of smooth muscle. Rarely, anaphylactic shock may occur.

Prophylaxis

When a patient gives a history of known allergies, or has had allergic transfusion reactions, an antihistamine may be given immediately before or at the beginning of the transfusion (e.g., diphenhydramine 50 mg orally or IM). It must never be mixed with the blood.

Treatment

The transfusion must be stopped immediately. An antihistamine is usually sufficient in mild cases (e.g., diphenhydramine 50 mg IM). For more severe reactions, epinephrine 0.5 to 1 ml of 1:1000 solution s.c. (or, in extreme emergencies,

0.05 to 0.2 ml diluted and injected slowly IV) should be given. A parenteral corticosteroid (e.g., dexamethasone sodium phosphate, 4 to 20 mg IV) may occasionally be required.

CIRCULATORY OVERLOADING

In heart disease with chronic anemia, when the cardiac musculature and reserve are likely to be deficient, transfusions may raise the venous pressure and cause heart failure, rapid pulse, falling blood pressure, rapid and shallow breathing, pulmonary edema, and cyanosis.

Prophylaxis

When such patients must be transfused, whole blood is **contraindicated**. A rise in venous pressure can be avoided by giving packed RBCs at a slow-to-moderate rate of infusion. The patient should be observed for evidence of increased venous pressure or pulmonary congestion. If the apparatus is available, direct observation of venous pressure during the course of the infusion is a useful precaution. If packed RBCs cause congestion, or must be given at an unduly slow rate (e.g., more than 2 h/u.), it is better to use washed RBCs. Prolonged transfusions pose a significant hazard of bacterial growth because the blood quickly reaches ambient temperature.

Treatment

The infusion should be discontinued, the patient's head elevated, and tourniquets applied to the extremities. Phlebotomy may be necessary (see in discussion of pulmonary edema in CONGESTIVE HEART FAILURE, §4, Ch. 4). Additional beneficial measures include O_2, morphine (except in cases of severe hypoxia), rapid digitalization when indicated, and warming the patient to increase the capacity of the vascular bed.

AIR EMBOLISM

Transmission of large amounts of air into the vein is potentially dangerous and can cause foaming of blood in the heart with consequent inefficiency of pumping, leading to heart failure. It is largely a complication of pressure infusion of blood from rigid glass bottles, but can also happen when changing IV sets or by erroneously venting a plastic blood bag.

Prophylaxis consists of avoiding air in tubing and being very careful with any pressure infusion and when changing IV sets. **Treatment** involves turning the patient on his left side, head down, to allow the air to escape a little at a time from the right atrium.

MICROAGGREGATES

Standard blood infusion sets include a filter that traps the few visible clots and fibrin shreds present in stored blood units. Recently it has been shown that blood also forms microaggregates during storage. These are microscopic collections of platelets, leukocytes, and fibrin that apparently begin forming during the first few days of blood storage and become more numerous in proportion to the duration of storage. These microaggregates can be detected in the lungs after massive transfusions and have been incriminated as a cause of the syndrome of posttraumatic pulmonary insufficiency, though direct evidence is lacking.

This potential hazard can be avoided by the use of special microaggregate filters which remove particles as small as 20 to 40 μ. Their use is advised only for patients likely to receive very large amounts of blood that has been stored more than 5 or 6 days. CAUTION: *Since these special filters also remove platelets, platelet transfusions should not be passed through them.*

EFFECTS OF COLD

Rapid transfusion of ice-cold blood can chill the patient's heart and cause arrhythmia or arrest. This can be avoided by the use of an IV set that includes a heat exchange device so that blood is warmed gently during delivery. In no case should blood be warmed above 37 C (98.6 F). Warming devices applied to the blood container itself, such as microwave warmers, are not recommended because (1) there is a high incidence of hemolytic effects, (2) any interruption in transfusion may result in warmed blood remaining connected while bacteria grow, and (3) the blood bank has no way of knowing if an unused unit of blood may have been warmed and rechilled.

MASSIVE TRANSFUSION COMPLICATIONS

When a patient receives a very large amount of stored blood in a short time (e.g., more than 20 u. in a day), his own blood is in effect washed out and the deleterious effects of storage on donor blood may become important, though such complications rather seldom occur.

Bleeding tendency is manifested by abnormal oozing and continued bleeding from raw and cut surfaces in association with a low platelet count. The patient has lost most of his platelets, and regular stored blood does not contain useful numbers. Clotting factors other than platelets are seldom involved. Platelet concentrates should therefore be given; four are usually enough for an adult. If these are not available, very freshly collected RBCs will usually be effective (see TABLE 3-4, p. 289). These should not be given to patients on extracorporeal circulation until the pump has been discontinued.

Citrate and potassium: Citrate is primarily of concern in patients with liver failure, who may be unable to metabolize it; potassium, in those with chronic renal disease. These are overrated hazards that are reduced by removal of plasma from donor blood. Potassium accumulation is insignificant in blood stored less than 1 wk (see FIG. 3-2).

OXYGEN AFFINITY

Older stored blood, particularly if collected in Acid Citrate Dextrose, has an increased affinity for O_2 and hence releases O_2 reluctantly to the tissues. This is caused by a decrease in RBC 2,3-diphosphoglycerate **(DPG)**. With the possible exception of exchange transfusions in erythroblastotic babies, there is little clinical evidence that DPG deficiency in stored blood has a significant effect on the recipient, and, in fact, it is rapidly restored after transfusion. RBCs collected in Citrate Phosphate Dextrose have adequate DPG during the first 2 wk of storage (see FIG. 3-1).

INVESTIGATION AND REPORTING OF REACTIONS

All transfusion reactions, even those that seem inconsequential, should be investigated and reported in writing. The investigation can be minimal in minor reactions (e.g., allergic), but should be full and complete for any suspected hemolytic reactions. A scheme of investigation is given in TABLE 3-6. The report may omit laboratory details, although the blood bank should keep a permanent record of these, but it should include an interpretation of results as well as recommendations regarding the handling of future transfusion therapy.

TABLE 3-6. SCHEDULE OF INVESTIGATION OF SUSPECTED TRANSFUSION REACTIONS

1. Specimens needed:
   a. Pretransfusion blood of recipient
   b. Post-transfusion blood of recipient
   c. Pilot samples of donor blood
   d. Blood from container implicated in reaction
   e. Post-transfusion urine

2. Investigation procedures* (letters refer to specimens listed above):

Immediate	Definitive	Corroborative
Examine for visible hemolysis (a, b, d, e)	Repeat cross-match (a, b, c) (major and minor)	Identification of any irregular antibody or incompatibility
Repeat ABO (a, b, c, d)	Repeat antibody screening (a, b, c)	Optional:
Repeat Rh (a, b, c, d)		Haptoglobin (a, b)
Direct antiglobulin test (a, b)	Use special and multiple technics if necessary; e.g., microscopic examination of negatives, prolonged incubation	Methemalbumin (a, b)
Also check cross-match report, donor and patient identification		Bilirubin (b)
		Urea (b)
	Bacteriologic smear and culture (d)	Hemosiderin (c)

* The procedures and specimens listed are applicable to most situations. Circumstances may, of course, vary and require different approaches in particular cases.

Modified from D. W. Huestis et al, Practical Blood Transfusion, ed. 2. Copyright 1976 by J. R. Bove, D. W. Huestis, and S. Busch. Used with permission of Little, Brown and Company and the author.

DISEASE TRANSMISSION

Virus B hepatitis may follow the infusion of whole blood, plasma, or other products prepared from human blood, notably fibrinogen. Serum albumin and plasma protein fraction, which have been heated to 60 C for 10 h during preparation, are, with rare exceptions, noninfectious. Depending on the geographic area and the methods used for testing, **hepatitis B surface antigen** is detectable in the blood of 0.05% to 1 or 2% of donors. In pooled human plasma products such as fibrinogen and antihemophilic factor, it is disseminated in accordance with the size of the pool. It is active in freshly frozen and liquid plasma.

New laboratory tests for hepatitis B surface antigen (now required on all donor blood) permit detection of 30 to 60% of carriers; the remainder are undetectable by present methods. This test will not detect **hepatitis A (infectious)** or other forms of viral hepatitis transmissible by transfusion. Since hepatitis is known to be more prevalent in certain population groups (e.g., drug addicts, commercial blood donors), avoidance of such donors and avoidance of unnecessary transfusions are important preventive measures.

Bacterial infection: Despite careful preparation, from 2 to 5% of all blood drawn contains a few bacteria, presumably from the skin of the donor. Fortunately, most organisms will not grow in blood if it is refrigerated properly (4 to 10 C), but some organisms, mainly the coli-aerogenes group, do grow at these temperatures. Transfusion of heavily contaminated blood may be fatal. Procedures such as allowing blood to reach room temperature, prolonged transfusions, or warming blood may greatly accelerate the growth of any bacteria, and are potentially hazardous.

Malaria is transmitted easily by infected donors, often armed forces or other personnel returning from endemic areas. Many donors are unaware that they have malaria, certain varieties of which may be latent and transmissible for 10 to 15 yr. All prospective donors must be asked whether they have ever had malaria or have been in a region where malaria is prevalent. Donors who have had malaria or suppressive antimalarial therapy are disqualified for 3 yr; those who have been exposed to malaria without suppressive therapy should be deferred for 6 mo. Storage does not render blood safe. Malarial symptoms should be treated appropriately if they appear.

Syphilis may be transmitted by fresh blood from a donor with the disease, but storing the blood for 96 h or more at 4 to 10 C kills the spirochete. An STS is required on all donor blood but, unfortunately, infective donors are often in a seronegative phase.

---

3. POLYCYTHEMIA

POLYCYTHEMIA VERA

A chronic, life-shortening, myeloproliferative disorder involving all bone marrow elements and characterized by an increase in RBC mass (erythrocytosis) and by hemoglobin concentration.

Etiology, Incidence, and Pathophysiology

Polycythemia vera is classified with chronic myelocytic leukemia, myelofibrosis, and thrombocythemia as a **myeloproliferative disease.** The average age at onset is 60 yr, but onset under age 40 occurs infrequently. The incidence is approximately 7:1 million population. Males are more frequently affected than females, and the disease is more common in Jews.

There is hyperplasia of all bone marrow elements (erythrocytes, megakaryocytes, granulocytes, and fibroblasts). Hypervolemia, increased cardiac output, and hyperviscosity and the resultant impaired blood flow are responsible for most clinical manifestations.

With myelofibrosis, a late development, anemia occurs and erythrokinetic patterns show that the total volume of red cells decreases as the result of shortened RBC survival, incompletely compensated by increased synthesis of red cells. Progressive sequestration of RBCs in the spleen is also contributory. As the disease progresses, the central marrow develops fibrosis, but the peripheral marrow (e.g., of the long bones), normally not involved in blood production, shows increased erythropoiesis; extramedullary hemopoiesis in the spleen, liver, and other sites becomes prominent.

Symptoms and Signs

Fatigability, decreased efficiency, difficulty in concentration, headache, drowsiness, forgetfulness, and vertigo are initial complaints, usually of recent onset (6 to 12 mo). Pruritus may be present, particularly after a hot bath. Rubor may be seen or patients may have normal skin color with only dusky redness of the mucous membranes, particularly the conjunctiva. Cyanosis is not present. The retinal veins may be dark red, full, and tortuous. The spleen is usually palpable. Some patients are asymptomatic.

Laboratory Findings

The RBC count ranges from 6 to 10 million/cu mm. Hb levels exceed 18 Gm/100 ml in men and 16 Gm/100 ml in women. The Hct is above 54% in men and 49% in women. The WBC count ranges from normal to 20,000/cu mm; basophilia may be present. The platelet count is usually increased to above 400,000/cu mm. When measured with ^{51}Cr, the RBC mass exceeds 36 ml/kg in men and 32 ml/kg in women, and is sometimes more than twice normal (normal, 28 to 33 ml/kg in men; 24 to 29 ml/kg in women). Since RBC mass is calculated on the basis of height, weight, and body surface area, 20% of the overweight should be added to the ideal weight of obese patients to obtain comparable values on a per kg body weight basis.

Sa$_{O_2}$ is normal. The leukocyte alkaline phosphatase score is above 100 in most patients (normal, 24 to 100). Blood and urine histamine levels are elevated and may be responsible for the pruritus and an increased frequency of peptic ulcer. Serum B$_{12}$ levels may exceed 900 pg/ml (normal, 200 to 900 pg/ml). Unsaturated B$_{12}$ binding capacity may exceed 2200 pg/ml (normal, 900 to 1700 pg/ml).

The bone marrow shows hyperactivity of the RBCs, granulocytes, megakaryocytes, and sometimes fibroblasts; marrow iron is frequently decreased or absent.

Uric acid metabolism is often increased. Serum uric acid levels may be 3 to 4 times normal (normal, 3 to 7 mg/100 ml). Most patients develop hyperuricemia and hyperuricosuria.

Clinical Course

Iron-deficiency anemia and absent marrow iron are common when polycythemia is first diagnosed. If phlebotomy is the only treatment, some degree of iron-deficiency anemia remains following therapy. The development of anemia after treatment indicates blood loss. Blood smears must be inspected for hypochromia and microcytosis, and serum iron levels and total iron-binding capacity should be determined.

Anemia without evidence of iron deficiency is usually an early sign of myelofibrosis, which develops in both untreated and treated patients. An enlarged spleen; distortion of the RBCs into ovoid, elliptical, or tear-shaped cells; leukocytosis of 20,000 to 50,000/cu mm with a shift to the left; appearance of giant platelets with or without thrombosis; and presence of reticulum fibers in the bone marrow are characteristic findings. Bone marrow aspiration may not be possible, but bone marrow biopsy will show fibrosis. Extramedullary hemopoiesis becomes increasingly prominent.

The transition to acute, usually myeloblastic (occasionally erythroblastic) leukemia occurs rarely. The incidence is greater in patients treated with ^{32}P than in those treated by phlebotomy. It occurs also in patients receiving chemotherapy, though reliable statistics are not yet available. Anemia may follow the development of acute leukemia. The blood smear shows many bizarre blast cells. The anemia becomes progressively more severe and the bone marrow shows diffuse infiltration with malignant cells. Death usually occurs in a few weeks.

Thromboses, CVAs, and gastrointestinal hemorrhages may develop, especially in untreated patients. The frequency of peptic ulcer is increased. Gouty arthritis occurs in less than 10% of the patients, mostly in the later stages of the disease, and may be accompanied by the development of uric acid kidney stones. Hemorrhage is a frequent surgical complication. If possible, patients should be in hematologic remission before surgery. Blood loss at surgery is replaced by whole blood transfusions.

Patients with polycythemia are medically (though not always legally) acceptable as blood donors. Recipients have the benefit of the relatively high Hcts.

Diagnosis

Polycythemia vera must be considered in any man with a Hct above 54% and any woman with a Hct above 49%. Before evaluation, patients should have been off diuretics for at least 2 wk, must not have been in congestive heart failure or living at altitudes above 7000 ft recently, and must not be taking male hormones. Minimal criteria for diagnosis are an elevated RBC mass, an Sa_{O_2} above 92%, and an enlarged spleen. If the spleen is not enlarged, leukocytosis (especially basophilia) and elevations in the platelet count, leukocyte alkaline phosphatase score, serum vitamin B_{12} level, or B_{12}-binding capacity should be present.

Prognosis

Treatment reduces symptoms and appears to prolong life by reducing the incidence of thrombosis and hemorrhage. Adequately treated patients may remain in complete clinical and hematologic remission for many years, but complications usually develop after 5 to 10 yr. Average survival time with treatment is about 13 yr. Death is usually due to myelofibrosis, acute leukemia, or diseases of old age.

Treatment

Phlebotomy is probably the safest therapy. It does not depress marrow function and is not mutagenic. Symptoms of hypervolemia are eliminated, but pruritus and symptoms of uric acid hypermetabolism remain. Iron-deficiency anemia may persist or develop following repeated phlebotomy. Phlebotomy is not as effective in patients with high iron absorption rates or greatly elevated platelet counts (more than 1.5 million/cu mm), and is inconvenient in patients with poor veins.

Usually, 3 to 6 phlebotomies are required to reduce the Hct to below 50% and to return the RBC mass to normal. Most patients can tolerate a 500-ml phlebotomy 3 times/wk, but elderly patients with advanced arteriosclerosis or cardiac complications should have no more than 250 ml of blood removed at a time. Following the initial series of phlebotomies, the Hct should be maintained at 42 to 47%, if possible. The number of phlebotomies needed depends on the patient's ability to absorb iron and thereby raise the Hct again. Since 1 pint of blood contains 250 mg of iron, a patient who absorbs 4 mg/day will need a phlebotomy every 2 mo; a patient who absorbs only 1.5 mg/day will need only 2 phlebotomies/yr. The average is 4/yr.

When phlebotomy is the only therapy, supplemental iron must *not* be given since it accelerates Hb production. A low-iron diet is impractical, but certain foods of very high iron content (e.g., clams, oysters, liver, legumes) should be avoided.

Phlebotomy followed by **radiophosphorus (^{32}P)** produces clinical and hematologic remission in almost all patients and eliminates all symptoms. Remissions usually last 18 mo, but vary from 6 mo to several years. Fewer follow-up visits are required and there are no immediate side effects, though about 10% of patients treated with ^{32}P develop acute leukemia, usually not until after more than 10 yr of treatment.

Initially, 3 to 5 mCi (or 2.3 mCi/sq m BSA) of ^{32}P are given IV; if given orally, the dose should be increased 25%. The patient is seen at 3- to 4-wk intervals until remission is achieved. Platelets should begin to decrease in 2 wk, reaching a low point in 3 to 5 wk; RBCs usually begin to decrease in 1 mo, reaching a low point 3 to 4 mo after treatment. If there is no decrease in platelets or RBCs within 3 mo of initial treatment, an additional 2 to 3 mCi of ^{32}P are given. A 25% increase in dose is given 6 mo after initial treatment if there is still no remission. Once the blood counts have returned to normal, patients are reexamined every 3 mo. The total initial effective dose is given at one time when relapse occurs.

Phlebotomy followed by **chemotherapy** relieves all symptoms and returns blood counts to normal in most cases. Great individual variations in response make frequent follow-up visits necessary, however, and the risk of overtreatment is greater than with ^{32}P or phlebotomy. Severe leukopenia and thrombocytopenia may develop before RBC values have fallen to normal levels.

Initially, therapy is given daily. When the Hct has stabilized between 45 and 50% for 2 mo without phlebotomy and the platelet count is less than 600,000/cu mm, maintenance therapy is instituted. Therapy is interrupted if remission is achieved (i.e., the Hct falls below 45%); remission may last for over a year without maintenance therapy. Chlorambucil 10 mg/day for 6 wk or cyclophosphamide 100 to 150 mg/day is given initially. Maintenance doses for chlorambucil are 6 to 10 mg/day for 4 wk, alternated with no therapy for 4 wk; those for cyclophosphamide are 50 to 75 mg/day. Another treatment schedule is melphalan 4 to 6 mg/day until a total of 1 mg/kg body wt has been reached. Thereafter, 2 mg or less are given daily.

Gouty arthritis is treated as for primary gout. Hyperuricemia requires treatment with allopurinol.

OTHER CAUSES OF POLYCYTHEMIA

For characteristic findings in some of the polycythemias, see TABLE 3-7.

In **stress polycythemia (stress erythrocytosis),** the Hct is persistently elevated to 55 to 60%. Plasma volume, measured with ^{131}I-labeled albumin, is usually decreased to 36 to 41 ml/kg (normal, 44 ml/kg in men; 43 ml/kg in women). The RBC mass, measured with ^{51}Cr, is at the upper limits of normal. Stress erythrocytosis is not true polycythemia and does not require therapy.

Erythrocytosis secondary to arterial hypoxemia (secondary polycythemia) may be due to an arteriovenous shunt, pulmonary fibrosis, altitude hypoxia, and the pickwickian syndrome. At rest, Sa_{O_2} may be slightly decreased in polycythemia vera and normal in cardiopulmonary disease or respiratory alkalosis. Measured after exercise however, Sa_{O_2} rises in patients with polycythemia vera and decreases in those with secondary polycythemia. After breathing 100% O_2, P_{O_2} values exceed 500 mm Hg in polycythemia vera but are under 400 mm Hg in secondary polycythemia. Sa_{O_2} may be particularly misleading in patients with respiratory alkalosis. Because the pH is above 7.4, the O_2 dissociation curve shifts to the left and Sa_{O_2} may be nearly normal despite depressed Pa_{O_2}. (See TABLE 3-8.) RBC mass is increased in both polycythemia vera and secondary polycythemia.

Tissue hypoxia and erythrocytosis occur in patients with some rare **hemoglobinopathies** associated with high O_2 affinity and a shift to the left in the O_2 dissocia-

TABLE 3-7. CHARACTERISTIC FINDINGS IN SOME OF THE POLYCYTHEMIAS

	Hct	RBC Mass	Plasma Volume	Spleen	Arterial Oxygen	Erythropoietin Production
Polycythemia vera	↑	↑	N	Enlarged	N	↓
Stress polycythemia	↑	N	↓	N	N	N
Secondary polycythemia (anoxia)	↑	↑	N	N	↓	↑
Secondary polycythemia (tumor)	↑	↑	N	N	N	↑

N = Normal; ↑ = increased; ↓ = decreased.

TABLE 3-8. ARTERIAL O_2 VALUES IN POLYCYTHEMIA VERA AND HYPOXIA

	Normal		Polycythemia Vera		Hypoxia	
	Mean	Range	Mean	Range	Mean	Range
Sa_{O_2}(%)						
Rest	96	93–97	94	90–96	85	71–92
Exercise	96	92–97	94.5	92–96	77	60–95
Pa_{O_2} (mm Hg)						
Rest	88	67–97	71	64–80	55	43–63
Exercise	88	67–100	75	66–83	44	32–59

tion curve. A patient with apparent polycythemia who is very young or has a family history of erythrocytosis should be suspected of having a hemoglobinopathy. The diagnosis can usually be confirmed by Hb electrophoresis.

Renal cysts and tumors are associated with erythrocytosis in less than 5% of patients with an increased RBC mass. Removal of the lesions is curative.

Rarer causes of erythrocytosis include large uterine myomas, cerebellar angioblastoma, and hepatoma. Platelet and WBC counts are not increased and the spleen is not enlarged. The increased production of RBCs is probably due to excessive elaboration of erythropoietin.

---

4. HEMORRHAGIC DISORDERS

Disorders characterized by a tendency to bleed.

The combined activity of vascular, platelet, and plasma factors is required for effective hemostasis. Counterbalancing mechanisms to inhibit or control coagulation are also necessary to prevent unwanted or excessive clotting. Abnormalities in any of these components or the presence of circulating inhibitors affect the clotting process and the ability to control hemorrhage.

Physiology

In the **vascular phase,** blood flow is reduced at the site of trauma by two mechanisms: (1) local vasoconstriction, which is an immediate reaction to injury, and (2) mechanical pressure on the injured vessels from the extravasation of blood into the surrounding tissues.

The **platelet phase** begins within seconds: the platelet plays a central role in hemostasis by adhering to and plugging sites of injury and releasing factors that initiate clotting via the intrinsic system. Circulating platelets are ordinarily nonadherent to each other or to normal endothelium. Their unique properties relate to changes which occur when the endothelium is broken. Under these circumstances, the platelets adhere to collagen and vascular surfaces; subsequently, adenosine diphosphate **(ADP)** is released from the platelet storage granules, resulting in platelet aggregation. This induces the formation of a small plug or platelet thrombus at the site of injury. During this phase, release of platelet phospholipids **(platelet factor 3)** initiates activation of the intrinsic system, and release of the platelet vasoactive substance **serotonin** produces a local vasoconstriction, slowing blood flow.

The **coagulation phase** involves interaction of a number of plasma proteins **(coagulation factors)** in addition to thromboplastin and calcium. The various factors are designated by Roman numerals as seen in TABLE 3-9, although earlier

TABLE 3-9. COAGULANTS AND PROCOAGULANTS*

Factor	Comments
I. Fibrinogen	Precursor of fibrin (polymerized protein) which forms the clot structure.
II. Prothrombin	Precursor of the proteolytic enzyme thrombin (converts fibrinogen to fibrin) and perhaps other accelerators of prothrombin conversion.
III. Thromboplastin	A tissue lipoprotein activator of prothrombin.
IV. Calcium	Necessary for prothrombin activation and fibrin formation. Magnesium and other ions may replace calcium.
V. Accelerator globulin (AcG)	Factor VI is assumed to be the active form. The rapid destruction of the factor (VI) by thrombin does not permit identification of the activity in serum.
VII. Serum prothrombin conversion accelerator (SPCA, convertin, stabile factor)	A serum factor, part of the prothrombin complex produced in the liver. Vitamin K-dependent. Accelerates prothrombin conversion by interaction with thromboplastin. Adsorbed with $BaSO_4$, decreased by dicumarol.
VIII. Antihemophilic globulin (Cofactor I, AHG)	A plasma factor interacting with platelet factor 3 and factor IX to initiate prothrombin activation. Labile on standing, destroyed by thrombin, not present in serum.
IX. Plasma thromboplastin component (PTC, Christmas factor)	A serum factor associated with platelet factor 3 and AHG. Activates prothrombin in the presence of thromboplastin. Stabile on standing, adsorbed with $BaSO_4$, decreased by dicumarol.
X. Stuart-Prower factor	A plasma and serum factor. Accelerator of prothrombin conversion, adsorbed with $BaSO_4$, decreased by dicumarol. (X_a, the active form, amplifies thrombin formation.)
XI. Plasma thromboplastin antecedent (PTA)	A plasma factor which is activated by Hageman factor, an accelerator of thrombin formation.
XII. Hageman factor (glass factor)	A plasma factor activated by glass, kaolin, perhaps fatty acids; activates PTA (XI).
XIII. Fibrin stabilizing factor	A plasma factor with transamidase activity. Produces a stronger fibrin that is insoluble in urea.
Fitzgerald factor (high mol wt kininogen)	Interacts with factor XII. Kinins are vasoactive and influence leukocyte migration.
Fletcher factor (prekallikrein)	Interacts with factor XII and Fitzgerald factor.

*The subscript ($_a$) designates the active forms of VII-XIII.

terminology remains in use for fibrinogen, prothrombin, thromboplastin, and calcium (factors I-IV). Several theories have been offered to describe the conversion of prothrombin to thrombin. One of these, the cascade or waterfall theory, depicts a sequence of events initiated by activation of factor XII (Hageman factor) to its active form, XII_a, by contact with foreign surfaces (collagen). A sequential activation of the other factors, XI, VIII, IX, X, and V in the presence of platelet factor 3 leads eventually to the activation of prothrombin to thrombin via what is known as the **intrinsic pathway**. Thrombin formation also is initiated by tissue substances outside the bloodstream released from areas of injury or tissue breakdown. This is referred to as the **extrinsic pathway** (see FIG. 3-3). Both pathways

Extrinsic System: (Prothrombin Time)

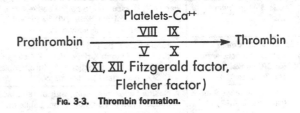

Intrinsic System: (Partial Thromboplastin Time)

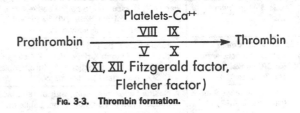

Fig. 3-3. Thrombin formation.

require calcium and factors V and X, and in final phase produce activation of factor X to factor X_a, which mediates thrombin formation. The intrinsic pathway also requires factors VIII and IX and is sensitive to the activated forms of XI and XII, and to two recently discovered factors, Fitzgerald and Fletcher factors, which interact with the kallikrein and kinin system. The extrinsic pathway is dependent upon factor VII and is not influenced by contact activation; i.e., factor XII.

Fibrin formation from fibrinogen is the next step in the coagulation phase. It is a thrombin-dependent reaction, as seen in Fig. 3-4, resulting from the separation of the small A and B peptides from the α, β, and γ double strands of the fibrinogen molecule produced by the proteolytic action of thrombin. The small fragments interfere with thrombin activity, acting as an antithrombin or inhibitor of blood coagulation. This tends to limit the size of the clot formed. The large fragments, the fibrin monomers, combine to form a gel which, in the presence of factor XIII (the fibrin stabilizing factor) and calcium, becomes a structured fibrin clot providing permanent hemostasis.

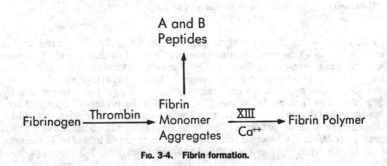

Fig. 3-4. Fibrin formation.

Clot retraction, which takes place subsequently, is produced by a contractile protein (thrombasthenin) contained in platelets entrapped in the clot. The retracted clot is less friable and less likely to be dislodged by circulation.

The **fibrinolysin system** becomes operative when the three phases of coagulation are completed. The purpose of the system is clot resolution. As seen in Fig. 3-5, circulating profibrinolysin (plasminogen) can be activated to the proteolytic enzyme fibrinolysin (plasmin) by a number of substances derived from tissues, by bacterial products (streptokinase), or by the plasma factor XII after contact with collagen. A potent activator, urokinase, is found in the urine and may represent an excretory product of the activator. (Concentrates of urokinase have been used therapeutically in thrombotic disorders to lyse clots.) Interaction of the fibrinolysin enzyme with fibrinogen or fibrin results in the breakdown of these molecules and formation of distinct fragments designated "X" and "Y" which have anti-

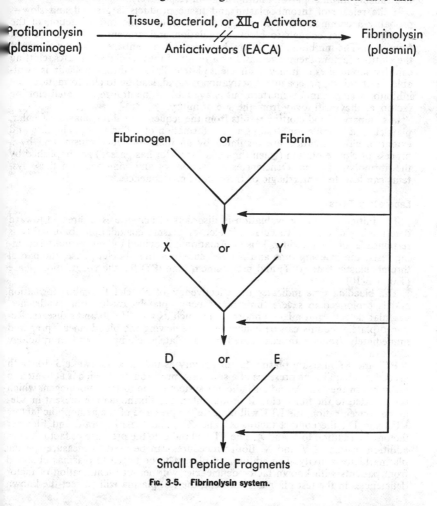

Fig. 3-5. Fibrinolysin system.

thrombin activity. This activity apparently exerts feedback inhibition on the original clot-promoting process. With further exposure to fibrinolysin the X and Y fragments are degraded into much smaller peptides designated "D" and "E."

Inhibitors of the coagulation system are naturally occurring and include **antithromboplastin, antithrombin,** and **antifibrinolysin.** The antithrombin (called antithrombin III) is the physiologic circulating inhibitor of thrombin and is present in sufficient quantities to neutralize all of the thrombin activity which can develop in plasma. Several other sources of antithrombin activity have been described. These are: (1) the adsorption of thrombin onto fibrin, (2) the activity of fibrinogen and fibrin degradation (split) products (see below), and (3) the heparin-facilitating plasma protein known as the **heparin cofactor.** The other naturally occurring inhibitors, antithromboplastin and antifibrinolysin, have similar capabilities for neutralizing thromboplastin and fibrinolysin respectively.

If the release of thromboplastin and tissue products is gradual and slow—probably a common occurrence *unrelated* to injury—the rate of action of the inhibitors is fast enough to block coagulation and prevent inappropriate clot formation. The inhibitors act slowly, however, when compared with the action of the clotting factors themselves, and as a result of these differential rates, clotting can develop at sites of injury if sufficient platelet lipid or thromboplastin is available. With injury, procoagulant activation is rapid, leading to clot formation; the inhibitor system cannot interfere but is available to neutralize activated clotting factors as they drift away from the site of injury.

In summary, blood clotting results from the sequence of three phases, vascular, platelet, and coagulation, leading to the formation of a fibrin clot. The rate and extent of clot formation are regulated by an inhibitory mechanism, and by a process of clot resolution (when the need for a clot has passed) accomplished by the fibrinolytic system. Deficiencies or excesses of any component of these systems can lead to hemorrhagic or thrombotic consequences.

Laboratory Tests

The initial laboratory evaluation in disorders of hemostasis is directed toward determining whether a vascular, platelet, or plasma coagulation abnormality is responsible for the bleeding. This information is provided by four primary screening tests: the **bleeding time** and **platelet count** for the platelet phase, the **partial thromboplastin time (PTT)** and **prothrombin time (PT)** for the coagulation phase (TABLE 3-10).

The **bleeding time** indicates the effectiveness of platelet thrombus formation and is prolonged in severe thrombocytopenia, platelet dysfunction syndromes, vascular defects, and mixed abnormalities such as von Willebrand's disease. Reduced platelet counts can be confirmed by reviewing the blood smear, prepared immediately from unanticoagulated blood. Platelet clumping and morphology also can be noted.

PTT and **PT** measure plasma factor activity as indicated in TABLE 3-10. Both procedures require the presence of a substrate, prothrombin (which is activated to thrombin in the assay), and an indicator system in the form of fibrinogen, which is converted to the fibrin clot. If prothrombin and fibrinogen are present in adequate concentration, the PTT will indicate the presence of the hemophilic factors VIII and IX, the contact factors XI and XII, and the Fitzgerald and Fletcher factors, in addition to V and X. The PT will indicate the presence of factor VII in addition to factors V and X. Both procedures can be used to measure specific plasma factor activity. The addition of plasma to be tested to plasmas obtained from patients with known factor deficiencies will permit identification of factor deficiencies in the test plasma. If present, the test plasma will correct the known

TABLE 3-10. CLASSIFICATION OF COAGULATION LABORATORY TESTS

Coagulation Function or Phase	Test	Comments
Vascular and/or platelet function	Tourniquet test (Rumpel-Leede)	May indicate vascular fragility or thrombocytopenia
	Bleeding time (Ivy)	Requires platelet function (both clot retraction and platelet factor 3 release)
	Platelet count (or estimate)	Quantitation of platelet number
	Clot retraction	Measures thrombasthenin-ATP* activity
	Platelet aggregation	Mechanical procedure to determine platelet response to added ADP**, collagen, and epinephrine
	Prothrombin consumption	Measures release of platelet factor 3
Plasma factor function	Prothrombin time (PT)	Measures extrinsic system activity (factors VII, X, V, II, and I)
	Partial thromboplastin time (PTT)	Measures intrinsic system activity (factors VIII, IX, XI, XII, V, X, II, I, Fitzgerald, and Fletcher)
	Specific assays for fibrinogen, factors V-XII	
	Two-stage prothrombin assay	Measures prothrombin quantitatively
Fibrinolytic activity	Euglobulin lysis time	Measures profibrinolysin and activators
	Fibrin plate lysis	Measures profibrinolysin, fibrinolysin, and activators
Antithrombin activity (heparin)	Thrombin clotting time (TCT)	Measures antithrombin activity (heparin) and can be modified to measure fibrinogen levels
Fibrin (fdp) and fibrinogen (FDP) degradation products (collectively designated as split products or FSP)	Protamine sulfate assay	Measures products of thrombin-induced degradation of fibrinogen
	Staphylococcal clumping	Measures products of thrombin- or fibrinolysin-induced degradation of fibrin or fibrinogen
	Immune assay	Also measures products of thrombin- or fibrinolysin-induced degradation of fibrin or fibrinogen

* Adenosine triphosphate.
** Adenosine diphosphate.

deficient plasma; if absent, it will not. It is possible by this means to obtain a quantitative measurement of each factor by determining the PT or PTT with varying mixtures of test and known deficient plasmas comparing values to a reference curve created by using mixtures of normal and deficient plasmas.

The terms **"fibrin split products"** (FSP) and **"fibrin, or fibrinogen, degradation products"** (fdp or FDP) are synonymous. They refer to any fragment resulting from the enzymatic cleavage of fibrin or fibrinogen by either fibrinolysin or thrombin. They include the fibrin monomer, X, Y, D, and E fragments, and many unnamed polypeptides. The *laboratory test* designated "FSP" (fibrin split products) customarily refers to detection of the fibrin monomer resulting from thrombin's action on fibrinogen, and as such, it is positive in, and pathognomonic of, DIC (see Disseminated Intravascular Coagulation, below). The presence of increased **fibrinolysin** activity is determined by measuring the lysis time of the euglobulin fraction of blood **(euglobulin lysis time)**. "Euglobulin" is an amorphous coagulum of various plasma proteins which precipitate out of plasma when the latter is acidified slightly with acetic acid. The euglobulin fraction contains most of the fibrinolysin originally present in the whole plasma, whereas the antifibrinolysin remains in the supernatant. With fibrinolytic activity separated from antifibrinolytic, the former can act quickly to degrade any adjacent proteins, in this case the euglobulin gel which has entrapped the fibrinolysin. The time for the euglobulin gel to visibly lyse is called the "lysis time," normally about 1½ to 2 h, and the test can measure increased fibrinolytic activity (shortened lysis times).

Other tests of blood coagulation of value for specific purposes are listed in Table 3-10. Further information on the bleeding time, clot retraction, coagulation time, platelet count, PTT, PT, FDP, and tourniquet test, including methods of performing these and other tests, can be found under Clinical Hematology in §24, Ch. 2. Table 3-10 in this section categorizes the coagulation studies in accordance with the function or phase of coagulation they test.

VASCULAR DISORDERS

These disorders seldom lead to serious blood loss. The tourniquet test may be positive, but other laboratory tests of hemostasis and blood coagulation are usually normal; diagnosis must frequently be made from associated clinical findings which are often characteristic.

Vascular Fragility

The most common vascular disorder leading to mild hemorrhagic manifestations is an increase in vascular fragility. This is an inherited condition and is more common in women, particularly after the menopause. It results in unsightly bruising tendencies, but rarely significant hemorrhage. The bleeding pattern is usually subcutaneous, and occasionally mucosal. Enhanced surgical or traumatic bleeding also can occur. Vascular fragility can appear transiently as a result of fever, generalized illness, or exposure to certain drugs, especially aspirin. The defect is in the small vessels; however, qualitative platelet disorders can produce apparent increased vascular fragility due to the very close association of platelet and small vessel function.

Laboratory findings reveal a positive tourniquet test and a normal or prolonged bleeding time. Other coagulation studies are normal. No effective therapy exists. Brief courses of corticosteroids may assist in reducing surgical or traumatic bleeding. Estrogen may be effective, particularly if the patient is postmenopausal.

ALLERGIC PURPURA
(Henoch-Schönlein or Anaphylactoid Purpura)

An acute or chronic vasculitis primarily affecting skin, joints, and the gastrointestinal and renal systems. It results from the effusion of blood and plasma into the subcutaneous, submucous, and subserous surfaces. The process is believed to be a result of an immune reaction, often following streptococcal infection, which damages the vascular endothelium. Skin lesions vary in appearance, but purpura is usually associated with erythema or urticaria. In contrast to other purpuras, the lesions may be pruritic. Fever and malaise are often present, and effusions into the joints or viscera may produce joint pain **(Schönlein's purpura)** or bouts of abdominal pain **(Henoch's purpura)**. The latter may mimic acute abdominal conditions. Acute glomerulitis associated with hematuria may lead to a severe renal disorder and death.

Laboratory findings are useful only to exclude other disorders. The diagnosis is largely based on recognition of the conglomerate of clinical findings. Except for the elimination of possible allergens, **treatment** is primarily symptomatic. Corticosteroids are usually disappointing. Immunosuppressive therapy (cyclophosphamide) has been used in a few cases with some success. The disease is often self-limited and carries a good prognosis.

HEREDITARY HEMORRHAGIC TELANGIECTASIA
(Rendu-Osler-Weber Syndrome)

A vascular anomaly characterized by telangiectatic lesions of the skin and mucosa, inherited as an autosomal dominant trait. The small red to violet lesions consist of thin, dilated vessels which blanch on pressure and tend to bleed spontaneously or as a result of trivial trauma; they are usually found on the lips, oral and nasal mucosa, tongue, and the tips of the fingers and toes. The symptoms are the result of bleeding and the consequent anemia, in general becoming progressively more severe with advancing age. Bleeding from superficial lesions may be profuse; bleeding from mucosal lesions (epistaxis and gastrointestinal bleeding) is more common and more serious. Rarely, involvement of visceral vessels may lead to systemic symptoms (e.g., pulmonary arteriovenous fistulas).

Laboratory studies are usually normal but may disclose evidence of acute hemorrhage or iron-deficiency anemia. Diagnosis depends on recognition of the characteristic lesions. If these are lacking or are overlooked, perplexing diagnostic problems may result, such as protracted and recurrent gastrointestinal bleeding of "unknown" etiology.

No specific **treatment** is known. However, estrogens administered systemically and corticosteroid nasal sprays have been effective, the latter for nasal mucosal bleeding. Accessible lesions may be treated with pressure, styptics, and topical hemostatics. Blood transfusions may be needed for acute hemorrhage. Iron therapy is frequently required on a continuous basis to correct the iron-deficiency anemia which develops with repeated bleeding.

MISCELLANEOUS VASCULAR PURPURAS

Hemorrhage may be a prominent manifestation of **scurvy.** Bleeding gums, perifollicular petechiae on the thighs and buttocks, and large IM or internal hemorrhages may be seen. Periosteal hemorrhages are characteristic in children. For therapy see VITAMIN C DEFICIENCY in §11, Ch. 3.

Autoerythrocyte sensitization (Gardner-Diamond syndrome) is characterized by spontaneous painful propagating ecchymoses which represent an immune reaction to the patient's erythrocyte stroma; they may be reproduced by the intradermal injection of the patient's erythrocytes. Psychoneurotic disorders have been found to be associated with this condition. Purpura associated with hypergammaglobulinemia also has been described and may be related to various collagen disorders or dysproteinemias. A vasculitis often is apparent. Correction of the underlying disease produces improvement. Corticosteroids may be helpful.

PLATELET DISORDERS

Platelet disorders can be considered in terms of a deficiency, either of numbers **(thrombocytopenia)** or of function **(thrombocytopathy).**

THROMBOCYTOPENIA

Disorders manifested by thrombocytopenia can be characterized by failure of production, increased destruction, increased utilization, or dilution, as outlined in TABLE 3-11. The **symptoms and signs** of all these conditions include bleeding into the skin (petechiae, ecchymoses) and mucosal bleeding (epistaxis; gastrointestinal tract, genitourinary, and vaginal bleeding). Bleeding into the CNS is uncommon as an early manifestation, while hemarthroses and delayed bleeding, characteristic of plasma factor deficiency, are rare. Splenomegaly, hepatomegaly, and lymphadenopathy are not ordinarily seen unless other disorders are responsible for the thrombocytopenia (Hodgkin's disease, lymphosarcoma, Gaucher's disease, etc.). As a result of bleeding, anemia may develop and lead to symptoms of weakness, fatigue, and signs of congestive heart failure. The clinical course is varied, ranging from mild petechial eruptions which may escape notice to severe and intractable bleeding. Placental transfer of maternal antiplatelet antibodies may cause thrombocytopenia and purpura in the neonate.

Laboratory findings are the same regardless of the etiology: a positive tourniquet test, a prolonged bleeding time, delayed prothrombin consumption, and deficient clot retraction. However, these tests are seldom necessary if an accurate platelet count has been obtained. Other coagulation assays are normal, unless the

TABLE 3-11. CHARACTERISTICS OF THROMBOCYTOPENIC DISORDERS

Production Failure (Megakaryocytopenia)	Increased Destruction (Megakaryocytosis)	Increased Utilization (Megakaryocytosis)	Dilution
Marrow hypoplasia: Idiopathic Irradiation Drugs (antineoplastic, benzene compounds, chloramphenicol, etc.) Infection (TB, septicemia, etc.)	**Immune:** ITP* Drugs (quinine, quinidine, thiazides, sulfonamides) Post-transfusion (antibodies to platelet antigen PL-A1)	**DIC† syndromes:** Gram-negative septicemia (Schwartzman-Sanorelli reaction) HUS‡ TTP§ Hemangiomas Neoplasms Burn injury Traumatic injuries	**Massive blood replacement or exchange transfusion** (stored blood rapidly becomes platelet-poor)
Marrow displacement: Fibrosis (agnogenic myeloid metaplasia) Neoplasm Lymphoma Granuloma (TB, sarcoid, etc.)	**Hypersplenic:** Lymphoma Leukemia Agnogenic myeloid metaplasia Gaucher's disease		
Marrow diversion and dyspoiesis: Leukemia Folic acid and B_{12} deficiency	**Toxic:** Alcohol Snake venom **Mechanical:** Extracorporeal circulation (renal dialysis, open heart procedures)		

* Idiopathic thrombocytopenia purpura.
† Disseminated intravascular coagulation.
‡ Hemolytic-uremic syndrome.
§ Thrombotic thrombocytopenic purpura.

thrombocytopenia is associated with another condition such as liver disease or disseminated intravascular coagulation.

The bone marrow aspirate is of value in excluding marrow failure due to a decrease or absence of megakaryocytes. Frequently the marrow will demonstrate displacement of megakaryocytes by tumor or fibrosis, or diversion of marrow production as seen in leukemia. More commonly seen, however, is a hypoplastic condition characterized by increased marrow fat and a marked decrease in all cellular elements. Some drugs which cause production failure (see TABLE 3-11) and various toxic or infectious agents may be implicated in the latter condition, although many cases without known exposure to toxic substances remain classified as idiopathic.

Management of thrombocytopenia caused by marrow damage or failure may require administration of platelet concentrates. Androgens have been advocated in hypoplastic disorders, primarily for stimulating erythropoiesis. Corticosteroids have not been shown to be effective in this form of thrombocytopenia.

IDIOPATHIC THROMBOCYTOPENIC PURPURA
(ITP; Purpura Hemorrhagica; Werlhof's Disease)

Thrombocytopenia in which no exogenous etiologic factor or underlying disease is readily apparent is the most common form of thrombocytopenia and is characterized by platelet destruction. No specific etiology has been identified, although occasionally an acute viral infection has been noted preceding the symptoms. Platelet antibodies have been identified, although not consistently. Infusions of plasma from patients with the disorder have produced thrombocytopenia in normal subjects. Symptoms, signs, and laboratory findings are as described above. The bone marrow aspirate generally reveals an abundance of megakaryocytes, most of which appear inactive or nonproductive.

The disorder occasionally is self-limited. Most of the adult forms, however, require therapy. About 25% will respond to corticosteroids (hydrocortisone 200 mg/day, or its equivalent, for 2 to 4 wk) and will not require continued steroid support. Splenectomy will achieve a remission in another 50%. Immunosuppressive therapy (cyclophosphamide and azathioprine) has been used effectively in some cases refractory to steroids and splenectomy. Recent reports also indicate vincristine to be of value. Administration of platelet concentrates may be necessary to control bleeding while awaiting the effects of more specific therapy.

OTHER FORMS OF THROMBOCYTOPENIA

Other forms of thrombocytopenia resulting from increased platelet destruction are noted in TABLE 3-11. Specific drugs (such as quinine, quinidine, and chlorothiazide) appear to mediate the formation of platelet antibodies. When the drug is stopped, platelet values return to normal usually within 1 wk. A direct toxic effect appears to be responsible for the thrombocytopenia of acute alcoholic intoxication. Specific viral disease such as measles, infectious mononucleosis, etc., may be responsible for the nonidiopathic type often seen in the younger age group in which spontaneous remissions can be expected; in some cases collagen disorders such as SLE can be identified.

Thrombocytopenia as a result of **hypersplenism** (destruction of sequestered platelets in the enlarged spleen) can be found in association with disorders which produce splenomegaly (see Ch. 9, below). Splenectomy is the only effective measure in these conditions although transient responses may be observed with therapy (irradiation, chemotherapy, corticosteroids) that reduces the size of the spleen.

Increased platelet destruction is prominent in the syndrome of **disseminated intravascular coagulation** (see below). This pattern appears in the **hemolytic-uremic syndrome (HUS)**, but is not as well-defined in **thrombotic thrombocytopenic purpura (TTP)** where antigen-antibody complex and complement appear to play a more prominent role. In both conditions, shortened erythrocyte survival can be demonstrated and occasionally the Coombs test for antiglobulins is positive. HUS and TTP differ primarily in the age of presentation and in organ system involvement. HUS is a disease of childhood, occurring with greatest frequency in infants less than 1 yr old. HUS is characterized by acute renal failure, with thrombocytopenia and hemolytic anemia developing a few days after the onset of gastrointestinal symptoms. Pallor, lethargy, hepatomegaly, and hypertension are common findings. The blood shows classic signs of fragmentation hemolysis. Although fibrin degradation products can be found in the urine and serum, major consumption of clotting factors does not occur. Hematuria and proteinuria are usually present. The major histologic findings in HUS are collapsed capillary loops in the glomeruli and partial to complete occlusion of vascular lumens. The vascular changes correlate well with the clinical presentation. When prolonged oliguria, anuria, and/or hypertension are present, renal vessels show severe lesions; in their absence, the vessels are normal. Renal function improves within 1 mo in most patients. The effect of glucocorticoids or anticoagulants has been controversial. Heparin therapy has been advocated by some clinicians.

TTP shows a predilection toward multiple organ involvement, whereas HUS involves the blood and the kidneys primarily. TTP occurs most commonly in young adults, with a higher incidence in women, and produces severe renal involvement in over 50% of cases. Neurologic complications are common, apparently the result of a diffuse vasculitis, and are a frequent cause of death. The disease is fulminant with death occurring in 80% of the cases within 3 mo. In contrast to HUS, renal failure occurs rather late in TTP. The hematologic findings are similar to those described for HUS although hemorrhagic complications are more common. Renal involvement is present in most patients and manifests as proteinuria, hematuria, and various casts.

The most conspicuous histologic feature is the presence of thrombi in renal afferent arterioles or, occasionally, in terminal intralobular arteries. Similar material may be found in the glomerular capillaries. Renal arterioles may show a conspicuous proliferation of endothelial cells. Tubular and interstitial changes are minimal and variable.

Unlike HUS, TTP is almost universally fatal. Recent studies have demonstrated that disseminated platelet thrombi are the underlying lesion and the blood clotting system is secondarily involved. Attempts at treatment of this lesion with corticosteroids, dextran, anticoagulants, and splenectomy have had limited success. Antiplatelet drugs (dipyridamole and aspirin) in large doses recently have been shown to be beneficial in some cases.

ABNORMALITIES OF PLATELET FUNCTION

In some patients the platelets are normal in number but functionally defective. Both congenital and acquired defects have been described; in addition, a variety of commonly used drugs has also been shown to inhibit platelet function. As a result, the bleeding time is usually prolonged. This finding in a patient who gives a history of easy bruising and bleeding after tooth extractions, tonsillectomy, and other surgical procedures should suggest the possibility of a qualitative platelet defect. Most other routine screening tests, such as the prothrombin, partial thromboplastin, and clotting times, will be normal and will help to differentiate these patients from those with defects in the coagulation mechanism. Since platelets play a role in the coagulation mechanism, an abnormal prothrombin consumption of clotted blood is sometimes found, and special studies may disclose that the platelet clotting activity (platelet factor 3) is defective. Special studies, which may not be performed in routine laboratories, may be required to demonstrate the presence of qualitative platelet defects.

Therapy

In most congenital disorders, transfusion of normal platelets, when required for bleeding episodes, is the only known form of therapy. When platelet dysfunction is associated with an acquired disorder, successful treatment of the underlying disease often results in improved platelet function. Drugs known to inhibit platelet function should be avoided when optimum hemostasis is desired. When a mild analgesic is required, acetaminophen may be used, as this drug does not inhibit platelet function.

CONGENITAL DEFECTS

Thrombasthenia: In this rare disorder, clot retraction is abnormal and the platelets are not aggregated by any concentration of adenosine diphosphate (ADP) or by most other agents known to cause platelet aggregation. The bleeding time is variable, often slightly prolonged. On direct blood smear (obtained without anticoagulant), the platelets appear isolated and no aggregates are seen.

Defects of collagen-induced platelet aggregation: In this group of disorders, aggregation by collagen is abnormal and in most cases is due to an inability to release endogenous ADP, the agent ultimately responsible for platelet aggregation. Unlike the findings in thrombasthenia, aggregation by ADP (added to the platelets) is normal. Two broad types of defects may account for this inability to release ADP. In one type of disorder, the platelets are deficient in the ADP which is normally found in the storage granules **(storage-pool disease)**; in another type, the platelets contain ADP but are unable to release it. These disorders are probably heterogeneous, and both familial and isolated cases have been described.

Platelet disorders associated with abnormal platelet morphology: In one congenital disorder **(Bernard-Soulier syndrome)**, unusually large platelets (some the size of RBCs) are a feature. Large platelets associated with functional abnormalities have also been described in association with the May-Hegglin anomaly, a thrombocytopenic disorder with abnormal leukocytes, and in the Chédiak-Higashi syndrome.

Platelet disorders associated with other congenital defects: In addition to those disorders with abnormal platelet morphology, abnormal platelet function has been found in the Wiskott-Aldrich syndrome and in Down's syndrome.

von Willebrand's disease: Although the prolonged bleeding time in these patients is probably due to an abnormality in platelet function during the primary arrest of bleeding, the basic defect appears to be the deficiency of a plasma factor (see discussion below).

ACQUIRED PLATELET DYSFUNCTION

Abnormalities of platelet function have been described in a wide variety of clinical disorders. The platelet defect which has been described in uremia has been attributed to some low-mol-wt substance which accumulates in uremic blood; the platelet defect usually disappears after dialysis. Other disorders in which qualitative platelet defects have been described are cirrhosis, dysproteinemias, scurvy, pernicious anemia, SLE, the myeloproliferative disorders, and leukemia. In many of these disorders, thrombocytopenia also occurs frequently.

Drug-induced platelet defects: Among drugs which may inhibit collagen-induced platelet aggregation are the nonsteroidal anti-inflammatory agents such as aspirin, indomethacin, and phenylbutazone. The inhibitory effects on platelet function obtained by ingesting a single dose (0.3 to 1.5 Gm) of aspirin may persist for 4 to 7 days. Aspirin also produces a modest prolongation of the bleeding time in normal subjects. The deleterious effect of dextran on hemostasis has also been attributed to an inhibitory effect on platelet function. Other drugs which may inhibit platelet aggregation include the tricyclic antidepressants, antihistamines, and phenothiazines.

HEREDITARY COAGULATION DISORDERS

THE HEMOPHILIAS

Bleeding disorders due to inherited deficiencies or abnormalities of coagulation factors. The most common forms, factor VIII or IX deficiencies, are termed hemophilia A and B respectively, and make up over 90% of these disorders. They are characterized by normal amounts of, but functionally inadequate, factors VIII and IX. They are inherited as sex-linked recessive traits and occur only in males, although female carriers transmit the abnormal gene. Inactivation of one of the two X chromosomes in the cell, as described in the "Lyon hypothesis" (see in SYNDROMES ASSOCIATED WITH SEX CHROMOSOME ABERRATIONS, in §10, Ch. 6), explains the low factor values and occasional bleeding problem which are seen in some female carriers. (Presumably they have a predominance of the abnormal X chromosome function.) A recent survey prepared for the National Heart and Lung Institute indicated a population of 25,000 hemophiliac patients in the USA, of whom over 80% have hemophilia A.

Symptoms and Signs

Symptoms of hemophilia begin in early childhood, often being noted at circumcision, and persist throughout life. The severity of the deficiency varies and frequently is characterized by serious hemorrhages which develop from trivial injuries and by bleeding manifestations which are virtually pathognomonic (e.g., hemarthrosis). Hematomas and hematuria also are common. Epistaxis, however, is more often seen in von Willebrand's disease; gastrointestinal bleeding suggests the presence of a specific lesion such as a peptic ulcer.

Laboratory Findings

Laboratory studies are required for diagnosis. The PTT is an effective screening assay for this condition and is abnormal in all severe cases. Occasionally a mild deficiency may be undetected by the procedure and therefore would require a specific assay. When an abnormality of PTT is observed in the presence of a normal PT, specific factor assay should be undertaken using commercially available plasma obtained from a patient who has the deficiency. Patients with severe manifestations of the disease have factor VIII or IX levels of < 1%; those who seldom have "spontaneous bleeding" are generally in a range of 5%; while values > 10% rarely are encountered and suggest the presence of von Willebrand's disease. Female carriers may be normal or as low as 2%. Values of < 60% are consistent with the carrier state.

Immune assays have been developed to identify the quantity of factor VIII as an antigen. A discrepancy between the amount of clotting factor and the antigenic activity indicates the presence of a functionally defective abnormal molecule. The immune assay can identify the carrier state with accuracy exceeding 90%.